pharmacology

The National Veterinary Medical Series for Independent Study

pharmacology

Franklin A. Ahrens, D.V.M., Ph.D.

Professor of Pharmacology
Department of Veterinary Physiology and Pharmacology
Iowa State University
College of Veterinary Medicine
Ames, Iowa

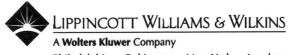

LIPPINCOTT WILLIAMS & WILKINS
A **Wolters Kluwer** Company
Philadelphia · Baltimore · New York · London
Buenos Aires · Hong Kong · Sydney · Tokyo

Senior Acquisitions Editor: Elizabeth A. Nieginski
Development Editor: Melanie Cann
Managing Editor: Amy G. Dinkel
Production Coordinator: Danielle Santucci
Editorial Assistant: Carol Loyd
Series Editor, Basic Sciences: John P. Kluge, DVM, PhD

The publisher gratefully acknowledges the support of the Iowa State University College of Veterinary Medicine in the initiation of the National Veterinary Medical Series.

The publisher gratefully acknowledges the Professional Examination Service (PES) for providing information about the format and content of the National Board Examination (NBE) for Veterinary Medical Licensing.

Copyright © 1996   Lippincott Williams & Wilkins

351 West Camden Street
Baltimore, Maryland 21201-2436 USA

Accurate indications, adverse reactions, and dosage schedules for drugs are provided in this book, but it is possible that they may change. The reader is urged to review the package information data of the manufacturers of the medications mentioned.

Printed in the United States of America

Library of Congress Cataloging-in-Publication Data

ISBN 0-683-00085-3

The Publishers have made every effort to trace the copyright holders for borrowed material. If they have inadvertently overlooked any, they will be pleased to make the necessary arrangements at the first opportunity.

02 03
3 4 5 6 7 8 9 10

Contents

Contributors

Donald C. Dyer, Ph.D.
Professor of Pharmacology
Department of Veterinary Physiology and Pharmacology
Iowa State University
College of Veterinary Medicine
Ames, Iowa

Walter H. Hsu, D.V.M., Ph.D.
Professor of Pharmacology
Department of Veterinary Physiology and Pharmacology
Iowa State University
College of Veterinary Medicine
Ames, Iowa

Dean H. Riedesel, D.V.M., Ph.D.
Professor
Department of Veterinary Clinical Sciences
Veterinary Teaching Hospital
Iowa State University
Ames, Iowa

Wendy A. Ware, D.V.M., M.S., Diplomate A.C.V.I.M. (Cardiology)
Associate Professor
Department of Veterinary Clinical Sciences and Physiology and Pharmacology
Staff Cardiologist
Veterinary Teaching Hospital
Iowa State University
Ames, Iowa

Preface

NVMS Pharmacology is intended as a concise review of pharmacology for students preparing for the National Board Examination (NBE) in veterinary medicine and for veterinary medical residents preparing for specialty board examinations. Students also will find the book to be a useful supplement to the textbooks used in pharmacology courses. The questions and complete explanations at the end of each chapter reinforce the basic and clinical concepts essential to rational drug use.

Pharmacology is generally taught in the preclinical years of the curriculum. The vast amount of information in the field and its ever-changing nature make preparation for the board examinations a daunting task for the senior student or resident. The authors hope that the concise but comprehensive review provided by *NVMS Pharmacology* will make this task less onerous.

Franklin A. Ahrens

Chapter 1

Principles of Drug Absorption, Disposition, and Action

Donald C. Dyer

I. **INTRODUCTION.** Pharmacology is the study of the properties of chemicals used as drugs for therapeutic and diagnostic purposes in medicine. Important areas of pharmacology are the study of drug absorption and drug disposition [distribution, biotransformation (metabolism), excretion, and pharmacokinetics], because these processes dictate the route of administration, dose, dose interval, and toxicity in animals receiving the drug. Also important is the study of the effects and mechanisms (biochemical and physiologic) by which drugs produce their action.

II. **DRUG ABSORPTION AND DISPOSITION**

A. **Reaching the site of action.** A drug usually must cross several tissue membranes from its locus of administration to reach its site of action and produce a drug response (Figure 1-1). The ways in which drugs cross membranes are fundamental processes that govern drug absorption, distribution, and excretion from the animal.

1. **Passive diffusion**
   a. Cell membranes have a **biomolecular lipoprotein layer** that may act as a barrier to drug transfer across the membrane. Cell membranes also contain pores. Thus, **drugs cross membranes based on their ability to dissolve in the lipid portion of the membrane and on their molecular size,** which regulates their filtration through the pores.
   b. **Weak acids and weak bases**
      (1) The majority of drugs are either weak acids or weak bases. The degree to which these drugs are lipid-soluble (nonionized, the form which is able to cross membranes) is determined by their pK_a and the pH of the medium containing the drug:

      pK_a = pH at which 50% of the drug is ionized and 50% is nonionized

      (a) In monogastric animals with a low stomach pH, weak acids such as aspirin (pK_a 3.5) tend to be better absorbed from the stomach than weak bases because of the acidic conditions.
      (b) Weak bases are poorly absorbed from the acidic environment of the stomach because they exist mostly in the ionized state (i.e., they have low lipid solubility). Weak bases are better absorbed from the small intestine where the environmental pH is more alkaline.
      (2) In order to use the **Henderson-Hasselbalch equation** to calculate the percent of a drug that exists in ionized form or to determine the concentration of a drug across a biologic membrane, one needs to know whether a drug is an acid or a base.
      (a) For weak acids use:

      $$pK_a = pH + \log \frac{\text{concentration of nonionized acid}}{\text{concentration of ionized acid}}$$

      (b) For weak bases use:

      $$pK_a = pH + \log \frac{\text{concentration of ionized base}}{\text{concentration of nonionized base}}$$

1

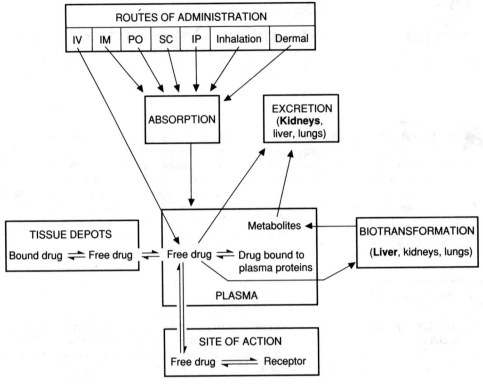

FIGURE 1-1. Routes of administration, absorption, deposition, and action of drugs. *IV* = intravenous; *IM* = intramuscular; *PO* = oral; *IP* = intraperitoneal; *SC* = subcutaneous.

(c) **Example calculation.** The Henderson-Hasselbalch equation can be used to determine the concentration ratio (plasma/gastric fluid) of unionized acetylsalicylic acid (HA), a weak acid (pK$_a$ 3.5), following achievement of equilibrium.

Biologic membrane

Plasma (pH 7.4)   Gastric fluid (pH 1.5)

Unionized HA (1) ⇌ HA (1)   Unionized

Ionized H$^+$ + A$^-$ (10,000)   H$^+$ + A$^-$ (0.01)   Ionized

10,001 units of the drug on this side of the membrane at equilibrium   1.01 units of the drug on this side of the membrane at equilibrium

$$pK_a = pH + \log \frac{\text{unionized (U)}}{\text{ionized (I)}}$$

$$pK_a = pH + \log \frac{\text{unionized (U)}}{\text{ionized (I)}}$$

$$3.5 = 7.4 + \log \frac{U}{I}$$

$$3.5 = 1.5 + \log \frac{U}{I}$$

$$-3.9 = \log \frac{U}{I}$$

$$2 = \log \frac{U}{I}$$

Take the antilog of both sides   Take the antilog of both sides

$$0.0001 = \frac{U}{I}$$

$$100 = \frac{U}{I}$$

If U = 1, then I = 10,000   If U = 1, then I = 0.01

$$\frac{\text{Plasma concentration (10,001)}}{\text{Gastric fluid (1.01)}} \approx 9,900$$

Therefore, at equilibrium:
- **(i)** The concentration of unionized drug (HA) is the same on both sides of the membrane.
- **(ii)** There is more total drug (unionized + ionized) on the side of the membrane where the degree of ionization is the greatest **(ion trapping).**

2. Filtration

- **a.** The fact that some low molecular weight chemicals (e.g., water, urea) cross membranes better than predicted by their lipid solubility suggests that membranes possess pores or channels.
- **b.** The glomerular filtration process in the kidney provides evidence for the existence of pores that are large enough to permit the passage of large molecular weight substances but small enough to retain albumin (mol. wt. ≈ 60,000).

3. Facilitated diffusion

- **a.** No cellular energy is required for facilitated diffusion, and it does not operate against a concentration gradient.
- **b.** Transfer of a drug across the membrane involves attachment to a carrier (i.e., a macromolecular molecule).
- **c.** Facilitated diffusion is not a major mechanism for drug transport. Examples of this type of process include reabsorption of glucose by the kidney and intestinal absorption of vitamin B_{12} along with intrinsic factor.

4. Active transport

- **a.** Active transport requires cellular energy and operates against a concentration gradient.
- **b.** The chemical structure of the drug is important in attaching to the carrier molecule. For example, the anticancer drug 5-fluorouracil is absorbed from the intestine by the same system used to absorb uracil.

5. Pinocytosis is a minor method for drug absorption, but it may be important in the absorption of some polypeptides, bacterial toxins, antigens, and food proteins by the gut.

B. **Routes of administration.** Many routes of administration involve an absorption process in which the drug must cross one or more tissue membranes before entering the blood stream. The intravenous route is an exception because the drug is placed directly in the circulation (see Figure 1-1). When administered subcutaneously or intramuscularly, most of the drug may enter the circulation through openings or fenestrations in the capillary wall and not penetrate any membrane.

1. Alimentary routes

a. Oral

- **(1)** **Advantages.** The oral route is the safest route. In addition, it is convenient and economical.
- **(2)** **Disadvantages**
  - **(a)** The acidic environment of the stomach and digestive enzymes may destroy the drug. In ruminants, the bacterial enzymes may inactivate the drug, or the digestive process may be altered by the drug (e.g., as occurs with antimicrobials).
  - **(b)** Some drugs may irritate the gastrointestinal mucosa.
  - **(c)** The presence of food may adversely alter absorption.
  - **(d)** Some drugs (e.g., propranolol) are extensively metabolized by the gastrointestinal mucosa and the liver before they reach the systemic circulation. This is referred to as the **first-pass effect.**
- **(3)** **Other considerations**
  - **(a)** **Antimuscarinic and narcotic drugs** may delay gastric emptying, and therefore, the rate of drug absorption, prolonging the drug onset time.
  - **(b)** A **hyperactive gut** may shorten the transit time and thus lessen the drug–gut contact time, leading to reduced absorption.

(c) **Enteric-coated tablets** may protect the drug from destruction by stomach acid and enhance absorption.

b. **Rectal.** The rectal route of administration can be used in an unconscious or vomiting animal.

2. **Parenteral routes** circumvent the gastrointestinal tract.

a. **Types**

(1) Intravenous
(2) Intramuscular
(3) Subcutaneous
(4) Intraperitoneal
(5) Intrathecal
(6) Intra-arterial

b. **Advantages. Rapid onset** (the intravenous route is faster than the intramuscular route, which is faster than the subcutaneous route) may be useful in an unconscious or vomiting animal, and **absorption is more uniform and predictable.** Because absorption from intramuscular and subcutaneous injection sites is determined in part by the amount of blood flow to that site, the absorption of local anesthetics is often purposely slowed by coadministration with epinephrine, which decreases the blood flow to the injection site.

c. **Disadvantages**

(1) Asepsis is necessary.
(2) Parenteral administration may cause pain, and there is a risk of penetrating a blood vessel during intramuscular injection.
(3) The speed of onset is so rapid (as with intravenous administration) that cardiovascular responses may occur to drugs that normally have minimal effects on the cardiovascular system.
(4) In food animals, discoloration of the meat or abscess formation may occur with intramuscular injection, which may devalue the carcass.

3. **Dermal or topical administration.** The degree of absorption is dependent on the lipid solubility of the drug. Abraded or sunburnt skin may absorb more drug than intact skin.

4. **Inhalation** is used for volatile or gaseous anesthetics. Response is rapid because of the large surface area of the lungs and the large blood flow to the lungs.

C. **Drug distribution** is the **reversible transfer of a drug** from one site in the body to another site. In much of the body, the junctions between the capillary endothelial cells are not tight, thereby permitting free drug (i.e., drug that is not bound to plasma proteins) to rapidly reach equilibrium on both sides of the vessel wall.

1. **Plasma–protein binding** of drugs can affect drug distribution because only the unbound drug is able to cross cell membranes freely (see Figure 1-1). The drug–protein binding reaction is **reversible** and obeys the laws of mass action:

$$\text{drug} + \text{protein} \rightleftharpoons \text{drug–protein}$$
$$\text{(free)} \qquad\qquad\qquad \text{(bound)}$$

a. Acidic drugs are bound primarily to **albumin,** and basic drugs are bound primarily to α_1-**acid glycoprotein.**

b. Binding does not prevent a drug from reaching its site of action, but it **slows the rate at which a drug reaches a concentration sufficient to produce a pharmacologic effect.**

c. **Effect on drug elimination**

(1) Drug–protein binding limits glomerular filtration as an elimination process, because bound drugs cannot be filtered.
(2) Binding does not typically limit the elimination of drugs that are actively secreted by the kidney or metabolized by the liver, because the fraction of the drug that is free is transported and metabolized. As the free drug concentration is lowered, there is rapid dissociation of the drug–protein complex to maintain the amount of drug in the free state.

(3) Sulfa drugs with a high affinity for binding to protein are eliminated more slowly in urine than those sulfa drugs with a lower binding affinity for plasma proteins.

d. **Drug interactions** may occur when two drugs are used that bind at the same site on the plasma proteins. Competition for the same site increases the percent of drug in the free form, thereby increasing the pharmacologic–toxicologic response to the displaced drug.

2. **CNS distribution.** Distribution of drugs into the central nervous system (CNS) and cerebrospinal fluid is **restricted.** There are three processes that contribute to keeping drug concentration in the CNS low.

a. **Blood–brain barrier.** In much of the CNS (except the area postrema, pineal body, and posterior lobe of hypothalamus), the capillary endothelial junctions are tight, and glial cells surround the precapillaries. These histologic features reduce filtration and require drugs to diffuse across cell membranes to leave the vascular compartment and enter the extracellular or cerebrospinal fluid.

b. **Active transport mechanisms** exist for organic acids and bases in the **choroid plexus,** allowing transport of drugs from the cerebrospinal fluid into the blood. For example, CNS concentrations of penicillin, a weak acid, are kept low by this active transport system.

c. **Cerebrospinal fluid** produced within the ventricles circulates through the ventricles and over the surface of the brain and spinal cord to flow directly into the venous drainage system of the brain. This process continuously dilutes the drug's concentration in the cerebrospinal fluid.

3. **Transplacental distribution**

a. Drug transfer across the placenta occurs primarily by simple diffusion, most easily if the drugs are lipid-soluble (i.e., nonionized weak acids or bases). Even when drugs with low lipid solubility are given to the mother, the fetus is exposed to some extent.

b. Drugs that affect the maternal CNS (e.g., anesthetics, analgesics, sedatives, tranquilizers) have the physical–chemical characteristics to freely cross the placenta and affect the fetus.

4. **Other distribution barriers.** The **prostate, testicles,** and **globe of the eye** contain barriers that prevent drug penetration, thus limiting drug concentration in these tissues.

5. **Drug redistribution** can terminate the drug response.

a. The biologic response to a drug is usually terminated by metabolism (biotransformation) and excretion; however, redistribution of a drug from its site of action to other tissues lowers its concentration at its site of action, thereby terminating the drug response.

b. Drugs exhibiting the redistribution phenomenon are highly lipid-soluble (e.g., thiopental).

D. **Drug metabolism (biotransformation)** is the chemical alteration of xenobiotics (e.g., drugs) and endogenous substances in the body.

1. **Function**

a. Following filtration at the renal glomerulus, most lipid-soluble drugs are reabsorbed from the filtrate. Biotransformation of drugs to more water-soluble (polar) chemicals **reduces their ability to be reabsorbed, thus enhancing their excretion and reducing their volume of distribution.**

b. Although drug biotransformation frequently reduces the biological activity of the xenobiotic, it is **not synonymous with drug inactivation** because the parent chemical may be transformed to a chemical with greater or significant biologic activity. For example, the inactive insecticide parathion is transformed to the active insecticide paraxon; codeine is biotransformed to the more active analgesic, morphine.

2. **Sites.** The **liver** is the most important organ for biotransformation, but the **lung, kidney,** and **gastrointestinal epithelium** also play a role.

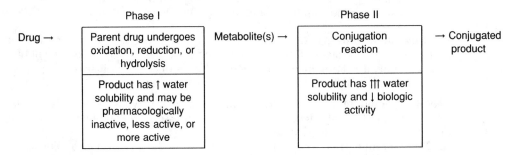

FIGURE 1-2. Phases of biotransformation.

3. **Phases.** Enzymatic reactions in biotransformation usually occur in two phases (Figure 1-2).

   a. **Phase I biotransformation enzymes** (also referred to as **microsomal enzymes** because they are found in the microsomal fraction following high speed centrifugation) are found in the **hepatic smooth endoplasmic reticulum.**

   (1) **Oxidation** is the addition of oxygen or the removal of hydrogen from the drug.

      (a) **Microsomal oxidation.** Most oxidation is carried out by the **cytochrome P-450 family of isozymes.**

         (i) The enzyme system is a **mixed function oxidase,** because one atom of oxygen is incorporated in the drug molecule and the other atom of oxygen combines with hydrogen to form water. Nicotinamide adenine dinucleotide phosphate (NADPH) provides the reducing equivalents.

         (ii) Examples of microsomal oxidation reactions are shown in Table 1-1.

      (b) **Nonmicrosomal oxidation.** A few chemicals are oxidized by enzymes found in the cytosol or mitochondria.

         (i) **Alcohol dehydrogenase** and **aldehyde dehydrogenase** oxidize ethanol and acetaldehyde.

         (ii) **Monoamine oxidase** oxidizes epinephrine, norepinephrine, dopamine, and serotonin.

         (iii) **Xanthine oxidase**

   (2) **Reduction** reactions, which usually involve the addition of hydrogen to the drug molecule, occur less frequently than oxidation reactions. Enzymes are located in both microsomal and nonmicrosomal fractions. Examples of chemicals biotransformed by reduction include chloramphenicol, prontosil, and naloxone.

   (3) **Hydrolysis.** Chemicals with either ester or amide linkages undergo hydrolysis.

      (a) **Esterases** occur primarily in nonmicrosomal systems and are found in the

TABLE 1-1. Microsomal Oxidation Reactions

Oxidation Reaction	Substrate
Side chain and aromatic hydroxylation	Pentobarbital, phenytoin, phenylbutazone
N- or O-dealkylation	Morphine, codeine, diazepam
N-oxidation	Acetaminophen, nicotine
S-oxidation	Phenothiazines (e.g., chlorpromazine)
Deamination	Amphetamine
Desulfuration	Thiopental, parathion

TABLE 1-2. Phase II Biotransformation

Conjugation Reaction	Substrate
Glucuronidation	Morphine, acetaminophen, sulfathiazole, digitoxin
Acetylation	Sulfonamides, clonazepam
Glutathione conjugation	Ethacrynic acid
Glycine conjugation	Salicylic acid, nicotinic acid
Sulfate conjugation	Catecholamines, acetaminophen
Methylation	Catecholamines, histamine

      plasma, liver, and other tissues. Examples of drugs hydrolyzed by ester-
ases include acetylcholine, succinylcholine, and procaine.

    (b) Amidases are nonmicrosomal enzymes found primarily in the liver. Exam-
ples of drugs hydrolyzed by amidases include procainamide and indomethacin.

  b. Phase II biotransformation (conjugation). A phase I metabolite or a parent chemical may undergo phase II biotransformation. This process involves the coupling of
an endogenous chemical to the drug metabolite (Table 1-2).

    (1) Enzyme systems are present in the microsomes, cytosol, and mitochondria.

    (2) Products of phase II biotransformation have greater water solubility and are
more readily excreted via the kidney.

4. Factors affecting drug metabolism

  a. Concurrent drug use. Certain drugs and chemicals (e.g., phenobarbital, pentobarbital, phenylbutazone, organochlorine pesticides, polycyclic hydrocarbons) increase the synthesis of liver cytochrome P-450 enzymes, increasing the rate of
drug biotransformation and reducing the magnitude and duration of the dose–response curve. Enzyme induction may explain some types of drug tolerance.

  b. Age. The ability to metabolize drugs is reduced in fetal, newborn, and aged animals.

  c. Sex. Male rats metabolize some drugs more rapidly than female rats. The extent
to which this phenomenon occurs in other animals is unclear.

  d. Disease. Liver pathology or dysfunction reduces the biotransformation ability of
the liver. Other diseases (e.g., congestive heart failure, renal disease) may alter
drug distribution, thereby influencing drug metabolism.

  e. Species differences

    (1) Aquatic amphibia and fish have low concentrations of drug metabolizing en-
zymes. The cytochrome P-450 system is primarily developed in terrestrial animals.

    (2) Cats have reduced glucuronyl transferase activity and metabolize drugs such
as aspirin slowly.

    (3) Dogs lack the ability to acetylate aromatic amino groups, such as those pres-
ent in sulfonamides.

    (4) Ruminants have low plasma pseudocholinesterase levels; therefore, drugs
such as succinylcholine have a longer duration of action in ruminants than in
horses, dogs, or cats.

E. **Drug excretion** refers to the processes by which a drug or drug metabolite is eliminated
from the body.

  1. Urine. The kidney is the primary organ for drug excretion.

    a. Glomerular filtration. All drugs that are not bound to plasma proteins are filtered.

    b. Active tubular secretion. In the **proximal tubule,** active transport mechanisms
exist for both **acid** and **base drugs** (Table 1-3). **Competition** between drugs for the
same carrier system can lead to adverse drug reactions or can be used to therapeutic advantage (e.g., probenecid inhibits the transport of penicillin, thereby enhancing the plasma concentration of penicillin).

TABLE 1-3. Actively Secreted Drugs

Acid Drugs	Base Drugs
Penicillin	Histamine
Ampicillin	Serotonin
Chlorothiazide	Procainamide
Ethacrynic acid	Neostigmine
Furosemide	Trimethoprim
Probenecid	Atropine
Salicylate	
Phenylbutazone	
Cephalosporins	

    c. Passive tubular reabsorption. Only **lipid-soluble drugs** are reabsorbed in this manner. Because most drugs are weak acids or weak bases, the pK_a of the drug and the pH of the urine in the tubular lumen affect how much of the drug is nonionized (i.e., reabsorbable).
      (1) Diet influences the urinary pH for both carnivores and herbivores.
        (a) In carnivores, the urinary pH ranges from 5.5–7.0.
        (b) In herbivores, the urinary pH ranges from 7.0–8.0.
      (2) Excretion can be enhanced for drugs eliminated primarily by the kidney by altering the pH of the urine. For practical purposes, this principle applies only to weak acidic or weak basic drugs with a pK_a of 5–8.
      (3) Quaternary drugs (R_4-N^+) are polar at all urine pHs. They are eliminated rapidly because they cannot be reabsorbed.

2. Bile and feces. Either the parent drug or the glucuronide form of the drug may be eliminated via the bile.
    a. Active transport processes exist in the liver for transporting acidic, basic, and neutral drugs into the bile. Because these drugs may eventually be reabsorbed from the gut lumen, biliary elimination processes tend to be less effective than renal excretion processes for eliminating a drug from the body.
    b. Enterohepatic circulation can significantly increase a drug's sojourn in the body.
      (1) Glucuronide metabolites can be hydrolyzed by bacterial β-glucuronidases, thereby releasing free drug that can then be reabsorbed.
      (2) Because a portion of the reabsorbed drug is eliminated by another route, the concentration of the free drug in the body progressively declines.

3. Breast milk
    a. Although this is not a significant route for drug excretion, it is important because drugs given to the mother can affect the newborn via the milk. For example, antimicrobial drugs given to the mother can affect the microflora of the newborn's gastrointestinal tract.
    b. Drugs that are bases are generally found in higher concentrations in milk than in plasma. Milk is acidic relative to plasma. Therefore, weak organic bases diffuse from the plasma into the milk, where they become more ionized, preventing passage back to the plasma. This is an example of **ion trapping.**

4. Saliva. Drugs enter the saliva by passive diffusion from the blood. Saliva is not a major route for excretion, but it is important in herbivores receiving parenteral antimicrobials, because swallowing antimicrobial drug–laden saliva may upset the digestive process in the rumen.

5. Expired air. This route of elimination is most important for volatile drugs (e.g., inhaled anesthetics).

6. Tears and **sweat** are minor routes of excretion.

F. **Pharmacokinetics** is the study of the time course of drug concentrations in the body. A basic concept of pharmacokinetics is that a relationship exists between a pharmacologic or toxicologic effect of a drug and the concentration of the drug in the body (e.g., blood). Pharmacokinetics is the basis for establishing withdrawal times for meats and milk-discard time for dairy products when drugs are administered to food-producing animals. Knowledge of pharmacokinetics parameters also permits the calculation of dose and dosing interval.

1. **Plasma concentration–time profile.** The processes of drug distribution and elimination are best understood by monitoring the plasma drug concentration over time following an intravenous injection.

   a. **Drug distribution and elimination.** The plasma concentration rapidly decreases as a result of both **distribution out of the vascular compartment** and **elimination.**

      (1) Immediately after injection, the **rapid decrease** in the blood concentration for most drugs is primarily the result of **distribution.**

      (2) Eventually, the plasma and tissue concentrations reach an **equilibrium** and the rate of decrease in the plasma from this point on is governed primarily by **elimination** processes.

      (3) If the drug distribution and elimination processes have significantly different rates, then the plasma drug concentration–time profile can be used to analyze these two processes.

   b. Mathematically, the **concentration–time curve** can be depicted as composed of two straight lines (Figure 1-3A).

      (1) During the **distribution phase,** the drug is transferred from the plasma. The line representing the distribution phase has an **intercept (A)** and a **slope (-α).**

      (2) During the **elimination phase,** the drug leaves the body. The line representing the elimination phase has an **intercept (B)** and a **slope (-β).** Most drugs are

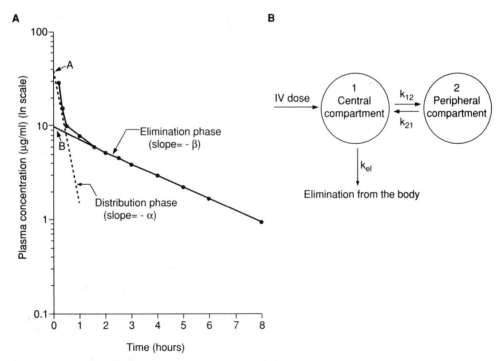

FIGURE 1-3. *(A)* The plasma concentration–time curve following intravenous injection of a drug exhibiting two-compartment pharmacokinetics. The distribution phase is represented by the line with intercept *A* and slope $-\alpha$. The elimination phase is represented by the line with intercept *B* and slope $-\beta$. *(B)* Two-compartment open model. The central compartment represents rapid equilibration and represents fluids such as the blood, interstitial fluid, and highly perfused organs (e.g., the lungs). The peripheral compartment reaches equilibrium more slowly and represents organs such as bone and fat. *IV* = intravenous; k_{el} = the rate constant of elimination from the central compartment; k_{12} and k_{21} = the rate constants of distribution between the central and peripheral compartments.

eliminated by a **first-order process** (i.e., a constant fraction of the drug is eliminated per unit of time).

(3) The theoretical plasma concentration at **time zero** (i.e., immediately following injection) equals A + B.

(4) The **area under the plasma concentration curve (AUC)** is the area under the plasma concentration–time curve from the first time drug concentration can be measured to the last time. The AUC can be calculated by the trapezoidal method or estimated as follows:

$$AUC = \left(\frac{A}{\alpha} + \frac{B}{\beta} \right)$$

c. Body compartments. Pharmacokinetic analysis frequently uses the **linear compartmental approach.** This method mathematically models the body as a series of interconnecting compartments in which drugs are distributed and eliminated (Figure 1-3B). These compartments do not correspond to physiologic or anatomic areas in the body; they are abstract mathematical entities that are useful for predicting drug concentrations.

(1) The distribution of drugs in the body is frequently depicted using a one-, two- or three-compartment model.

(2) Because many drugs used in veterinary medicine can be described by a two-compartment open model (see Figure 1-3B), this is the only model described here.

d. Apparent volume of distribution (V_d). The apparent volume of distribution is a proportionality constant relating the plasma drug concentration to the total amount of drug in the body. It is a theoretical volume into which an injected dose of a drug would have to disperse if it were to be present throughout that volume in the same concentration as occurs in plasma immediately following the injection (i.e., time zero). The mathematical expression for the apparent volume of distribution is:

$$V_d = \frac{Dose}{\left(\dfrac{A}{\alpha} + \dfrac{B}{\beta} \right) \beta},$$

where dose is the amount (mg or g) administered; A and α are the intercept and slope of the distribution phase, respectively; and B and β are the intercept and slope of the elimination phase, respectively. Because the apparent volume of distribution can be used to calculate the amount of a drug needed to achieve a desired plasma concentration, it is common to divide the apparent volume of distribution by the animal's weight so that the units are ml/kg or L/kg.

2. The **half-life ($t_{1/2}$)** of a drug is the time needed to reduce the drug concentration by half. This value is determined during the elimination phase of the drug:

$$t_{1/2} = \frac{\ln 2}{\beta} = \frac{0.693}{\beta}$$

a. The half-life encompasses the processes of distribution, biotransformation, and renal excretion.

b. It indicates the time required to attain or lose 50% of the **steady state concentration** (i.e., the plasma concentration that remains constant because the rate of drug absorption equals the rate of drug elimination).

c. The half-life has limited value as an indicator of drug elimination or distribution.

3. Total body clearance (Cl_B) is the volume of blood that is effectively cleared of a drug in a specified period of time:

$$Cl_B = \beta \cdot V_d = \frac{0.693 \, V_d}{t_{1/2}}$$

a. Clearance expresses the rate of drug removal from the body.

b. Disease and infection may alter drug distribution and clearance, but not the half-life. In other words, the volume of distribution and clearance can be altered, and thus the half-life will be altered, but altering the half-life will not necessarily affect the volume of distribution or clearance. Therefore, **clearance is a more important pharmacokinetic term than half-life.**

4. Bioavailability (F) is the amount of drug reaching the systemic circulation intact.

    a. By definition, the bioavailability of an intravenous dose is 100%, or 1. All other routes of administration have a bioavailability of less than 1. Bioavailability is calculated as follows:

$$F = \frac{(AUC)^{nIV} \cdot dose^{IV} \cdot \beta^{nIV}}{(AUC)^{IV} \cdot dose^{nIV} \cdot \beta^{IV}},$$

    where AUC = the area under the plasma concentration curve; nIV = nonintravenous route of administration; IV = intravenous route of administration; and β = slope of the elimination phase.

    b. Determination of dosage

        (1) Knowledge of bioavailability for an **oral dosage** is particularly important, because it indicates what the extravascular dose must be multiplied by to obtain an equivalent intravenous dose. The **presence of food may alter the bioavailability of some drugs.**

        (2) A dose may be calculated if the drug's bioavailability (F), clearance (Cl_B), and the average steady state concentration ($\overline{C}_p\infty$) of the drug needed to produce the pharmacologic response are known:

$$\frac{F \cdot dose}{dosing\ interval} = \overline{C}_p\infty \cdot Cl_B$$

III. PHARMACODYNAMICS: MECHANISMS OF DRUG–RECEPTOR INTERACTIONS

A. **Receptors** bind ligands (e.g., drugs) and transduce signals (a process referred to as **signal transduction**).

    1. Many drug receptors are macromolecules present in cell membranes, which, when activated, initiate a biochemical change within the cell or tissue to produce a pharmacologic response.

    2. Drug binding to receptors uses **chemical bonds** similar to those used for enzyme–substrate interactions: hydrogen bonds, coordinate covalent bonds, and van der Waals forces. Covalent bonds in drug–receptor interactions are rare but significant, because they produce a long-lasting response.

B. **Drugs** have two identifiable properties: **affinity** for the receptor and **intrinsic activity.**

    1. Affinity is a proclivity to bind to a receptor.

    2. Intrinsic activity is the property of the drug that permits it to initiate postreceptor processes that lead to a response.

        a. Agonists are drugs that have both **affinity** and **intrinsic activity.** Examples include acetylcholine, xylazine, epinephrine, histamine, angiotensin, and prostaglandin $F_{2\alpha}$.

        b. Antagonists are drugs that have an **affinity** for the receptor site but lack intrinsic activity. They block or reduce the effects of agonists.

            (1) Examples include atropine, yohimbine, phentolamine, and chlorpheniramine.

            (2) Antagonists may act in a **competitive** or **noncompetitive** manner.

            (3) Antagonists may be **reversible** or **irreversible.**

TABLE 1-4. Receptor Antagonism

Agonist	Antagonist
Isoproterenol	Propranolol
Epinephrine	Phentolamine
Histamine	Chlorpheniramine
Acetylcholine	Atropine

C. **Antagonism.** There are three types of antagonism in pharmacology: **receptor, physiologic,** and **chemical.**

1. In **receptor antagonism,** two drugs, an agonist and an antagonist, compete for the same receptor (Table 1-4).

2. In **physiologic antagonism,** receptors in opposing physiologic systems are activated simultaneously. For example, epinephrine increases heart rate while acetylcholine (ACh) decreases heart rate.

3. In **chemical antagonism,** a drug forms chemical bonds with two or more molecules. For example, dimercaprol (British antilewisite, BAL) chelates mercury and D-penicillamine chelates copper, lead, and mercury, leading to increased excretion of the metals. This type of antagonism often does not require a cellular receptor. ·

D. **Signal transduction.** There are four well-known mechanisms by which receptors produce a pharmacologic response.

1. **Ligand-gated ion channels** regulate the flow of ions through the cellular plasma membrane channels.
   a. Once the drug (ligand) binds to the receptor, the response occurs within milliseconds.
   b. Examples of synaptic transmitters that act via ion channels include acetylcholine (at nicotinic receptors), γ-aminobutyric acid (GABA), glycine, and glutamate.

2. **G proteins** couple the binding of the ligand on the cell surface receptor with intracellular **second messengers** (Figure 1-4).
   a. An agonist binds to a receptor, causing guanosine diphosphate (GDP) to be displaced from the G protein and replaced with guanosine triphosphate (GTP).
   b. The G protein–GTP complex regulates the activity of enzymes or ion channels to produce a response.
      (1) Hydrolysis of the GTP to GDP halts the activity of the enzyme or ion channels.
      (2) The G protein–GTP complex may last for as long as 10 seconds, whereas the initial agonist–receptor complex may have lasted for only a few milliseconds. Therefore, **amplification** of the original agonist–receptor signal is possible.
   c. G proteins may elicit either **stimulatory** or **inhibitory** responses. Each cell may have more than one G protein type.

3. **Intracellular receptors** are activated by a group of hormones [**corticosteroids, mineralocorticoids, estrogens, progesterone, triiodothyronine (T_3), thyroxine (T_4), vitamin D**] that are highly lipid-soluble and thus, are able to cross the cellular plasma membrane.
   a. Glucocorticoid receptors are located in the cytoplasm. They combine with the drug and then move to the nucleus. Receptors for T_3, T_4, and the estrogens are in the nucleus. The receptor–drug complex increases binding of ribonucleic acid (RNA) polymerase, leading to transcription of target genes.
   b. The **response time** can range from minutes to hours because new proteins must be synthesized. Similarly, the **offset time** is long once drug treatment is stopped. Effects may persist for hours to days.

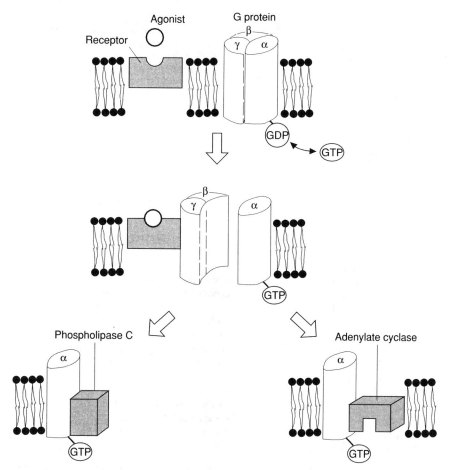

FIGURE 1-4. When an agonist binds to a receptor that is linked to a G protein–mediated second messenger system, the conformation of the receptor in the membrane is changed, enabling it to encounter a G protein complex. When the activated receptor encounters the G protein, it induces the G protein to exchange the guanosine diphosphate *(GDP)* molecule for a guanosine triphosphate *(GTP)* molecule. The presence of GTP causes the α subunit to separate from the G protein and diffuse within the membrane until it encounters the enzyme (e.g., phospholipase C, adenylate cyclase) that initiates the second messenger response. This second messenger response may involve regulation of enzymatic activity or activation of ion channels. Hydrolysis of the GTP to GDP halts the activity of the enzyme or ion channels. (Modified with permission from Bullock J, Boyle J III, and Wang MB: *NMS Physiology,* 3rd ed. Baltimore, Williams & Wilkins, 1994, p 29.)

    4. Protein tyrosine kinases mediate the responses of insulin, epidermal growth factor (EGF), platelet-derived growth factor (PDGF), and other trophic hormones.

      a. Receptors are proteins, found in the cell membrane, consisting of an extracellular portion that binds the ligand, a transmembrane portion that transmits the signal through the cell membrane, and a cytoplasmic portion that terminates in the cytoplasm.

      b. The cytoplasmic portion of the receptor possesses tyrosine kinase activity. The enzyme catalyzes the phosphorylation of substrate proteins, which produces a biologic response.

E. **Dose–response relationships**

    1. Graded dose–response relationships. Increases in the dose produce increases in response. Graded dose–response curves have four characteristic variables (Figure 1-5).

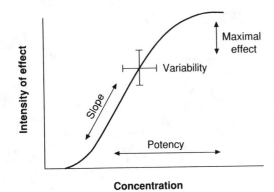

FIGURE 1-5. Log dose–effect curve, showing the four characteristic variables. (Redrawn with permission from Goodman Gilman A, Rall TW, Nies AS, and Taylor P: *Goodman and Gilman's The Pharmacological Basis of Therapeutics,* 8th ed. New York, Pergamon Press, 1990, p 67.)

    a. Potency refers to the dose (concentration) of a drug needed to produce an effect. The smaller the dose to produce the effect, the greater the potency.
        (1) Potency is not an important property of a drug, provided the formulated form of the drug can be conveniently administered.
        (2) If two drugs have similar pharmacologic activity, the more potent drug is not necessarily the drug of choice. Consideration must also be given to other factors, such as side effects, toxicities, cost, and duration of action.
    b. Slope is of both practical and theoretical importance.
        (1) Drugs that act on a common receptor (e.g., norepinephrine and phenylephrine both act on the α_1-adrenoceptor) have dose–response curves with parallel slopes.
        (2) Drugs that have steep dose–response curves are potentially more difficult to use because small increases in the dose may produce toxicity.
    c. Variability in the response can be expected from a specific dose, and variation in dosage may be required to produce a given response.
    d. Maximal effect is the maximum response possible for the effector.

  2. Quantal dose–response relationships are based on an **all-or-none response.** The assumption is made that individual animals respond to the maximum possible or not at all.
    a. Quantal dose–response relationships are used to establish the useful drug effect and the toxic drug effect curves.
    b. The graph of a quantal dose–response relationship does not show the intensity of the effect, but rather, the **frequency** with which any dose produces the all-or-none response (Figure 1-6A).
        (1) The **therapeutic index** (Figure 1-6B) is a ratio used to evaluate the safety of the drug:

$$TI = \frac{LD_{50}}{ED_{50}},$$

        where TI = the therapeutic index; LD_{50} = the dose necessary to kill 50% of a population (the **lethal dose**); and ED_{50} = the dosage that produces the desired effect in 50% of the population (the **effective dose**). Theoretically, the larger the therapeutic index, the safer the drug. However, if the LD_{50} and ED_{50} curves are not parallel, the therapeutic index may be misleading.
        (2) The **standard safety margin** is a more conservative measure of a drug's safety than the therapeutic index. It is the percent by which the ED_{99} (i.e., the dosage that produces the desired effect in 99% of the population) must be increased before an LD_1 is reached (i.e., the dose necessary to kill 1% of the population):

$$\text{Standard safety margin} = \frac{LD_1 - ED_{99}}{ED_{99}} \cdot 100$$

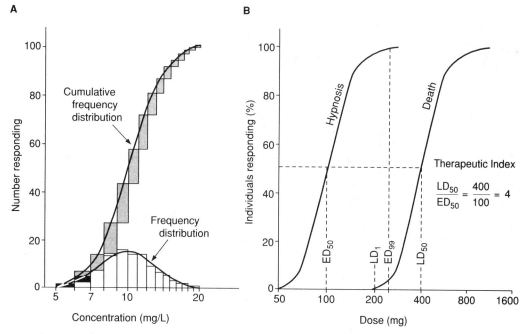

FIGURE 1-6. *(A)* The effective concentration to produce a quantal response was determined in each of 100 subjects. The number of subjects who required each dose is plotted, giving a lognormal frequency distribution *(white bars).* The *stippled bars* demonstrate that the normal frequency distribution, when summated, yields the cumulative frequency distribution—a sigmoid curve that is a quantal concentration–effect curve. *(B)* Quantal dose–response curves for the useful action and toxic action of a drug. ED_{50} is the dose necessary to produce the desired effect in 50% of the population. LD_{50} is the dose that will kill 50% of the population. (Redrawn with permission from Goodman Gilman A, Rall TW, Nies AS, and Taylor P: *Goodman and Gilman's The Pharmacological Basis of Therapeutics,* 8th ed. New York, Pergamon Press, 1990, p 69.)

For example, if 10 mg/kg of a drug is effective in 99% of the animal population, and a dose of 100 mg/kg will cause toxicity in 1% of the same population, then:

$$\text{Standard safety margin} = \frac{100 - 10}{10} \cdot 100$$

The dose that is effective in 99% of the population must be increased by 900% to produce a toxic effect in 1% of the population.

STUDY QUESTIONS

DIRECTIONS: Each of the numbered items or incomplete statements in this section is followed by answers or by completion of the statement. Select the **one** numbered answer or completion that is **best** in each case.

1. The same dose of a drug is given by two different routes of administration (A,B), and the plasma concentration is followed over time, as shown in the graph below. Which one of the following statements is true?

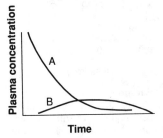

(1) Curve A results from intramuscular administration.
(2) Curve B results from intravenous administration.
(3) Curve A results from oral administration.
(4) Curve A results from intravenous administration.
(5) Curve B represents the drug with the greatest bioavailability.

2. The first-pass effect is most apt to occur following administration of a drug by which route?

(1) Intravenous
(2) Intramuscular
(3) Subcutaneous
(4) Oral
(5) Inhalation

3. The maximal effect achieved by a drug is a measure of:

(1) the drug's potency.
(2) the drug's efficacy (intrinsic activity).
(3) the drug's antagonistic magnitude.
(4) the drug's therapeutic index.
(5) the drug's lipid solubility at its pK_a.

4. A drug is eliminated by first-order processes. Assume 50 mg of the drug is administered intravenously and after 6 hours, 25 mg remain in the body. Approximately how much of the drug will remain in the body at 24 hours?

(1) 18 mg
(2) 15 mg
(3) 10 mg
(4) 6 mg
(5) 3 mg

5. A client brings a severely dehydrated dog in renal failure to your practice. The dog's glomerular filtration rate is 25% of the normal rate. The antibiotic of choice is cleared solely by glomerular filtration. The drug's volume of distribution (V_d) is only in the extracellular fluid, and it is 50% of normal in this dog. In a healthy animal, the antibiotic's half-life ($t_{1/2}$) is 60 minutes. What would the half-life of this drug be in this animal?

(1) 30 minutes
(2) 60 minutes
(3) 90 minutes
(4) 120 minutes
(5) 240 minutes

6. The mechanism by which most drugs are absorbed following an intramuscular injection is:

(1) simple diffusion.
(2) active transport.
(3) pinocytosis.
(4) facilitated diffusion.

7. Drug X is a weak acid with a pK_a of 4. Approximately what percent of the drug is ionized in an environment with a pH of 2?

(1) 10%
(2) 5%
(3) 1%
(4) 0.1%
(5) 0.5%

8. Treatment with phenobarbital for several days before the administration of pentobarbital decreases pentobarbital's duration of action. The mechanism by which this occurs involves:

(1) stimulation of synthesis of microsomal enzymes in the liver.
(2) neutralization by phenobarbital of naturally occurring inhibitors.
(3) acceleration of the excretion of pentobarbital.
(4) competition for receptor sites in the central nervous system (CNS).
(5) increased binding of pentobarbital to plasma proteins.

9. Which of the following drug characteristics tends to favor a low apparent volume of distribution (V_d)?

(1) Extensive plasma protein binding
(2) High molecular weight
(3) High water solubility
(4) All of the above

10. The two curves below were obtained for drug A and drug B. The ordinate represents the percent of animals responding to the beneficial effect of the drug.

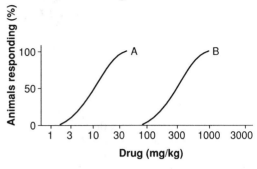

Which of the following statements is true?

(1) Drug A is 30 times more potent than drug B.
(2) Drug A is 300 times more potent than drug B.
(3) Drug B is 30 times more potent than drug A.

11. Acidifying the urine would be expected to increase the rate of elimination for:

(1) a weak acid with a pK_a of 7.
(2) a weak base with a pK_a of 6.
(3) both a weak acid with a pK_a of 7 and a weak base with a pK_a of 6.

ANSWERS AND EXPLANATIONS

1. The answer is 4 [II B 2 b, F].
Curve A results from intravenous administration, as evidenced by the lack of an absorption phase. Curve B shows an ascending plasma concentration phase (i.e., the absorption phase), followed by a descending plasma concentration phase (i.e., the elimination phase). Curve B could not represent the drug with the greatest bioavailability because, by definition, the bioavailability of an intravenous dose is 100% or 1; all other routes of administration have a bioavailability of less than 100%.

2. The answer is 4 [II B 1 a (2) (d)].
The first-pass effect is most apt to occur following oral administration of a drug. The first-pass effect refers to the loss of a significant amount of drug during the absorption process, so that a large quantity of the drug is then unavailable for distribution. Usually, the first-pass effect is evident for drugs that are metabolized significantly by the gut epithelium and liver prior to distribution via the systemic circulation.

3. The answer is 2 [III E 1].
The maximal effect achieved by a drug is a measure of the drug's ability to produce an effect (i.e., its efficacy or intrinsic activity). The potency of a drug is related to the dose required to produce a given effect, not the maximal effect. A drug's therapeutic index is a measure of the safety of a drug. The lipid solubility and maximal effect of a drug are not related.

4. The answer is 5 [II F 2].
Approximately 3 mg of the drug will remain in the body 24 hours following administration. Because the drug is eliminated by a first-order process, a constant fraction of the drug is eliminated per unit of time. If 25 mg remains in the body after 6 hours, then the half-life ($t_{1/2}$) is 6 hours. Using this reasoning, the answer can be determined:

50 mg in body at time zero

25 mg in body 6 hours after administration

12.5 mg in body 12 hours after administration

6.25 mg in body 18 hours after administration

3.12 mg in body 24 hours after administration

5. The answer is 4 [II F 2–3].
The drug's half-life ($t_{1/2}$) is influenced by the volume of distribution (V_d) and body clearance (Cl_B) according to the following formula:

$$t_{1/2} = \frac{0.693 \cdot V_d}{Cl_B}$$

Because clearance is reduced to 25% of normal and the volume of distribution is 50% of normal, the half-life is doubled:

Normal: $t_{1/2} = \dfrac{0.693 \cdot 1}{1}$

$= .693$ (the units are not important)

Therefore, when the volume of distribution changes from 1 to 0.5 and the body clearance changes from 1 to 0.25, the half-life equals 1.386:

$$t_{1/2} = \frac{0.693 \cdot 0.5}{0.25} = 1.386$$

In other words, the half-life doubles. If the normal half-life is 60 minutes, then the expected half-life in this dog would be 120 minutes.

6. The answer is 1 [II A 1 a, B 2].
Most drugs that are injected intramuscularly are absorbed by simple diffusion. The drug diffuses from the injection site into the vascular compartment, where it is distributed systemically. Diffusion of the drug through the capillary membrane or capillary channels (pores) permits its absorption.

7. The answer is 3 [II A 1 b (2)].
Approximately 1% of the drug is ionized. Using the Henderson-Hasselbalch equation for weak acids:

$$pK_a = pH + \log \frac{\text{nonionized acid (U)}}{\text{ionized acid (I)}}$$

$$4 = 2 + \log \frac{U}{I}$$

$$2 = \log \frac{U}{I}$$

Taking the antilog of both sides: $100 = \frac{U}{I}$

If U = 1 drug unit, then I = 0.01 unit of drug. Therefore, the total drug units (U + I) are 1.01. By definition, U + I = 100%; therefore, 1.01 units of drug = 100%. Thus:

$$\frac{0.01 \text{ ionized drug}}{1.01 \text{ total drug}} = \frac{x\%}{100\%}$$

x = 0.99%, or approximately 1%.

8. The answer is 1 [II D 4 a].
Pentobarbital is oxidized by the cytochrome P-450 enzyme system present in the endoplasmic reticulum (microsomes) of the liver. Pretreatment with phenobarbital induces the liver cells to synthesize more cytochrome P-450 enzymes. Thus, animals pretreated with phenobarbital for several days have a greater capacity to metabolize pentobarbital.

Weak acid

$$pK_a = pH + \log \frac{\text{nonionized (U)}}{\text{ionized (I)}}$$

$$7 = 5 + \log \frac{U}{I}$$

$$2 = \log \frac{U}{I}$$

Taking the antilog of both sides:

$$100 = \frac{U}{I}$$

If U = 1 drug unit, then:

$$I = 0.01$$

1.01 drug units = 100%.

$$\frac{.01}{1.01} = \frac{X\%}{100\%}$$

X = 0.99% ionized (approx. 1%)

9. The answer is 4 [II F 1 a–d].
Extensive plasma protein binding, a high molecular weight, and high water solubility all favor a low apparent volume of distribution (V_d). Both a high percentage of binding to plasma proteins and a high molecular weight keep the majority of the drug in the vascular compartment. Drugs with a high degree of water solubility generally have low lipid solubility; therefore these drugs cross biologic membranes poorly, limiting their distribution.

10. The answer is 1 [III E 1 a; Figure 1-5].
Drug A is 30 times more potent than drug B. Potency refers to the amount of drug required to produce a specified effect or response. The dosage that produces the desired effect in 50% of the population (i.e., the ED_{50}) for drug A is 10 mg/kg, whereas the ED_{50} for drug B is 300 mg/kg.

11. The answer is 2 [II A 1 b (2), E 1 c].
The rate of elimination of a weak base with a pK_a of 6 is likely to increase if the urine is acidified. The Henderson-Hasselbalch equation can be used to ascertain the percent of the drug that exists in ionized form. (The ionized form is not subject to passive reabsorption following the filtration process and therefore is excreted more readily.) Assume acidification of urine to pH 5:

Weak base

$$pK_a = pH + \log \frac{\text{ionized (I)}}{\text{nonionized (U)}}$$

$$6 = 5 + \log \frac{I}{U}$$

$$1 = \log \frac{I}{U}$$

Taking the analog of both sides:

$$10 = \frac{I}{U}$$

If U = 1 drug unit, then:

$$I = 10$$

11 drug units = 100%.

$$\frac{10}{11} = \frac{X\%}{100\%}$$

X = 90.9% ionized

Because a larger portion of the base will be ionized at pH 5, the base will be eliminated faster than the acid.

Chapter 2

Drugs Affecting Peripheral Neurohumoral Transmission
Donald C. Dyer

I. **INTRODUCTION TO THE PERIPHERAL EFFERENT NERVOUS SYSTEM**

A. The **somatic nervous system** innervates **skeletal muscle** and controls motor functions of the body. Axons originate from the spinal cord and release the neurotransmitter acetylcholine (ACh) at the neuromuscular junction. Some drugs can affect both the somatic and the autonomic nervous systems because ACh is a transmitter in both systems. The somatic nervous system is discussed in more detail in Chapter 4.

B. The **autonomic nervous system** regulates the activity of the **heart, glands,** and **smooth muscle.** Two neurons are involved in the transmission process. The first neuron originates in the central nervous system (CNS) and synapses in a ganglion outside the CNS. A second neuron then innervates the target (effector) tissue.

1. **Organization** (Figure 2-1)
   a. **Sympathetic nervous system**
      (1) **Preganglionic neurons** originate from the thoracic and lumbar portions of the spinal cord and terminate in the para- or prevertebral ganglia, or they directly innervate the adrenal medulla. Functionally, the adrenal medulla responds as if it were a ganglion.
      (2) **Postganglionic neurons** originate from the ganglia and innervate the effector tissue.
   b. **Parasympathetic nervous system**
      (1) **Preganglionic neurons** originate from either the midbrain, the medulla oblongata, or the sacral portion of the spinal cord. They terminate on postganglionic neurons. The terminals of the preganglionic neurons and ganglia are located in or close to the effector tissue.
      (2) **Postganglionic neurons** innervate the tissue.

2. **Neurotransmitters** are chemical substances that transmit impulses across junctions such as synapses (e.g., nerve to nerve, nerve to effector tissue).
   a. **Sympathetic nervous system**
      (1) **Preganglionic neurons** release **ACh** onto **nicotinic receptors** of postganglionic neurons or the adrenal medulla.
      (2) **Postganglionic neurons** release **norepinephrine** onto **adrenergic receptors (adrenoceptors)** in the effector tissue.
   b. **Parasympathetic nervous system**
      (1) **Preganglionic neurons** release **ACh** onto **nicotinic receptors** of postganglionic neurons.
      (2) **Postganglionic neurons** release **ACh** onto **muscarinic receptors** in the effector tissue.

3. **Receptors** (Table 2-1)
   a. **Cholinergic receptors** mediate the effects of **ACh.** They are muscarinic or nicotinic, named after the plant alkaloids responsible for the physiologic effects of poisonous mushrooms and tobacco, respectively.
      (1) **Muscarinic** receptors have at least five subtypes.
      (2) **Nicotinic** receptors have two subtypes.
   b. **Adrenergic receptors (adrenoceptors)** mediate the effects of **norepinephrine** and **epinephrine.**
      (1) α-**Adrenoceptors:** α_1, α_2
      (2) β-**Adrenoceptors:** β_1, β_2

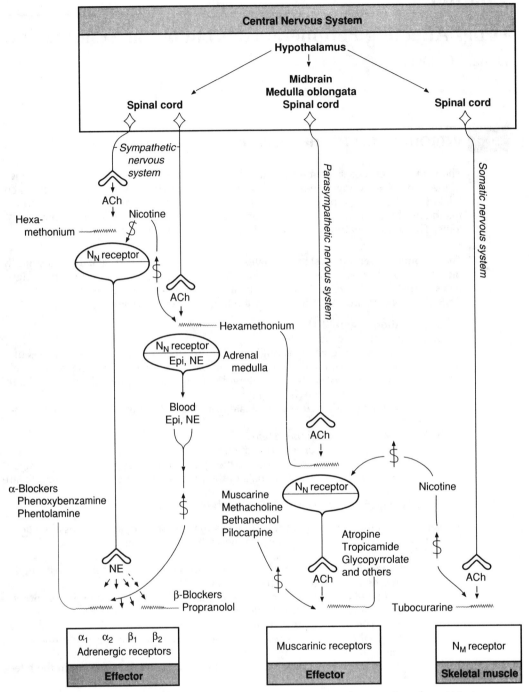

FIGURE 2-1. Effector neurons of the peripheral nervous system. Drugs that stimulate (⚡) and block (〰〰〰) receptors are also shown. N_N = ganglionic nicotine receptor; N_M = skeletal muscle nicotine receptor; NE = norepinephrine; Epi = epinephrine; ACh = acetylcholine.

Table 2-1. Tissue Receptors and Response to Stimulation

Effector Organ	Sympathetic		Parasympathetic	
	Receptor Type	Response to Stimulation	Receptor Type	Response to Stimulation
Heart				
S-A node	β_1	↑ Heart rate	M_2	↓ Heart rate
Atria	β_1	↑ Contractility	M_2	↓ Contractility
		↑ Conduction velocity		↑ Conduction velocity
A-V node	β_1	↑ Automaticity ↑ Conduction velocity	M_2	↓ Conduction velocity A-V block
Ventricles	β_1	↑ Contractility ↑ Conduction velocity ↑ Automaticity	M_2	↓ Contractility
Arteries				
Coronary	α	Contraction	. . .	Little or no effect
	β_2	Dilation		
Mesenteric and renal	α β_2	Constriction Dilation	. . .	No effect
Skin	α	Constriction	. . .	Little or no effect
Skeletal muscle	α	Constriction		
	β_2	Dilation	. . .	Little or no effect
Veins	α	Constriction	. . .	No innervation
	β_2	Dilation	. . .	No innervation
Eye				
Iris				
Radial muscle	α_1	Constriction (mydriasis)	. . .	No innervation
Circular muscle			M_3	Contraction (miosis)
Ciliary muscle	β	Relaxation	M_3	Contraction
Salivary glands	α_1	Secretion	M	Secretion
Bronchi	β_2	Dilation	M_3	Constriction
Urinary bladder	α, β	Retention	M_3	Contraction

A-V = atrioventricular; M = muscarinic; S-A = sinoatrial; ↑ = increase or stimulation; ↓ = decrease or inhibition.

II. ADRENERGIC AGONISTS (SYMPATHOMIMETIC AMINES). An overview is presented in Table 2-2.

A. Catecholamines

1. **Epinephrine, norepinephrine,** and **dopamine** are endogenous substances that serve as hormones and neurotransmitters. They are also used therapeutically as drugs.
   a. **Chemistry and biosynthesis** are illustrated in Figure 2-2.
   b. **Mechanism of action** (Figure 2-3)

Table 2-2. Adrenergic Pharmacology—An Overview

	Adrenergic Receptors			
	α_1	α_2	β_1	β_2
Agonists	←--- Epinephrine ---→			
	←-- Norepinephrine -----------------------------------→			←---- Metaproterenol ----→
	←----- Methoxamine -----→		←-------------------------- Isoproterenol --------------------------→	
	←---- Phenylephrine ----→	←-------- Xylazine --------→	←----- Dobutamine ------→	←------- Terbutaline -------→
Response	Arterioles (↑)	Arterioles (↑)	Heart (PIA, ↑ HR)	Arterioles (↓)
	Veins (↑)	Presynaptic adrenergic terminal (↓ NE release)	Juxtaglomerular cells (↑ renin release)	Bronchi (↓)
	Eye radial muscle (↑)	CNS (sedation)		Presynaptic adrenergic terminal (↑ norepinephrine release)
	Pilomotor muscle (↑)	Presynaptic cholinergic terminal (↓ ACh release)		
	Heart (PIA)			Uterus (↓)
	Gut (↓ via ↑ K⁺ channels)			Gut (↓)
Antagonists	←- Phenoxybenzamine -→	←------ (weak action) -----→	←-------- Atenolol --------→	
	←-------- Prazosin --------→	←------ Yohimbine ------→		
	←-------------------------- Phentolamine --------------------------→		←-------------------------- Propranolol --------------------------→	

ACh = acetylcholine; CNS = central nervous system; HR = heart rate; NE = norepinephrine; PIA = positive inotropic action; ↑ = vasoconstriction, contraction, stimulation; ↓ = vasodilation, relaxation, inhibition.

(1) **Epinephrine** is a potent agonist of all adrenoceptors (i.e., α_1, α_2, β_1, β_2).
(2) **Norepinephrine** is a potent agonist of α_1, α_2, and β_1 adrenoceptors. It has little effect on β_2 receptors.
(3) **Dopamine**
    (a) Dopamine causes the release of norepinephrine from adrenergic neurons, which activates β_1 adrenoceptors and α adrenoceptors.
    (b) Dopamine activates specific dopamine receptors.
        (i) **D_1 receptors** are present in the renal, mesenteric, and coronary circulation and are activated by low concentrations of dopamine. Activation produces vasodilation that is blocked by specific dopamine antagonists (e.g., haloperidol), but not by β adrenoceptor antagonists.
        (ii) **D_2 receptors** are present in the ganglia, the adrenal cortex, and certain areas of the CNS.

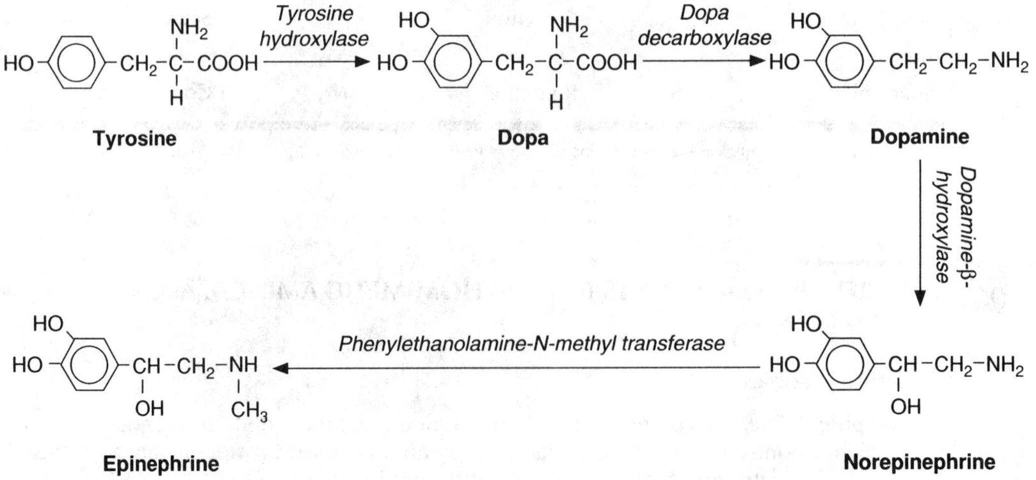

FIGURE 2-2. Biosynthesis of dopamine, norepinephrine, and epinephrine.

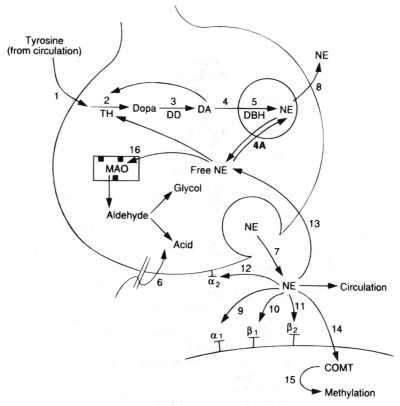

FIGURE 2-3. Site of action of drugs affecting the sympathetic nervous system. The figure depicts the events taking place at the junction of a sympathetic nerve terminal and an end-organ cell.

Tyrosine from the circulation enters the nerve terminal **(1)** and is converted, first **(2)** via tyrosine hydroxylase (*TH*) into dopa and then **(3)** via dopa decarboxylase (*DD*) into dopamine (*DA*). Dopamine enters the vesicles of the nerve terminal **(4)**, where it is converted **(5)**, via dopamine β-hydroxylase (*DBH*), into norepinephrine (*NE*), which is stored in the vesicles. Free NE in the axoplasm also enters and leaves the vesicles **(4A)**.

In the process of nerve impulse transmission across the neuroeffector junction, the nerve terminal is depolarized **(6)** by an action potential. The storage vesicle fuses with the plasma membrane, and the neurotransmitter NE is released into the junction **(7)** by exocytosis. Indirect-acting sympathomimetics can also cause NE to leave the vesicles and enter the neuroeffector junction **(8)**.

Once released from the nerve cell, NE activates the postsynaptic α_1, β_1, and β_2 receptors **(9, 10, 11)** on the effector cell, thereby producing the effector response. NE also activates the presynaptic α_2 receptors **(12)** on the nerve terminal itself.

Several mechanisms terminate the action of NE. Most important is the reentry of NE into the nerve terminal (a process known as uptake-1) **[13]**. Some of the NE enters the effector cell (uptake-2) **[14]**, and some enters the circulation.

Two enzymes play a role in the metabolism of NE. The NE that enters the effector cell is methylated **(15)** by catechol-O-methyltransferase (*COMT*) to normetanephrine. The NE in the axoplasm of the nerve terminal is converted **(16)** by monoamine oxidase (*MAO*) in the nerve cell's mitochondria, first to the aldehyde, and then to the glycol or to 3-methoxy-4-hydroxymandelic acid (vanillylmandelic acid, or VMA). The glycol and the acid are the major metabolites excreted in the urine. (Reprinted with permission from Jacob LS, *NMS Pharmacology*, 4th ed. Baltimore, Williams & Wilkins, 1996, p 22.)

c. Pharmacokinetics

(1) Absorption

    (a) Catecholamines are poorly absorbed following oral administration, partly because the drugs are rapidly conjugated and oxidized.

    (b) They are absorbed from the respiratory tract when nebulized and inhaled.

    (c) Subcutaneous absorption is slow because of vasoconstriction.

(2) Fate

    (a) Distribution. Catecholamines do not cross the blood–brain barrier readily.

    (b) Deactivation (see Figure 2-3)

        (i) Tissue uptake mechanisms remove the drug from the receptor site, thereby decreasing the number of receptors being occupied and decreasing the response.

            Uptake$_1$ is the active uptake of the drug into the presynaptic sympathetic nerve terminal. Cocaine produces a sympathomimetic effect by blocking uptake$_1$.

            Uptake$_2$ is the uptake of catecholamines into the effector tissue. Effector tissue contains monoamine oxidase (MAO) and catechol O-methyltransferase (COMT), which metabolize catecholamines to inactive products.

        (ii) The liver and kidneys, which are rich in **MAO** and **COMT,** inactivate circulating catecholamines.

    (c) Excretion. The metabolites are excreted in the urine.

d. Pharmacologic effects. The pharmacologic response to an agonist is a function of the **affinity of the agonist for the receptor,** the **number of receptors,** and the **efficacy of the agonist.**

    (1) Epinephrine

        (a) Blood pressure effects

            (i) Low doses may cause little change in blood pressure. They increase skeletal muscle blood flow via activation of β_2 adrenoceptors and increase heart rate and force of contraction via activation of β_1 adrenoceptors. β_2 adrenoceptors have a higher affinity than α adrenoceptors for epinephrine, producing a preferential activation at low doses.

            (ii) Higher doses. Increasing the dose of epinephrine leads to the activation of α adrenoceptors, which causes vasoconstriction and reduces the blood flow to the skeletal musculature. Because α adrenoceptors predominate in the cutaneous, mesenteric, and renal vascular beds, the net result is an increase in blood pressure.

              Activation of the α adrenoceptors increases total peripheral resistance and counters the β_2 receptor-induced vasodilation. In addition, the larger dose of epinephrine activates more β_1 receptors in the heart, which increases cardiac output and contributes to the increase in blood pressure.

              As the blood pressure increases, baroceptors in the arch of the aorta and carotid sinus are activated. They, in turn, activate the vagus and increase vagal tone on the heart to reduce cardiac output, lowering the systemic blood pressure.

        (b) Vascular effects

            (i) Skin. Activation of α adrenoceptors causes vasoconstriction, decreasing blood flow.

            (ii) Skeletal muscle. At low concentrations, β_2 adrenoceptors are activated, increasing blood flow to skeletal muscle. At higher concentrations, activation of α adrenoceptors reduces blood flow.

            (iii) Mesentery and kidneys. Activation of α adrenoceptors leads to a decreased blood flow.

            (iv) Lungs. Decreased blood flow results from vasoconstriction of arteries and veins.

            (v) Heart. Blood flow increases, largely because of the metabolic products created by the increase in cardiac work.

        (c) Cardiac effects. β_1 adrenoceptors predominate in the heart, but α and β_2 adrenoceptors are also present. Epinephrine causes:

            (i) Increased force of contraction (positive inotropic effect)

            (ii) Increased rate of contraction (positive chronotropic effect)

            (iii) Increased output

            (iv) Increased excitability

(v) Increased automaticity

(vi) Increased potential for arrhythmias

(vii) Decreased efficiency (greater oxygen consumption)

(d) Smooth muscle effects

(i) Gastrointestinal tract. Epinephrine relaxes smooth muscle via activation of α_2 and β adrenoceptors, and increases contraction of the sphincters by activating α adrenoceptors.

(ii) Uterus. Contraction (mediated by α receptors) or relaxation (mediated by β receptors) may occur, depending on the state of estrus, pregnancy, and species.

(iii) Urinary bladder. Urinary retention occurs when the fundus relaxes (as a result of β adrenoceptor stimulation) and the trigone and sphincter contract (as a result of α adrenoceptor stimulation).

(iv) Bronchioles. Relaxation occurs via activation of β_2 adrenoceptors.

(v) Eye. Mydriasis (pupillary dilation) results when α adrenoceptors in the radial muscles of the iris are stimulated. **Intraocular pressure may be reduced** by a local vasoconstrictor action that decreases the production of aqueous humor.

(vi) Spleen. Contraction (mediated by α adrenoceptors) increases blood erythrocyte levels, particularly in dogs.

(vii) Pilomotor muscles. Contraction (mediated by α adrenoceptors) erects the hairs on the skin, particularly in carnivores during fear or rage reactions.

(e) Metabolic effects

(i) Blood concentrations of glucose, free fatty acids, and lactic acid increase when β adrenoceptors in the liver, skeletal muscle, and adipose tissue are stimulated.

(ii) Some of the effects of epinephrine on glucose concentrations are secondary (e.g., inhibition of insulin secretion via activation of α_2 receptors and stimulation of glucagon secretion via activation of β_2 receptors).

(2) Norepinephrine elicits all of the effects produced by epinephrine that are mediated via α_1, α_2, and β_1 adrenoceptors, with the following exceptions:

(a) At similar doses, norepinephrine will increase the mean blood pressure more than epinephrine because it is not able to relax the skeletal blood vessels via β_2 receptors.

(b) Baroreceptor activation and vagal reflex will occur at lower doses for norepinephrine than epinephrine. This reflex can be strong enough to decrease cardiac output despite the direct activation of cardiac β_1 receptors.

(3) Dopamine has unique pharmacologic actions. The release of norepinephrine from the sympathetic postganglionic nerve terminal by dopamine contributes to its pharmacologic effects.

(a) Activation of D_1 receptors causes vasodilation of the renal and mesenteric vasculature at low rates of infusion. Natriuresis and diuresis result from the increased glomerular filtration rate and renal blood flow.

(b) Activation of D_2 receptors in the CNS decreases blood pressure and heart rate, and causes vasodilation in the renal and mesenteric vascular beds. It is unlikely that CNS D_2 receptors are activated when dopamine is infused, because dopamine does not cross the blood–brain barrier.

(c) Activation of β_1 receptors, which occurs at somewhat greater concentrations, produces a positive inotropic effect on the heart.

(d) Activation of α_1 receptors causes vasoconstriction; however, very high concentrations are necessary to produce this effect.

e. Therapeutic uses

(1) Epinephrine

(a) Epinephrine will reduce **bronchospasm.**

(b) Epinephrine is used to treat **hypersensitivity reactions** and **anaphylactic shock** that is characterized by bronchospasm and hypotension.

      (c) Epinephrine reduces cutaneous blood flow, which makes it useful for **prolonging local anesthetic effects.**

      (d) Applied topically, it can be used to control **localized hemorrhage.**

      (e) Epinephrine promotes the outflow of aqueous humor, making it useful for the treatment of **open-angle glaucoma.**

      (f) Epinephrine is used to restore cardiac activity following **cardiac arrest.**

   (2) Norepinephrine may be used to correct the **hypotension induced by spinal anesthesia.** It is not useful for correcting hypotension in most types of shock, because sympathetic activity is already high and further vasoconstriction may compromise the renal and mesenteric circulations.

   (3) Dopamine may be used to treat:

      (a) Cardiogenic shock

      (b) Septic shock

      (c) Acute heart failure (usually as supportive therapy)

f. Adverse effects

   (1) Epinephrine

      (a) Anxiety, fear, restlessness

      (b) Palpitations

      (c) Cerebral hemorrhage

      (d) Cardiac arrhythmias (especially in hyperthyroid patients)

   (2) Norepinephrine. Adverse effects are similar to those of epinephrine. In addition, extravasation following intravenous injection may cause necrosis and sloughing at the site because of intense vasoconstriction.

   (3) Dopamine. Adverse effects include those of epinephrine and norepinephrine, but they are short-lived because dopamine is rapidly metabolized.

2. Isoproterenol

  a. Mechanism of action. Isoproterenol, a potent **nonselective β-adrenoceptor agonist,** increases tissue cyclic adenosine monophosphate (cAMP) levels as β_1 and β_2 receptors activate adenyl cyclase. Isoproterenol has low affinity for α adrenoceptors.

  b. Pharmacokinetics

   (1) Absorption. Isoproterenol is readily absorbed parenterally or as an aerosol.

   (2) Fate. It is principally metabolized by COMT and MAO, but MAO is less effective than with epinephrine or norepinephrine.

   (3) Excretion. Metabolites are excreted in urine.

  c. Pharmacologic effects

   (1) Intravenous infusion **decreases mean blood pressure** by reducing peripheral resistance, primarily in skeletal muscle.

   (2) Cardiac output increases, owing to increases in cardiac contractility and heart rate.

   (3) Tissues possessing β_2 adrenoceptors (e.g., bronchiolar, gastrointestinal smooth muscle) **are relaxed.**

   (4) Antigen-induced release of histamine (a β_2-receptor effect) **is inhibited.**

  d. Therapeutic uses

   (1) Acute bronchial constriction

   (2) Complete atrioventricular (A-V) block

  e. Adverse effects

   (1) Tachycardia

   (2) Arrhythmias (as a result of general stimulation of cardiac tissues)

B.   Noncatecholamines

1. Phenylephrine

  a. Mechanism of action. Phenylephrine is a **direct α_1-receptor agonist** (Figure 2-4). It also has some β-adrenergic stimulatory properties at high doses.

  b. Pharmacologic effects. Phenylephrine **increases blood pressure** (primarily by vasoconstriction).

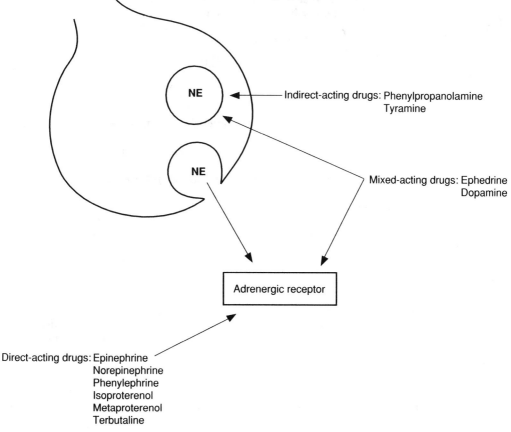

Direct-acting drugs: Epinephrine
Norepinephrine
Phenylephrine
Isoproterenol
Metaproterenol
Terbutaline

FIGURE 2-4. Comparison of direct-, mixed-, and indirect-acting sympathomimetic amines. Direct-acting drugs are able to elicit a pharmacologic response independently of the sympathetic neuron. Indirect-acting drugs produce a response by releasing norepinephrine (*NE*) from the neuron after they are transported into the neuron. Mixed-acting drugs stimulate the adrenergic receptor directly and by inducing the release of norepinephrine from the neuron.

    c. Therapeutic uses
        (1) Phenylephrine has an advantage over epinephrine as a **vasopressor** in situations where cardiac stimulation is undesirable, such as during general anesthesia with halothane.
        (2) Phenylephrine is used as a **topical nasal decongestant.**
        (3) It is used in ophthalmology as a **mydriatic agent** (during examinations), to reduce posterior **synechiae** formation, and to relieve the pain associated with **uveitis.**
    d. Adverse effects
        (1) Phenylephrine may elicit a **reflex bradycardia** when administered intravenously.
        (2) **Hypertension,** especially in geriatric, hyperthyroid, or hypertensive patients, may occur.
        (3) **Nasal irritation** and **rebound congestion** may occur following long-term nasal use.

  2. Dobutamine (see also Chapter 6 I D 2)
    a. Chemistry. The clinically used formulation of dobutamine is the racemic mixture of two enantiomeric forms, the negative and positive isomers.
    b. Mechanism of action. Dobutamine activates α and β adrenoceptors.

    (1) The **negative isomer** is an α_1- and β_1-**receptor agonist.**

    (2) The **positive isomer** is an α_1-**receptor antagonist,** which can block the effects of the negative isomer, and a β_1-**receptor agonist** that is ten times more potent than the negative isomer.

  c. Pharmacokinetics

    (1) Absorption. Dobutamine is not absorbed orally and is given by intravenous infusion.

    (2) Metabolism. Its half-life is short.

  d. Pharmacologic effects

    (1) Dobutamine produces an **inotropic effect,** which is greater than its chronotropic effect.

    (2) It **increases cardiac output** by increasing cardiac contractility and stroke volume.

  e. Therapeutic uses. Dobutamine is used for the **short-term treatment of heart failure.**

  f. Adverse effects

    (1) Dobutamine may increase oxygen use; therefore, it should be used with care after myocardial infarction to avoid increasing infarct size.

    (2) It may induce arrhythmias.

    (3) Other adverse effects may include those described for epinephrine [see II A 1 f (1)].

3. Ephedrine

  a. Mechanism of action. Ephedrine is a **mixed-acting agent** (i.e., it has direct and indirect actions); however, its primary action is indirect. Thus, a significant portion of its action results from the norepinephrine released from the adrenergic nerve terminal.

  b. Pharmacokinetics

    (1) Absorption. Ephedrine is absorbed from the gastrointestinal tract and can be administered orally.

    (2) Fate. It is resistant to metabolism by MAO and is not a substrate for COMT, so it has a prolonged action.

  c. Pharmacologic effects

    (1) Ephedrine **increases blood pressure** by causing peripheral vasoconstriction and cardiac stimulation.

    (2) It causes **bronchodilation** by activating β_2 adrenoceptors.

    (3) It causes **urinary bladder sphincter constriction** by activating adrenergic receptors.

  d. Therapeutic uses. Ephedrine is a scheduled drug [i.e., additional regulations for its use are imposed by the Food and Drug Administration (FDA)].

    (1) It is used to treat **asthma-like conditions.**

    (2) It is used as a **mydriatic.**

    (3) It is used to treat **primary urinary bladder sphincter incompetence.**

  e. Adverse effects are similar to those of epinephrine [see II A 1 f (1)].

    (1) Hypertension and **cardiac arrhythmias** may occur with systemic use.

    (2) CNS stimulation may cause **insomnia, nervousness, nausea,** and **agitation.**

    (3) Tachyphylaxis (i.e., diminished response following repeated administration) may occur. It is thought to be caused by a depletion of norepinephrine in the adrenergic nerve terminals susceptible to ephedrine.

4. Phenylpropanolamine

  a. Chemistry and mechanism of action. Phenylpropanolamine is an **indirect-acting sympathomimetic amine.**

  b. Pharmacokinetics

    (1) Absorption. Phenylpropanolamine is absorbed from the gastrointestinal tract and can be administered orally.

    (2) Fate. Phenylpropanolamine is resistant to metabolism by MAO and is not a substrate for COMT.

  c. Pharmacologic effects. The effects of phenylpropanolamine are similar to those of ephedrine, except phenylpropanolamine has little CNS stimulatory activity.

  d. Therapeutic uses
  - **(1)** Phenylpropanolamine is used for **primary urinary bladder sphincter incompetence.** Tachyphylaxis has not been documented when it is used for this purpose.
  - **(2)** It is also an orally acting **nasal decongestant.**
  e. Adverse effects are similar to those of ephedrine. In addition, anorexia may occur.

5. Terbutaline is an orally effective **direct-acting β_2-receptor agonist** used as a bronchodilator. It is the bronchodilator of choice for animals with heart disease, hyperthyroidism, or hypertension; however, it should be administered with caution because high doses may stimulate β_1 receptors.

III. ADRENERGIC ANTAGONISTS (see Table 2-2)

A. α-**Adrenergic antagonists**

1. Phenoxybenzamine
  a. Mechanism of action
  - **(1)** Phenoxybenzamine differs from most α-receptor antagonists in that it **binds covalently to the α receptor.** This is a stable chemical bond that produces a long-lasting and irreversible block of the receptor.
  - **(2)** Phenoxybenzamine is more effective in blocking α_1 than α_2 adrenoceptors.
  b. Pharmacologic effects
  - **(1)** Phenoxybenzamine decreases total peripheral resistance, causing hypotension.
  - **(2)** Heart rate may be increased via activation of the baroreceptor reflex or by blocking of the presynaptic α_2 receptors in the heart.
  - **(3)** Phenoxybenzamine can block pupillary dilation, lid retraction, and contraction of the nictitating membrane.
  c. Therapeutic uses
  - **(1)** In dogs and cats, it reduces **hypertonus at the urethral sphincter.**
  - **(2)** In horses, phenoxybenzamine has been used to treat **laminitis** and **secretory diarrhea.**
  d. Adverse effects
  - **(1) Hypotension** may be enhanced in hypovolemic animals.
  - **(2)** Phenoxybenzamine **should not be used in horses with colic.**

2. Prazosin
  a. Mechanism of action. Prazosin is a **competitive** and **selective α_1-receptor antagonist.**
  b. Pharmacologic effects
  - **(1)** Prazosin relaxes arterial and venous smooth muscle.
  - **(2)** There is a decrease in total peripheral resistance, but little tachycardia because α_2 adrenoceptors are not blocked.
  c. Therapeutic uses
  - **(1)** Prazosin is used in the treatment of **congestive heart failure.** It decreases arterial pressure, which improves movement of blood out of the heart.
  - **(2)** It is also used in the treatment of **hypertension.**
  d. Adverse effects include **diarrhea, tachycardia, hypotension,** and **fluid retention.**

3. Phentolamine
  a. Mechanism of action. Phentolamine is a competitive α_1- and α_2-adrenoceptor antagonist.
  b. Pharmacologic effects
  - **(1) Heart rate** may be increased by activation of the baroreceptor reflex or by blocking of the presynaptic α_2 receptors in the heart.

(2) **Blood pressure** is lowered by inhibition of α_1 and α_2 adrenoceptors in vascular smooth muscle and by direct relaxation of smooth muscle.

c. **Therapeutic uses.** Phentolamine is used to treat **hypertension** and to control high blood pressure resulting from **sympathomimetic amine overdose.**

d. **Adverse effects. Tachycardia** is frequently observed.

4. **Yohimbine**
   a. **Mechanism of action.** Yohimbine is a competitive α_2-adrenoceptor antagonist that promotes the formation of cAMP by blocking α_2-receptor activation.
   b. **Pharmacologic effects**
      (1) Yohimbine may increase insulin blood levels in animals with type II diabetes, because α_2 receptors inhibit insulin release.
      (2) Yohimbine can cause CNS stimulation, increased heart rate, and increased blood pressure.
   c. **Therapeutic uses.** Yohimbine is used to reverse the effects of **xylazine,** and may be effective in reversing the toxic effects of **amitraz,** which has α_2-agonist actions.
   d. **Adverse effects** are primarily CNS stimulation.

B. *β*-**Adrenergic antagonists**

1. **Propranolol** (see also Chapter 6 II B 2 c)
   a. **Pharmacokinetics**
      (1) **Absorption.** Propranolol is well absorbed following oral administration.
      (2) **Fate.** There is a significant first-pass effect, which reduces the systemic bioavailability. In dogs, only 2%–27% of an oral dose reaches the blood. Rapid metabolism occurs in the liver.
   b. **Mechanism of action.** Propranolol is a nonselective *β*-adrenoceptor antagonist that competitively blocks both β_1 and β_2 receptors.
   c. **Pharmacologic effects**
      (1) Propranolol decreases the sinus heart rate and depresses A-V conduction.
      (2) It decreases cardiac output.
      (3) It decreases myocardial oxygen demand.
      (4) It decreases the automaticity of cardiac tissue.
      (5) It increases airway resistance.
   d. **Therapeutic uses**
      (1) Propranolol is used to treat **hypertension associated with thyrotoxicosis** and **pheochromocytoma.**
      (2) It is used to treat **arrhythmias** (e.g., atrial and ventricular premature complexes, supraventricular and ventricular tachycardia).
   e. **Adverse effects**
      (1) Up-regulation of *β* receptors (i.e., an increased number of receptors) occurs with long-term therapy.
      (2) Abrupt cessation of therapy may lead to excessive stimulation of *β* receptors, thereby exacerbating the symptoms.
   f. **Contraindications**
      (1) Propranolol may cause bronchospasm and is contraindicated in asthmatic animals.
      (2) Propranolol is contraindicated in animals with heart failure or sinus bradycardia.
      (3) It is contraindicated in animals with hepatic disease or insufficiency.

2. **Atenolol**
   a. **Mechanism of action.** Atenolol is a **competitive β_1-selective adrenoceptor antagonist.**
   b. **Pharmacologic effects.** Atenolol decreases heart rate, cardiac output, and systolic and diastolic pressures.
   c. **Therapeutic uses.** Atenolol is used to treat **supraventricular arrhythmias, hypertrophic cardiomyopathy in cats,** and **hypertension.**
   d. **Adverse effects**

Table 2-3. Cholinergic Receptor Pharmacology—An Overview

	Cholinergic Receptors				
	Nicotinic Receptors		**Muscarinic Receptors**		
	N_M	N_N	M_1	M_2	M_3
Agonists	←-- Acetylcholine --→				
	←------------------- Nicotine ---------------------→			←------------------------	←-------- Bethanechol --------→
	←Succinylcholine→				
Response	Neuromuscular junction (↑)	Autonomic ganglia (↑) Adrenal medulla (↑ release of Epi, NE) CNS (still under investigation)	Myenteric plexus (↑) Autonomic ganglia (↑) CNS (still under investigation)	S-A node (↓ HR, slowed spontaneous depolarization) Atrium (NIA, shortened duration of action potential) A-V node (↓ conduction velocity, ↑ refractory period) Ventricle (NIA)	Eye ciliary muscle (↑) Iris circular muscle (↑) Bronchi smooth muscle (↑) GI smooth muscle (↑) Urinary bladder wall (↑) Sphincters GI tract (↓) Urinary bladder (↓) Vascular endothelium (↑ EDRF)
Antagonists	←Tubocurarine→	←Hexamethonium→	←-- Atropine --→		
			←------- Pirenzepine -------→		

A-V = atrioventricular; CNS = central nervous system; EDRF = endothelium-derived relaxing factor; Epi = epinephrine; GI = gastrointestinal; HR = heart rate; NE = norepinephrine; NIA = negative inotropic action; S-A = sinoatrial; ↑ = vasoconstriction, contraction, stimulation; ↓ = vasodilation, relaxation, inhibition.

(1) Although atenolol is selective for β_1 receptors, it should be used cautiously in animals with asthma or a history of bronchospasm.

(2) Excessive β_1 blockade can greatly reduce cardiac output.

IV. CHOLINERGIC AGONISTS (Table 2-3)

A. ACh

1. **Chemistry and biosynthesis** (Figure 2-5). ACh is a quaternary chemical, synthesized by the enzyme choline acetyltransferase from choline and acetyl coenzyme A (acetyl CoA).

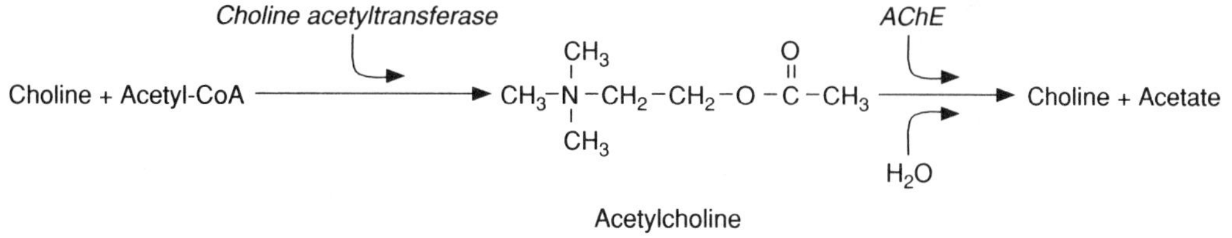

FIGURE 2-5. Synthesis and hydrolysis of acetylcholine (ACh). *Acetyl CoA* = acetyl coenzyme A; *AChE* = acetylcholinesterase.

2. **Mechanism of action.** ACh stimulates muscarinic and nicotinic receptors.

3. **Pharmacologic effects** (see Table 2-2)
   a. **Cardiovascular.** The actions of ACh on the heart are similar to the effects produced by vagal stimulation. ACh **decreases systemic blood pressure** following intravenous injection. Possible mechanisms include negative inotropic or chronotropic action and vasodilation.
      (1) Vasodilation in response to nerve-released ACh is of little physiologic importance in the maintenance of blood pressure, because most peripheral blood vessels are not cholinergically innervated. However, drugs that are analogs of ACh are capable of producing vasodilation via activation of muscarinic receptors in the blood vessels.
      (2) Vasodilation is thought to be caused by two processes:
         (a) Inhibition of the release of norepinephrine from the sympathetic nerve terminal
         (b) Interaction with muscarinic receptors on the endothelial cells to release nitric oxide, which initiates the relaxation of vascular smooth muscle
   b. **Smooth muscle and glands**
      (1) Stimulation of muscarinic receptors **increases gastrointestinal motility and secretion.**
      (2) ACh causes smooth muscle **contraction in the uterus, ureters, bladder, bronchi,** and **sphincter muscles of the iris.**
      (3) Activation of muscarinic receptors **increases salivary** and **lacrimal gland secretions.**

4. **Therapeutic uses.** ACh has little or no use as a therapeutic drug.

5. **Antagonists. Atropine** is a specific antagonist at muscarinic receptors.

B. **Methacholine (acetyl-β-methylcholine).** The addition of a methyl group to the β position of choline in ACh results in methacholine. Methacholine is hydrolyzed much more slowly than ACh, and therefore, is more useful as a drug.

C. **Carbachol (carbamylcholine)**

1. **Chemistry.** Carbachol has a carbamic acid–ester bond that is not hydrolyzable by cholinesterase.

2. **Mechanism of action.** Carbachol activates both muscarinic and nicotinic receptors.

3. **Therapeutic use.** Carbachol is used topically to **produce miosis** in ophthalmology.

D. **Bethanechol**

1. **Chemistry.** Bethanechol chemically resembles methacholine and carbachol. It is resistant to hydrolysis by cholinesterase.

2. **Pharmacologic effect.** Bethanechol is an agonist of muscarinic receptors.

3. **Therapeutic uses.** It is used to treat **abdominal distention, esophageal reflux,** and **distention of the urinary bladder.**

E. **Pilocarpine**

1. **Chemistry.** Pilocarpine is a tertiary amine alkaloid.

2. **Pharmacologic effects.** Pilocarpine resembles methacholine in actions; however, because it does not contain a quaternary nitrogen, it can cross biologic membranes more easily.

3. **Therapeutic uses.** Pilocarpine is primarily used to **produce miosis** and to **lower intraocular pressure in glaucoma.**

V. ANTICHOLINESTERASE AGENTS (INDIRECT CHOLINERGIC AGONISTS)

A. **Mechanism of action.** These agents act indirectly by preventing the hydrolysis of ACh by acetylcholinesterase **(AChE).** Therefore, at synaptic junctions, more cholinergic receptors are occupied by ACh, causing increased muscarinic and nicotinic responses. Anticholinesterase agents prevent the hydrolysis of ACh via three primary mechanisms:

1. **Reversible AChE inhibition.** The quarternary nitrogen of the drug reversibly binds to the active center of the enzyme at the anionic site.

2. **Carbamylation of AChE.** These agents are substrates for AChE and occupy the active site for an extended period of time, thereby increasing the ACh concentration at synapses.

3. **Phosphorylation of AChE.** These drugs form a stable covalent bond with the enzyme, and their effects are long-lasting.

B. **Preparations**

1. **Physostigmine**
   a. **Chemistry.** Physostigmine is a tertiary amine.
   b. The **mechanism of action** is carbamylation of AChE.
   c. **Pharmacokinetics.** Physostigmine is well absorbed from the gastrointestinal tract, subcutaneous tissues, and mucous membranes. It crosses the blood–brain barrier.
   d. **Pharmacologic effects.** The pharmacologic effects mimic those of ACh.
      (1) Physostigmine produces miosis, salivation, and increased gastrointestinal motility.
      (2) In large doses, it causes fasciculation followed by paralysis of skeletal muscle (caused by the accumulation of ACh at the skeletal neuromuscular junction).
   e. **Therapeutic uses.** Physostigmine is used to treat simple and secondary **glaucoma,** and to counteract **intoxication by atropine** and other antimuscarinic drugs.

2. **Neostigmine**
   a. **Chemistry.** Neostigmine contains a quaternary nitrogen.
   b. The **mechanism of action** is carbamylation of AChE.
   c. **Pharmacokinetics**
      (1) **Absorption.** Typical of quaternary nitrogens, neostigmine is not well absorbed orally, nor does it cross the blood–brain barrier.
      (2) **Fate.** Neostigmine is hydrolyzed by plasma esterases.
      (3) **Excretion.** It is excreted in the urine.
   d. **Pharmacologic effects**
      (1) The pharmacologic effects of neostigmine mimic those of ACh, causing effects similar to those of physostigmine.
      (2) Neostigmine reverses the neuromuscular block produced by tubocurarine-like drugs by:
         (a) Inhibition of AChE
         (b) Increasing the release of ACh from nerve endings
         (c) Acting directly on the skeletal neuromuscular junction
   e. **Therapeutic uses**
      (1) Reversal of tubocurarine-like blockade at the skeletal neuromuscular junction
      (2) Paralytic ileus
      (3) Atony of the urinary bladder
      (4) Myasthenia gravis-like conditions
   f. **Contraindications.** Neostigmine is contraindicated in the presence of bowel or bladder obstruction.

3. **Edrophonium**
   a. The **mechanism of action** is reversible inhibition of AChE.
   b. **Pharmacokinetics.** Edrophonium is administered parenterally and has a short duration of action (10–15 minutes).
   c. **Pharmacologic effects.** Its actions are similar to those of neostigmine.
   d. **Therapeutic uses.** Edrophonium is used to diagnose myasthenia gravis-like disease and antagonize tubocurarine-like drugs.

4. **Pyridostigmine** and **demecarium** are similar to physostigmine and neostigmine; however, they have longer half-lives. Pyridostigmine is used to treat myasthenia gravis, and demecarium is used to treat glaucoma.

5. **Carbaryl** is a carbamate anticholinesterase, similar to physostigmine and neostigmine, used to control fleas. The effects of overdose are similar to organophosphate poisoning and are treatable with atropine.

6. **Organophosphates**
   a. **Preparations**
      (1) **Diisopropyl fluorophosphate (DFP)** is an irreversible inhibitor that phosphorylates the esteratic site of AChE. It has a long duration of action and is used topically in the treatment of glaucoma.
      (2) **Echothiophate.** The mechanism of action resembles that of DFP. It has a long duration of action and is used topically in the treatment of glaucoma.
      (3) **Malathion** and **parathion.** These insecticides are metabolized by cytochrome P-450 enzymes to malaoxon and paraoxon, respectively. The metabolites are the active cholinesterase inhibitors. Their actions are similar to those of DFP.
      (4) **Dichlorvos** is a broad-spectrum anthelmintic used to treat infections in horses, cats, dogs, and pigs. It is used to control fleas, lice, and ticks in dogs and cats.
   b. **Toxicity** (see also Chapter 15 III I)
      (1) **Clinical signs**
         (a) **SLUD** (i.e., **s**alivation, **l**acrimation, **u**rination, and **d**efecation) refers to a constellation of signs that are related to muscarinic stimulation. In addition, **miosis** and **bradycardia** may be seen.
         (b) **Anorexia** and **vomiting** may occur.
         (c) **Neurologic signs** include convulsions and fasciculations of skeletal muscle. Respiratory failure caused by **weakness of the respiratory muscles** ultimately leads to **death.**
      (2) **Treatment**
         (a) **Detoxification**
            (i) **Dermal exposure.** The skin should be washed with soap and water to remove unabsorbed toxin. These chemicals are highly lipid-soluble and are readily absorbed via the skin; therefore, personnel should wear protective gear to prevent contact with the toxin.
            (ii) **Oral exposure.** Gastric lavage should be considered if the organophosphates have been ingested.
         (b) **Stabilization**
            (i) **Respiratory assistance** may be required.
            (ii) **Anticonvulsants** may be administered.
         (c) **Antidotal therapy** (see Chapter 15 III I 4)
            (i) **Atropine** will reduce the muscarinic effects.
            (ii) **Pyridine-2-aldoxime methiodide (2-PAM, pralidoxime)** reactivates AChE.

VI. PARASYMPATHETIC ANTAGONISTS (ANTIMUSCARINIC DRUGS)

A. **Atropine**

1. **Chemistry.** Atropine, a tertiary amine, is the prototype for all antimuscarinic drugs. It is an alkaloid obtained from the plant *Atropa belladonna* (deadly nightshade).

2. Mechanism of action

  a. Atropine is a competitive and nonselective antagonist of ACh at muscarinic receptors.

  b. It has a high affinity for muscarinic receptors and has little effect in blocking receptors for other substances such as histamine, serotonin, or norepinephrine.

3. Pharmacokinetics. Atropine is rapidly and well absorbed when given orally.

4. Pharmacologic effects

  a. Heart

  (1) Heart rate. The effect of atropine on the heart rate is variable.

   (a) The rate may slow initially or following a low dose, possibly as a result of central vagal stimulation.

   (b) As the muscarinic receptors on the sinoatrial (S-A) node are blocked by higher concentrations of atropine, tachycardia results.

  (2) The PR interval is shortened.

  b. Vasculature. Because blood vessels are regulated primarily by the sympathetic nervous system, atropine at usual doses has a small to modest effect on the systemic blood pressure.

  c. CNS. Toxic doses of atropine produce CNS stimulation, possibly followed by depression as the toxicity progresses.

  d. Smooth muscle

  (1) Gastrointestinal peristaltic contractions are reduced in amplitude and frequency. Muscle tone is also reduced.

  (2) Biliary tract smooth muscle is relaxed.

  (3) Urinary bladder and ureter tone are reduced.

  (4) Bronchodilation occurs in the large bronchi.

  e. Eye

  (1) Mydriasis. Atropine blocks the muscarinic receptors for ACh on the sphincter smooth muscle of the iris.

  (2) Cycloplegia is the inability to accommodate for near vision. Atropine inhibits cholinergic control of the ciliary muscle of the lens.

  f. Secretion

  (1) Salivary and bronchial secretions are reduced.

  (2) Sweat gland secretions are reduced.

  (3) Gastric secretions are reduced at high doses.

5. Therapeutic uses

  a. Atropine is used as a **preanesthetic agent** to reduce salivary and respiratory secretions.

  b. Antimuscarinics are used in ophthalmology to **produce cycloplegia and mydriasis;** however, because atropine has a long duration of action, its usefulness in this capacity is limited.

  c. It may be used to treat **renal** and **biliary colic** when combined with opioids.

  d. It is used to counter **anticholinesterase overdose** or **toxicity.**

  e. It may be useful in treating **mushroom toxicity** if muscarine is the toxic agent.

6. Adverse effects include tachycardia, photophobia (from mydriasis), xerostomia, increased body temperature (caused by a decrease in sweating), restlessness, disorientation, and CNS stimulation.

7. Treatment of toxicity. An anticholinesterase agent (e.g., neostigmine, physostigmine) should be administered to increase the concentration of ACh at muscarinic receptor sites. CNS stimulation may be controlled by benzodiazepines.

B. **Scopolamine (hyoscine),** an alkaloid resembling atropine in chemical structure and pharmacologic properties, may produce excitement or sedation. It is effective against motion sickness.

C. **Propantheline**

  1. Chemistry. Propantheline is a synthetic quaternary ammonium antimuscarinic drug.

2. Mechanism of action. Its antimuscarinic properties are similar to those of atropine.

3. Therapeutic uses
   a. In small animals, propantheline has been used as an antispasmodic and antise-
   cretory drug in the treatment of **diarrhea.**
   b. In horses, it has been **used to relax the rectum** prior to rectal examination.

4. Adverse effects are similar to those of atropine, except propantheline does not effectively enter the CNS.

D. **Glycopyrrolate**

1. Chemistry. Glycopyrrolate is a synthetic quaternary ammonium.

2. Pharmacokinetics
   a. Glycopyrrolate does not effectively enter the CNS or eye.
   b. It is eliminated primarily via the kidney; metabolism plays a small role in its
   elimination.

3. Pharmacologic effects. Glycopyrrolate has antimuscarinic properties similar to
those of atropine.

4. Therapeutic uses
   a. Glycopyrrolate is used as a **preanesthetic drug.**
   b. Glycopyrrolate has been used to treat **sinus bradycardia, S-A arrest,** and **incomplete A-V block.**

E. **Tropicamide,** a synthetic antimuscarinic drug, is used in ophthalmology to induce mydriasis and cycloplegia. It has an advantage over atropine in that its duration of action
is much shorter.

F. **Pirenzepine** is an investigational antimuscarinic drug with selectivity for M_1 muscarinic receptors. It reduces gastric acid secretion.

VII. **GANGLIONIC NICOTINIC AGONISTS AND ANTAGONISTS.** Ganglionic nicotinic agonists and antagonists are of limited use in veterinary medicine. Skeletal neuromuscular junction nicotinic antagonists (see VIII) have more therapeutic uses.

A. Nicotine is a **nicotinic receptor (N_N) agonist.**

1. Mechanism of action (see Figure 2-1; Table 2-3)
   a. Nicotine acts on nicotinic receptors in both the sympathetic and parasympathetic ganglia, where it stimulates the postganglionic neuron. It mimics the actions of ACh in this aspect.
   b. Nicotine stimulates the adrenal medulla to release epinephrine and norepineph-
   rine·into the blood stream.
   c. In the somatic nervous system, nicotine stimulates the skeletal neuromuscular
   junction at N_M nicotinic receptors.

2. Pharmacokinetics
   a. Absorption. Nicotine is absorbed by all routes, including the dermal route.
   b. Fate. It is metabolized by the liver.
   c. Excretion. It is eliminated by the kidneys.

3. Pharmacologic effects
   a. CNS. Stimulation of the motor cortex by nicotine produces tremors.
   b. Respiratory. Respiration may be initially stimulated and then depressed.
   c. Cardiovascular. Increases in blood pressure, heart rate, and peripheral resistance result from stimulation of sympathetic ganglia and the adrenal medulla.
   d. Smooth muscle and glands. Stimulation of parasympathetic ganglia may increase gastrointestinal motility and salivary secretion.

4. Therapeutic uses. Nicotine has no therapeutic use but is available for use as an insecticide.

5. Adverse effects
   a. Use of nicotine as an insecticide and ingestion of tobacco have resulted in toxicity in animals.
   b. Convulsions may occur with high doses.
   c. Vomiting and muscle fasciculations may occur.

B. **Hexamethonium, trimethaphan,** and **mecamylamine** are **N_N antagonists.** These drugs have limited use in veterinary medicine. The primary disadvantage to their use is that they are not selective (i.e., they block transmission in both sympathetic and parasympathetic ganglia).

   1. Trimethaphan has been used to lower blood pressure during surgery.

   2. Mecamylamine has been used to treat hypertension in human medicine.

VIII. NEUROMUSCULAR BLOCKING DRUGS

A. **Mechanism of action.** These drugs act on N_M receptors via two different mechanisms to relax skeletal muscle.

   1. Depolarizing drugs (e.g., **succinylcholine**). Succinylcholine acts like ACh to depolarize the neuromuscular junction, but it is hydrolyzed by AChE less rapidly.
   a. Phase I. The sodium channel associated with the N_M receptor is opened and the receptor is depolarized. Persistent binding of succinylcholine to the N_M receptor transforms the receptor so that it is incapable of transmitting further impulses. This phase is associated with muscle fasciculations.
   b. Phase II. Over time, the sodium channel closes and repolarization occurs, rendering the neuromuscular junction resistant to depolarization. Flaccid paralysis ensues.

   2. Competitive blocking drugs (e.g., **tubocurarine, gallamine, pancuronium, alcuronium, atracurium, vecuronium**). These drugs occupy the N_M receptor but do not activate it. By reducing the number of N_M receptors available for ACh, the endplate potential is reduced, the threshold required to excite the muscle is not reached, and the muscle relaxes.

B. **Pharmacokinetics**

   1. Depolarizing drugs
   a. Following intravenous administration, succinylcholine has a rapid onset of action. The duration of action varies according to species: pigs (2–3 minutes), horses and cats (5 minutes), cattle and sheep (6–8 minutes), and dogs (25 minutes).
   b. Succinylcholine is hydrolyzed by pseudocholinesterase. Animals that have been exposed to an organophosphate cholinesterase inhibitor (e.g., in flea collars, eyedrops, or anthelmintics) up to 30 days before succinylcholine administration may experience a prolonged duration of action caused by a reduced rate of hydrolysis.

   2. Competitive blocking drugs. Each drug has a specific duration of action that varies according to species (Table 2-4).
   a. Tubocurarine is not significantly metabolized in animals. Approximately 50% is excreted unchanged in the urine and 50% in the bile. Caution should be taken not to administer tubocurarine to animals with liver or kidney disease.
   b. Gallamine is not metabolized and is excreted unchanged in the urine.
   c. Pancuronium is metabolized by the liver, but the kidney is the major route for elimination.

Table 2-4. Duration of Action of Competitive N_M Blockers*

Animal	Tubocurarine		Gallamine		Alcuronium		Pancuronium		Atracurium		Vecuronium	
	Dose (mg/kg)	Duration (min)	Dose (mg/kg)	Duration (min)	Dose (mg/kg)	Duration (min)	Dose (mg/kg)	Duration (min)	Dose (mg/kg)	Duration (min)	Dose (mg/kg)	Duration (min)
Horse	0.3	60	1	20–25	0.05	60	0.06	40	0.15	30	0.1	30
Cow	0.06	30	0.5	30–40	...	...	0.04	40	...	...	...	...
Sheep	0.04	30	0.4	>120	...	...	0.025	45	0.5	30	0.04	15
Pig	0.4	30	1	30	...	...	0.1	30	...	...	...	...
Dog	...	...	1	30	0.1	70	0.06	30	0.5	40	0.1	25
Cat	...	...	1	15–20	...	...	...	...	0.5	40	0.1	25

Based on data in Einstein R, Jones RS, Knifton A, and Starmer GA: *Principles of Veterinary Therapeutics*. Essex, England, Longman Scientific and Technical Publishers, 1994, pp 162–165.
* Following intravenous administration.

    d. Atracurium undergoes spontaneous degradation in the plasma (Hoffmann process). It is also hydrolyzed by esterases, which do not involve the liver or kidneys, making it the drug of choice for relaxing skeletal muscle in animals with liver or kidney disease.

    e. Vecuronium is eliminated by the kidney (approximately 15%) and by metabolism and biliary excretion.

C. **Factors influencing the effects of neuromuscular blockers**

    1. Genetic or cholinesterase inhibitor-induced decreases in plasma cholinesterase activity will prolong the duration of action of succinylcholine.

    2. Hepatic disease may prolong the duration of action of succinylcholine because the liver synthesizes plasma cholinesterase.

    3. Aminoglycoside antibiotics, which inhibit ACh release, exhibit neuromuscular blocking activity.

    4. Halogenated hydrocarbon general anesthetics such as halothane enhance neuromuscular blockade by stabilizing the postjunctional membrane.

D. **Therapeutic uses.** Neuromuscular blockers promote and enhance skeletal muscle relaxation. Muscle relaxation facilitates endotracheal intubation and allows surgery to be performed with less general anesthetic, enhancing safety. Neuromuscular blocking agents do not block pain (i.e., they do not affect sensory mechanisms).

E. **Adverse effects**

    1. All neuromuscular blocking drugs may produce **apnea,** possibly necessitating artificial respiration.

    2. Succinylcholine. Adverse effects associated with succinylcholine include **painful muscle contractions, bradycardia,** and **increases in bronchiolar and salivary secretions. Malignant hyperthermia** may occur in pigs and horses.

    3. Tubocurarine may **reduce blood pressure** by causing **histamine release** and by blocking transmission in autonomic ganglia. Dogs and cats are prone to histamine release by tubocurarine, which precludes its use in these species. Histamine release may also cause **bronchospasm, increased bronchial secretions,** and **salivation.**

    4. Gallamine increases heart rate by blocking muscarinic receptors on the heart. Gallamine should be avoided in animals that cannot tolerate **tachycardia.** It releases less histamine than tubocurarine.

    5. Alcuronium does not significantly release histamine or block autonomic ganglia. Because it is eliminated primarily by the kidneys, it should not be used in animals with renal disease.

    6. Pancuronium causes a small increase in heart rate.

    7. Atracurium does induce histamine release, but less so than tubocurarine.

F. **Reversal of neuromuscular blockade**

    1. Depolarizing drugs. No good antagonists exist for succinylcholine. Artificial respiration should be provided until recovery occurs.

    2. Competitive neuromuscular blockers can be antagonized by cholinesterase inhibitors such as **edrophonium** and **neostigmine.**

STUDY QUESTIONS

DIRECTIONS: Each of the numbered items or incomplete statements in this section is followed by answers or by completion of the statement. Select the **one** numbered answer or completion that is **best** in each case.

1. α_1 Receptors are associated with which one of the following effects?

(1) Cardioacceleration
(2) Vasodilation
(3) Pupillary dilation
(4) Bronchodilation
(5) Pupillary constriction

2. What is the most likely cause of death in organophosphate poisoning?

(1) Gastrointestinal bleeding
(2) Hypertension
(3) Respiratory failure
(4) Congestive heart failure
(5) Cardiac arrhythmia

Questions 3–5

Assume that the diagram can represent either the parasympathetic or the sympathetic nervous system.

3. Which one of the following drugs acts at site 5?

(1) Phenylpropanolamine
(2) Prazosin
(3) Atenolol
(4) Nicotine

4. Tropicamide is a useful drug for inducing dilation of the pupil and paralysis of accommodation. At which one of the following sites on the diagram does tropicamide exert its effects?

(1) Site 3
(2) Site 4
(3) Site 5
(4) Site 6
(5) Site 7

5. Acetylcholine (ACh) interacts at all of the following sites in the diagram *except:*

(1) site 2.
(2) site 4.
(3) site 5.
(4) site 6.
(5) site 7.

6. Which one of the following drugs produces dilation of vessels in muscle, constriction of cutaneous vessels, and positive intropic and chronotropic effects on the heart?

(1) Metaproterenol
(2) Norepinephrine
(3) Acetylcholine (ACh)
(4) Epinephrine
(5) Isoproterenol

7. Which of the following drugs produces pupillary dilation without causing cycloplegia?

(1) Scopolamine
(2) Pilocarpine
(3) Isoproterenol
(4) Tropicamide
(5) Phenylephrine

8. Which bronchodilator is considered the most safe for use in an animal with cardiac disease?

(1) Isoproterenol
(2) Terbutaline
(3) Propranolol
(4) Epinephrine
(5) Atenolol

DIRECTIONS: Each of the numbered items or incomplete statements in this section is negatively phrased, as indicated by an italicized word such as *not, least, or except.* Select the **one** numbered answer or completion that is **best** in each case.

---

9. Nicotinic receptor sites are found in all of the following locations *except:*

(1) parasympathetic ganglia.
(2) sympathetic ganglia.
(3) skeletal muscle.
(4) bronchial smooth muscle.

10. When placed in the eye, echothiophate can cause all of the following *except:*

(1) miosis.
(2) ciliary spasm.
(3) reversal of cycloplegia.
(4) mydriasis.
(5) reduction in intraocular pressure.

ANSWERS AND EXPLANATIONS

1. The answer is 3 [Table 2-1].
Sympathetic stimulation causes the α_1 adrenoceptors in the iris to contract, causing pupillary dilation (mydriasis). An increased heart rate is associated with β_1 adrenoceptors. Vasodilation and bronchodilation are associated with β_2 adrenoceptors. Miosis (i.e., constriction of the pupils) is associated with stimulation of muscarinic cholinergic receptors.

2. The answer is 3 [V B 6 b (1) (c)].
Organophosphate cholinesterase inhibitors prevent the hydrolysis of acetylcholine (ACh). ACh accumulates at cholinergic synapses. All autonomically innervated tissues may be affected by the excess ACh, but excess ACh at the skeletal muscle neuroeffector junction ultimately leads to paralysis of the respiratory muscles, the primary cause of death.

3–5. The answers are: 3-1 [II B 4; III A 2, B 2; VII A; Figure 2-1], **4-4** [VI E; Figure 2-1]; **5-1** [IV A; Figure 2-1].
Phenylpropanolamine is an indirect-acting sympathomimetic amine that acts on the postganglionic sympathetic neuron to release norepinephrine. Prazosin and atenolol are α_1- and β_1-adrenoceptor antagonists; therefore, they act at site 6. Nicotine, a nicotinic-receptor agonist, acts at site 4 in the parasympathetic and sympathetic nervous systems.

Tropicamide, a short-acting muscarinic antagonist, acts at site 6 on the diagram. It antagonizes acetylcholine (ACh) at the muscarinic receptors of the sphincter muscle in the iris and ciliary muscles, producing mydriasis and cycloplegia.

ACh does not have receptors on the axon (site 2). It does react with cholinergic receptors at sites 4, 5, and 6, and with acetylcholinesterase (AChE) at site 7.

6. The answer is 4 [II A 1 b; Table 2-1].
Activation of β_2 adrenoceptors, α_1 adrenoceptors, and β_1 adrenoceptors produces vasodilation in muscle, constriction of skin vasculature, and positive inotropic and chronotropic effects on the heart, respectively. The only

drug listed that activates α_1, β_1, and β_2 adrenoceptors is epinephrine.

7. The answer is 5 [II B 1; Table 2-1].
Phenylephrine, an α_1-adrenoceptor agonist, constricts the radial muscles of the iris to produce dilation. Scopolamine and tropicamide are muscarinic antagonists that produce dilation; however, they also produce cycloplegia. Pilocarpine is a direct-acting muscarinic antagonist that produces miosis when placed in the eye. Activation of β adrenoceptors in the eye, such as that caused by isoproterenol, does not cause dilation.

8. The answer is 2 [II B 5].
Terbutaline would be the drug of choice when it is necessary to induce bronchodilation in an animal with heart disease. A drug with β_2 agonistic activity is necessary to produce bronchodilation. Although isoproterenol and epinephrine are β_2 agonists, they are also strong β_1 agonists and thus would be expected to excite the heart. Propranolol is a β_1- and β_2-antagonist and blocking β_2 adrenoceptors causes bronchoconstriction. Atenolol is a β_1-adrenoceptor antagonist. Although terbutaline is the drug of choice in this situation, caution is warranted because at high doses, terbutaline may stimulate β_1 adrenoceptors.

9. The answer is 4 [VII A 1, Figure 2-1].
Bronchial smooth muscle contains muscarinic cholinergic receptors, not nicotinic receptors. Both the parasympathetic and sympathetic ganglia contain N_N-nicotinic cholinergic receptors, and the skeletal neuromuscular junction contains N_M-nicotinic cholinergic receptors.

10. The answer is 4 [V B 6 b; Table 2-1].
Echothiophate, a cholinesterase inhibitor, is an indirect-acting cholinergic agonist. The buildup of acetylcholine (ACh) causes miosis, ciliary spasm, reversal of cycloplegia, and reduced intraocular pressure. Mydriasis can be caused by blocking muscarinic receptors in the sphincter smooth muscle of the iris or by contracting the radial muscles of the iris via α_1 adrenoceptors.

Chapter 3

Autacoids and Their Antagonists

Donald C. Dyer

I. INTRODUCTION

A. Definitions

1. **Autacoids** are substances that are synthesized and function in a localized area. They participate in responses to injury. They normally do not function as typical circulating hormones.

2. **Autacoid antagonists** inhibit autacoid synthesis, release, or effects on tissue receptors.

B. Functions. The physiologic roles of many autacoids remain unknown.

1. Autacoids modulate blood flow in specific tissues.

2. Some autacoids modulate secretory processes.

C. Major classes*

1. **Biogenic amines** include **histamine** and **serotonin (5-hydroxytryptamine, 5-HT).**

2. **Phospholipid-derived autacoids**
   a. **Eicosanoids** include **prostaglandins (PGs), leukotrienes (LTs),** and **thromboxanes (TXs).**
   b. **Platelet-activating factor (PAF)**

3. **Polypeptides** include **angiotensin** and **kinin.**

II. BIOGENIC AMINES

A. Histamine (Table 3-1)

1. **Agonists**
   a. **2-Methylhistamine** is the prototypic H_1 **agonist.**
   b. **4-Methylhistamine** and **impromidine** are prototypic H_2 **agonists.**

2. **Biosynthesis, storage, and catabolism** (Figure 3-1). The concentration and rate of synthesis of histamine vary greatly from tissue to tissue.
   a. **Biosynthesis.** Dietary **histidine** is decarboxylated by L-histidine decarboxylase to form **histamine.**
   b. **Storage.** Histamine is widely distributed in tissues.
      (1) **Bound histamine.** The histamine content of many tissues is dictated by the number of mast cells and basophils they contain.
         (a) The storage granules of **mast cells** and **basophils** contain histamine in a complex with heparin sulfate and chondroitin sulfate E. The rate of histamine synthesis and turnover in mast cells is low.
         (b) Most histamine is stored in the **lungs, skin,** and **intestinal mucosa.**
            (i) Allergic responses in the skin and lungs are due in part to histamine release.

---

* Not all known autacoids are discussed in this text. The reader should consult a standard pharmacology text for information about vasoactive intestinal polypeptide, substance P, and the cytokines.

TABLE 3-1. Histamine Pharmacology—An Overview

	Histamine Receptors		
	H_1	H_2	H_3
Agonists	←————————————Histamine (of no clinical use)————————————→		
	←2-Methylhistamine→	←———Betazole———→	No therapeutic drugs yet available
		←4-Methylhistamine→	
		←———Impromidine———→	
Response	GI and bronchial smooth muscle (↑)	Gastric acid secretions (↑)	Histamine, norepinephrine, serotonin, and acetylcholine release (↓)
	Small arteries (↓)	Small arteries (↓)	
	Large arteries (↑)	Positive inotropic effect on heart	
	Positive inotropic effect on heart	Increased heart rate	
	Increased coronary blood flow	Increased coronary blood flow	
	Sedation	Sympathetic nervous system transmission (↓)	
	Contraction of endothelial cells (increased vascular permeability)		
Antagonists	←———Pyrilamine———→	←———Cimetidine———→	No therapeutic drugs yet available
	←Tripelennamine→	←———Ranitidine———→	
	←Chlorpheniramine→		
	←Dimenhydrinate→		
	←Diphenhydramine→		
	←———Promethazine———→		
	←———Terfenadine———→		
	←———Astemizole———→		

↑ = vasoconstriction, contraction, stimulation; ↓ = vasodilation, relaxation, inhibition; HR = heart rate.

       (ii) Food and vagal stimulation can release histamine from the stomach mucosal cells. The released histamine then initiates gastric acid secretion.

    (2) Free histamine. The **hypothalamus** contains histamine that acts as a neurotransmitter in the endocrine system.

  c. Catabolism. Two enzymes are involved in the degradation of histamine.

    (1) Histamine-N-methyltransferase acts on histamine to form N-methylhistamine.

    (2) Diamine oxidase (histaminase) acts on histamine to form imidazoleacetic acid.

3. Release mechanisms

  a. Physical injury. Heat, cold, or trauma can disrupt the mast cells, thereby releasing histamine. In addition, histamine release is an important component of the physiologic reaction to insect or animal venoms (i.e., erythema, pain, itching).

  b. Immune-mediated release. When sensitized mast cells or basophils are coupled to immunoglobulin E (IgE) antibodies and then exposed to the proper antigen, the mast cells degranulate, releasing histamine.

  c. Drug-induced release. Drugs, especially strong bases (e.g., morphine, poly-

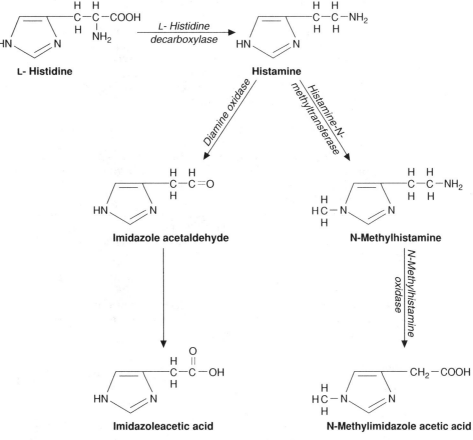

FIGURE 3-1. Synthesis and catabolism of histamine.

myxin, tubocurarine), or their vehicles are capable of inducing histamine release; however, this release does not involve degranulation or mast cell injury. These drugs displace or compete with histamine for the binding sites with heparin.

4. Receptors
    a. H_1 receptors mediate contraction of bronchiolar and intestinal smooth muscle, vasodilation of small arteries and veins, capillary permeability, and pruritus.
    b. H_2 receptors mediate gastric acid secretion and vasodilation.
    c. H_3 receptors are located presynaptically on neurons and modulate transmitter release. There are no drugs used in veterinary medicine that specifically activate or block these receptors.

5. Pharmacologic effects
    a. Cardiovascular system
        (1) Decreased blood pressure. Histamine dilates arterioles, capillaries, and venules and increases cardiac contractility and heart rate by activating both H_1 and H_2 receptors. The decrease in peripheral resistance cannot be overcome by the increase in cardiac output; therefore, the blood pressure drops.
        (2) Edema. Increased capillary permeability results when endothelial cells contract, exposing the basement membrane. Fluid and protein cross the basement membrane, producing edema.
    b. Respiratory system
        (1) H_1-receptor activation causes respiratory smooth muscle contraction in most

species (except in cats, where activation of H_1 and H_2 receptors causes bronchodilation). Asthmatics are generally more sensitive to histamine.

(2) Histamine also stimulates glandular secretion and PG formation.

c. Glandular tissue

(1) Histamine increases gastric acid and pepsin secretion from the gastric mucosa via H_2 receptors on the parietal cells.

(2) Histamine also increases the release of catecholamines from the adrenal medulla and stimulates salivary secretion.

d. Intradermal tissue

(1) **Triple response.** Intradermal injection of histamine, such as occurs with an insect sting, produces a typical response:

(a) **Reddening.** Histamine dilates small arterioles at the site of injection.

(b) **Flare.** Dilation of the arterioles extends beyond the injection site. The flare is thought to involve an axon reflex, because cutting the nerves abolishes the reflex.

(c) **Wheal.** At the injection site, increased capillary permeability causes separation of the endothelial cells and edema.

(2) **Pain and itching.** Histamine stimulates H_1 receptors on sensory nerve endings.

6. Therapeutic uses. Histamine analogs are used occasionally for diagnostic purposes (i.e., to test gastric acid secretion).

a. Histamine phosphate. Profound side effects limit its use as a diagnostic tool.

b. Betazole is an analog of histamine with a ten-fold selectivity for stimulation of gastric acid production over vasodilation.

B. **Serotonin**

1. Chemistry (Figure 3-2)

2. Biosynthesis, storage, and catabolism

a. Biosynthesis. Tryptophan hydroxylase acts on dietary tryptophan to form 5-hydroxytryptophan. L-Aromatic acid decarboxylase acts on the 5-hydroxytryptophan to form serotonin.

b. Storage

(1) **Central nervous system (CNS).** Serotonin is synthesized and stored in the CNS, where it is thought to act as a neurotransmitter.

(2) **Gastrointestinal tract. Enterochromaffin cells** in the gastrointestinal tract store approximately 90% of the body's serotonin. The function of serotonin in the gastrointestinal tract is unknown; it may regulate motility.

(3) **Blood. Platelets** actively transport and store serotonin. The function of serotonin in platelets is unknown.

c. Catabolism. Serotonin is deaminated by monoamine oxidase (MAO) to form 5-hydroxyindoleacetaldehyde, which is then oxidized to 5-hydroxyindoleacetic acid.

3. Receptors. There are more receptors for serotonin than for any other biogenic amine. The major categories of serotonin receptors include $5\text{-}HT_1$, $5\text{-}HT_2$, $5\text{-}HT_3$, $5\text{-}HT_4$, $5\text{-}HT_5$, $5\text{-}HT_6$ and $5\text{-}HT_7$.

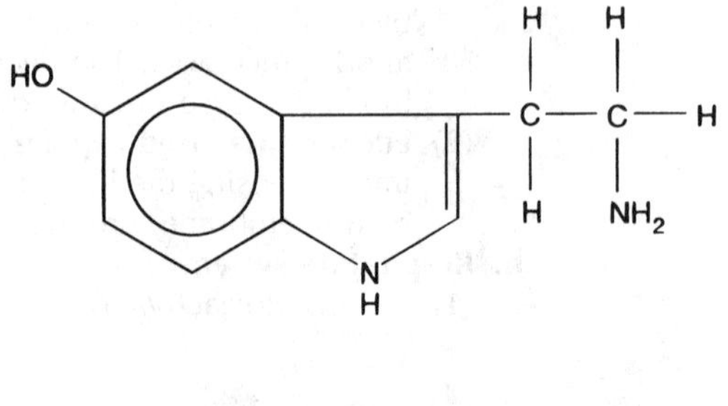

FIGURE 3-2. Serotonin.

4. **Pharmacologic effects**
   a. **Vascular changes.** Serotonin may produce vasoconstriction or vasodilation, depending on the vascular bed and the species.
   b. **Smooth muscle contraction.** Many types of smooth muscle (e.g., bronchial, uterine, gastrointestinal) contract in response to serotonin.
   c. **Pain.** Serotonin, which is found in plant, animal, and insect venoms, causes pain and pruritis by stimulating sensory nerve endings.
   d. **Other effects.** Serotonin may be involved in regulating gut motility, body temperature, sleep, aggression, pain, mood, and endocrine function.

5. **Therapeutic uses.** Serotonin has no therapeutic use.

III. PHOSPHOLIPID-DERIVED AUTACOIDS

A. Eicosanoids (PGs, TXs, and LTs)

1. **General considerations**
   a. **Biosynthesis** (Figure 3-3). Eicosanoids are derived from polyunsaturated acids.
      (1) **Arachidonic acid (5,8,11,14-eicosatetraenoic acid),** a 20-carbon essential fatty acid with four double bonds, is the primary substrate. It is released from membrane phospholipids, primarily by phospholipase A_2 in response to physical, chemical, hormonal, and neurotransmitter stimuli.
      (2) **Metabolism of arachidonic acid** can take place via three pathways.
         (a) The **cyclooxygenase pathway** produces **PGs,** such as prostacyclin (PGI_2), and **TXs.**
         (b) The **5-lipoxygenase pathway** synthesizes **LTs.**
         (c) The **cytochrome P-450–dependent monooxygenase pathway** synthesizes several **epoxides,** such as epoxyeicosatetraenoic acid (5,6-EETE).
   b. **Nomenclature**
      (1) **PGs** were originally detected in seminal fluid. They have since been shown to originate from the seminal vesicles.
      (2) **TXs** are synthesized in thrombocytes and contain an oxane ring, as opposed to the cyclopentane ring of the PGs.
      (3) **LTs,** conjugated trienes, were first detected in leukocytes.

2. **PGs and TXs**
   a. **Chemistry** (Figure 3-4)
      (1) PGs are divided into 10 specific molecular groups, A through J. Each group is characterized by the substituent attached to positions 9 and 11 of the cyclopentane ring.
      (2) The subscript numbers 1, 2, and 3 denote the number of double bonds in the aliphatic side chains attached to the cyclopentane ring.
      (3) For the PGF series of PGs, the subscript α or β refers to the configuration of the hydroxyl group at carbon 9.
   b. **Biosynthesis, storage, and catabolism** (see Figure 3-3)
      (1) **Biosynthesis.** PGs can be synthesized from three fatty acids:
         (a) PGE_1 is derived from **dihomo-γ-linoleic acid.**
         (b) PGE_2 is derived from **arachidonic acid.**
         (c) PGE_3 is derived from **eicosapentaenoic acid.**
      (2) **Storage.** PGs and TXs are not stored; instead, they are synthesized de novo in response to appropriate stimuli.
      (3) **Catabolism**
         (a) **PGs**
            (i) Degrading enzymes are located in the lungs (which remove 90% of PGE_2 and $PGF_{2\alpha}$), kidney, spleen, adipose tissue, and intestine.
            (ii) **Prostacyclin (PGI_2)** is spontaneously hydrolyzed in body fluids to the biologically inactive 6-keto-$PGF_{1\alpha}$.

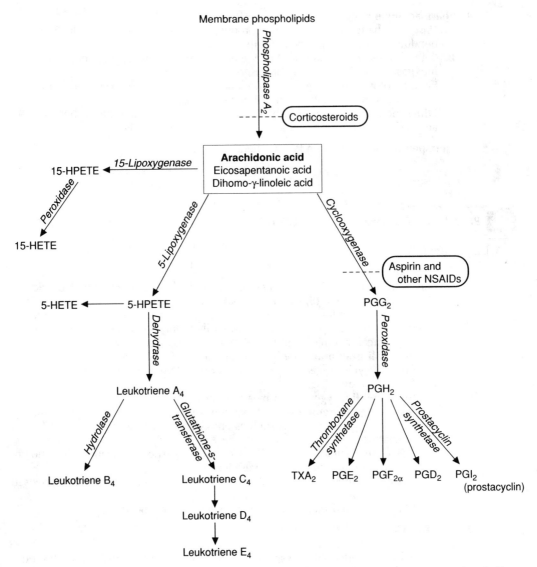

FIGURE 3-3. Eicosanoid biosynthesis. Various stimuli, including certain hormones, activate phospholipase A_2, causing the release of arachidonic acid from membrane phospholipids. Other substrates for eicosanoid synthesis include eicosapentanoic acid and dihomo-γ-linoleic acid. There are three pathways of arachidonic acid metabolism that produce biologically active products. Which pathway is followed appears to depend on the enzyme concentration and local environmental conditions in each tissue. The 15-lipoxygenase pathway produces epoxides. The 5-lipoxygenase pathway leads to the formation of the leukotrienes. The cyclooxygenase pathway ultimately leads to the synthesis of thromboxane (TXA_2), prostacyclin (PGI_2), and three prostaglandins (PGE_2, $PGF_{2\alpha}$, and PGD_2). HETE and HPETE = hydroxy and hydroxyperoxy derivatives of eicosatetraenoic acid; NSAIDs = nonsteroidal anti-inflammatory drugs.

        (b) **TXA$_2$** is spontaneously hydrolyzed in blood fluids to the biologically inactive TXB$_2$.

    c. **Pharmacologic effects.** PGs and TXs affect smooth muscle, platelet aggregation, the reproductive system, and the peripheral and central nervous systems (Table 3-2).

        (1) **Smooth muscle effects.** PGs and TXs affect smooth muscle in the blood vessels, gastrointestinal tract, and lungs.

        (2) **Platelet aggregation.** Prostacyclin (PGI$_2$) and TXA$_2$ inhibit and promote plate-

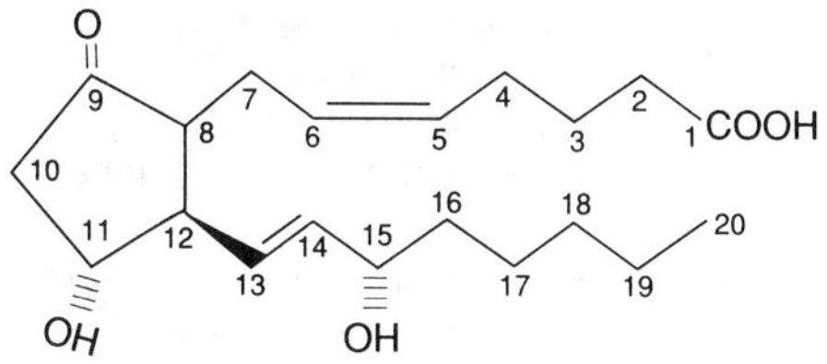

FIGURE 3-4. Chemical structure of two prostaglandins, PGE_2 and $PGF_{2\alpha}$.

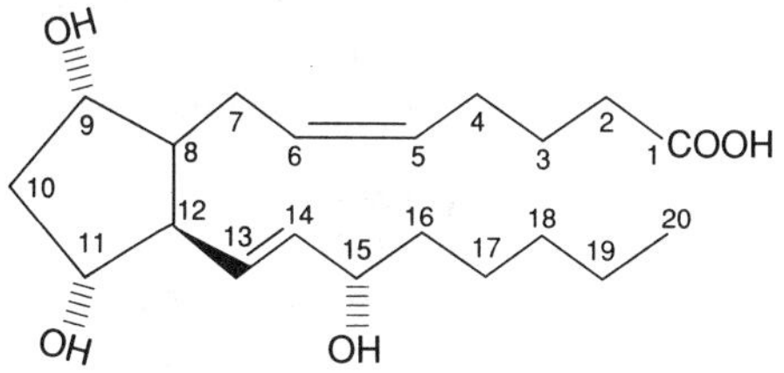

let aggregation, respectively. PGI_2 is synthesized by vascular endothelial cells, and TXA_2 is synthesized by platelets.

   (a) Small daily doses of aspirin are used to permanently inhibit platelet cyclooxygenase in animals with cardiovascular disease, thereby preventing TXA_2 formation. Aspirin may prevent thromboembolism in cats with cardiomyopathy.
   (b) Endothelial cell damage may cause a hemostatic plug to form as a result of a decrease in PGI_2 synthesis and an increase in TXA_2 synthesis.
(3) **Reproductive system effects.** The uterus produces $PGF_{2\alpha}$, a luteolytic hormone.
(4) **Central and peripheral nervous system effects**
   (a) **Fever.** Instillation of PGE_1 or PGE_2 into the cerebral ventricles increases body temperature. Pyrogens initiate the release of interleukin-1, which promotes PGE_2 formation. The antipyretic activity of aspirin and other nonsteroidal anti-inflammatory drugs is by inhibition of PGE_2 synthesis.
   (b) **Sleep.** Infusion of PGE_2 into the cerebral ventricles induces sleep.
   (c) **Neurotransmission.** PGE-type prostaglandins inhibit the release of norepinephrine from sympathetic neurons. The physiologic importance of this action is not known.

TABLE 3-2. Pharmacologic Effects of Prostaglandins and Thromboxanes

Effect	TXA_2	PGE_1	PGE_2	$PGF_{2\alpha}$	PGI_2
Vasodilation			✓		✓
Vasoconstriction	✓			✓	
Contraction of GI longitudinal muscle			✓	✓	
Contraction of GI circular muscle				✓	✓
Bronchodilation		✓	✓		✓
Bronchoconstriction	✓			✓	
Platelet aggregation	✓				
Inhibition of platelet aggregation					✓
Luteolysis				✓	
Fever		✓	✓		

GI = gastrointestinal; PGE_1 = prostaglandin E_1; PGE_2 = prostaglandin E_2; $PGF_{2\alpha}$ = prostaglandin $F_{2\alpha}$; PGI_2 = prostaglandin I_2 (prostacyclin); TXA_2 = thromboxane A_2.

(5) Neuroendocrine effects. PGE-type prostaglandins enhance the release of growth hormone (GH), prolactin, thyroid-stimulating hormone (TSH), adrenocorticotropic hormone (ACTH), follicle-stimulating hormone (FSH), and luteinizing hormone (LH). The significance of these actions remains uncertain.

d. Therapeutic uses. $PGF_{2\alpha}$ derivatives (e.g., cloprostenol sodium, prostaglandin $F_{2\alpha}$ tromethane, fenprostalene, fluprostenol sodium) are used most frequently in veterinary medicine. Therapeutic uses include:

    (1) Induction of luteolysis and synchronization of estrus

    (2) Treatment of pyometra or chronic endometritis

    (3) Expulsion of mummified fetuses

    (4) Induction of abortion after mismating

    (5) Scheduling of estrus and ovulation (e.g., for a controlled breeding program)

    (6) Induction of abortion in feedlot heifers fewer than 150 days pregnant

    (7) Induction of parturition

e. Administration

    (1) $PGF_{2\alpha}$ derivatives should not be administered intravenously.

    (2) Skin absorption necessitates caution in handling of PG preparations by pregnant women and people with asthma or respiratory disease.

f. Adverse effects include unintended parturition, bronchoconstriction, gastrointestinal stimulation, and exacerbation of cardiovascular effects (in older animals).

3. LTs

  a. Biosynthesis (see Figure 3-3)

    (1) LTs are synthesized by the enzyme **5-lipoxygenase** in neutrophils, monocytes, macrophages, mast cells, and keratinocytes, as well as the lungs, spleen, brain, and heart.

      (a) 5-Lipoxygenase reacts with arachidonic acid to form 5-hydroxyperoxyeicosatetranoic acid (5-HPETE), an intermediate that is reduced by a dehydrase to LTA_4. (The subscript indicates the number of double bonds present.)

      (b) LTA_4 is either hydrolyzed to LTB_4 or converted to LTC_4 in the presence of glutathione s-transferase. Removal of the glutamic acid moiety by γ-glutamyl transpeptidase yields LTD_4. Removal of the glycine by a dipeptidase forms LTE_4.

    (2) Stimuli for LT production include:

      (a) Phagocytosis and the presence of immune complexes in macrophages

      (b) Mast cell anti-IgE antibodies

      (c) Release of PAF by basophils and mast cells

  b. Pharmacologic effects

    (1) The **slow-reacting substance of anaphylaxis (SRS-A)** is now known to be a mixture of LTC_4, LTD_4, and LTE_4. These LTs have the following effects:

      (a) Smooth muscle contraction. LTs contract most smooth muscle and are potent **vaso-** and **bronchoconstrictors.**

      (b) Increased capillary permeability

      (c) Increased mucous secretion

    (2) Chemotaxis. LTB_4 is a potent chemotactic chemical for leukocytes, eosinophils, and monocytes. It promotes neutrophil adhesion to and migration through the vascular endothelium.

B. PAF

1. Biosynthesis

  a. Phospholipase A_2 acts on 1-O-alkyl-2-acyl-glycerophosphocholine to yield **1-O-alkyl-2-lyso-glycerophosphocholine (lyso-PAF).** Lyso-PAF is acetylated by acetyl coenzyme A in the presence of lyso-PAF acetyltransferase to form PAF.

  b. Activation of phospholipase A_2 in the synthesis of PAF also releases arachidonic acid, which is the substrate for the eiconosanoids. Because the eiconosanoids all have significant biological activity, it is difficult to delineate the pathophysiologic functions of PAF.

2. **Pharmacologic effects**
   a. **Marked vasodilation**
   b. **Increased vascular permeability.** PAF is approximately 1000-fold more potent than histamine or bradykinin in this respect.
   c. **Aggregation of platelets, polymorphonuclear leukocytes, and monocytes**
   d. **Contraction of gastrointestinal, uterine, and small bronchiolar smooth muscle**
   e. **Other.** PAF may be involved in ovulation, implantation, parturition, inflammation, and allergic responses.

IV. POLYPEPTIDES

A. **Angiotensins** are polypeptides that elevate blood pressure.

1. **Biosynthesis and metabolism**
   a. **Angiotensinogen,** an α_2 plasma globulin synthesized in the liver, is the precursor for all angiotensins.
   b. **Renin,** an enzyme secreted by juxtaglomerular cells in the kidney, metabolizes angiotensinogen to form the decapeptide **angiotensin I.**
   c. **Angiotensin converting enzyme (ACE),** an enzyme found in large amounts in lung capillary endothelial cells and other vascular beds, metabolizes angiotensin I to the biologically active octapeptide **angiotensin II.**
   d. **Angiotensin II** is metabolized by an aminopeptidase to **angiotensin III,** which retains some biologic activity. Other peptidases metabolize angiotensin II to inactive products.

2. **Receptors.** Two receptor subtypes for angiotensin II have been identified.
   a. **Angiotensin$_1$ receptors** mediate most of the actions of angiotensin II.
      (1) Angiotensin$_1$ receptors are G-protein coupled and activate phospholipase C, which mediates the generation of inositol triphosphate (IP$_3$) and diacylglycerol (DAG) from phosphatidyl inositol.
      (2) IP$_3$ induces Ca^{2+} release from the endoplasmic reticulum while DAG activates protein kinase C. Both events contribute to the contraction of smooth muscle.
   b. **Angiotensin$_2$ receptors** and their signal transduction pathways remain under study.

3. **Pharmacologic effects**
   a. **Regulation of blood pressure and fluid and electrolyte balance** are important functions of the renin–angiotensin system.
      (1) **Vasoconstriction.** Angiotensin II is 40 times more potent as a vasoconstrictor than norepinephrine.
      (2) **Aldosterone production.** Angiotensin II promotes the synthesis and secretion of aldosterone by the adrenal cortex zona glomerulosa. Aldosterone promotes sodium and water retention and potassium loss.
      (3) **Increased thirst.** Angiotensin II has a centrally mediated dipsogenic action.
   b. **Sympathetic nervous system stimulation.** Angiotensin II facilitates the release of norepinephrine from sympathetic neurons and inhibits the uptake of norepinephrine back into the neurons. Both mechanisms increase the effect of sympathetic stimulation.

4. **Therapeutic uses.** Angiotensin II is not approved for clinical use.

5. **Adverse effects.** Hypertension, edema, and electrolyte imbalances can occur from overactivity of the renin–angiotensin system.

B. **Kinins (bradykinin** and **kallidin)** are polypeptides that dilate blood vessels.

1. **Chemistry**
   a. **Bradykinin** is a nonapeptide.

b. Kallidin (lysyl-bradykinin) is a decapeptide.
2. **Biosynthesis and catabolism**
   a. Biosynthesis. Kallikreins are two distinct enzymes (one from plasma and the other from tissue) that catalyze the formation of bradykinin and kallidin from α_2-**globulins.**
   b. Catabolism. Kinases, especially **peptidyl dipeptidase (ACE),** inactivate both bradykinin and kallidin.
3. **Receptors.** Specific receptors have been identified, but no therapeutic receptor antagonists are available.
4. **Pharmacologic effects.** Several types of snake and insect venoms exert their toxic effects by inducing kinin formation.
   a. Effects of kinins include:
      (1) Vasodilation of resistance arteries
      (2) Contraction of nonvascular (e.g., bronchial, intestinal) smooth muscle
      (3) Venous contraction
      (4) Increased vascular permeability and edema
      (5) Induction of pain
   b. Kinins may initiate the formation of PGs, which also have pronounced biologic effects.

V. AUTACOID ANTAGONISTS

A. **Biogenic amine antagonists**
   1. **Histamine antagonists**
      a. Histamine-receptor antagonists (Table 3-3). Therapeutically useful histamine antagonists block either H_1 or H_2 receptors. At present, there are no clinically useful H_3 antagonists.
         (1) H_1-**receptor antagonists** (see Table 3-3) are sometimes referred to as the classic antihistaminics because they were the first to be discovered.

TABLE 3-3. H_1-Receptor Antagonists

Class	Substituent at X*	Typical Members	Comments
Ethylenediamines	N	Tripelennamine Pyrilamine	Moderate sedation
Phenothiazines	N	Promethazine	Strong sedation, antiemetic, antimuscarinic effects
Alkylamines	C	Chlorpheniramine	Slight sedation
Piperazines	C—N	Cyclizine Meclizine	Slight sedation, prevents motion sickness
Ethanolamines	C—O	Diphenhydramine Dimenhydrinate Carbinoxamine	Strong sedation, antiemetic, antimuscarinic effects
Piperidines	...	Terfenadine Astemizole	Low incidence of sedation
Other	...	Cyproheptadine	Moderate sedation

C = carbon; N = nitrogen; O = oxygen.
*

(a) **Preparations.** Prototypic H_1 antagonists include pyrilamine, tripelennamine, chlorpheniramine, dimenhydrinate, and diphenhydramine.

(b) **Mechanism of action.** Most H_1-receptor antagonists inhibit histamine in a competitive manner.

(c) **Pharmacokinetics**

    (i) All H_1-receptor antagonists are effectively absorbed following oral administration.

    (ii) Many of the H_1-receptor antagonists are capable of inducing the hepatic cytochrome P-450 system.

(d) **Pharmacologic effects**

    (i) H_1 blockers **relax contracted bronchiolar** and **intestinal smooth muscle.**

    (ii) They **inhibit histamine-induced vasodilation** and **increased capillary permeability.**

    (iii) They **inhibit pruritis** and **pain sensations** by preventing stimulation of sensory nerves. Some H_1 blockers exert a potent local anesthetic action, which may contribute to their inhibition of itching and pain.

    (iv) **Sedation** is a common, and often undesirable, effect. Terfenadine and astemizole do not cross the blood–brain barrier and so lack sedative properties; however, these two drugs have had limited use in veterinary medicine.

    (v) **Antimuscarinic effects** are prominent for some H_1 antagonists (e.g., diphenhydramine, promethazine).

(e) **Therapeutic uses**

    (i) **Treatment of allergy.** Conditions effectively treated by H_1 blockers include **urticaria** and **pruritis, allergic reactions to drugs,** and **systemic anaphylaxis.**

    (ii) **Prevention of motion sickness.** Diphenhydramine, dimenhydrinate, cyclizine, and meclizine are useful for this application.

    (iii) **Sedation.** Promethazine and diphenhydramine are the most potent sleep-inducers.

(f) **Adverse effects**

    (i) **CNS depression** (e.g., lethargy, somnolence, ataxia) is the most common adverse effect, but may diminish with time. Antihistamines may adversely affect the performance of working dogs.

    (ii) **Antimuscarinic effects** (e.g., xerostomia, urinary retention) occur with many H_1 antagonists. These agents should be used with caution in animals with angle closure glaucoma.

    (iii) **CNS stimulation** may occur with high doses in certain species (e.g., pyrilamine in horses).

(2) **H_2-receptor antagonists** (Figure 3-5). These drugs, which have little effect on H_1 receptors, are inhibitors of gastric acid secretion. H_2-receptor antagonists inhibit gastric acid secretion stimulated by histamine as well as secretion stimulated by gastrin, acetylcholine (ACh), and food. This phenomenon explains why H_2-receptor antagonists are effective therapy for peptic ulcers.

(a) **Cimetidine**

    (i) **Mechanism of action.** Cimetidine competitively inhibits H_2 receptors.

    (ii) **Pharmacokinetics.** Cimetidine is well absorbed—in dogs, the oral bioavailability is approximately 95%. Cimetidine is metabolized by the liver, and the parent drug is excreted unchanged by the kidneys.

    (iii) **Pharmacologic effects.** Cimetidine decreases gastric acid production during basal conditions and when stimulated by food, vagal activity, pentagastrin, gastrin, or histamine.

    (iv) **Therapeutic uses.** Cimetidine is used in treating gastric, abomasal, and duodenal ulcers, drug-induced erosive gastritis, duodenal gastric reflux, and esophageal reflux.

    (v) **Adverse effects** are uncommon in animals. However, aged animals

FIGURE 3-5. Chemical structure of two H$_2$-receptor antagonists, cimetidine and ranitidine.

Cimetidine

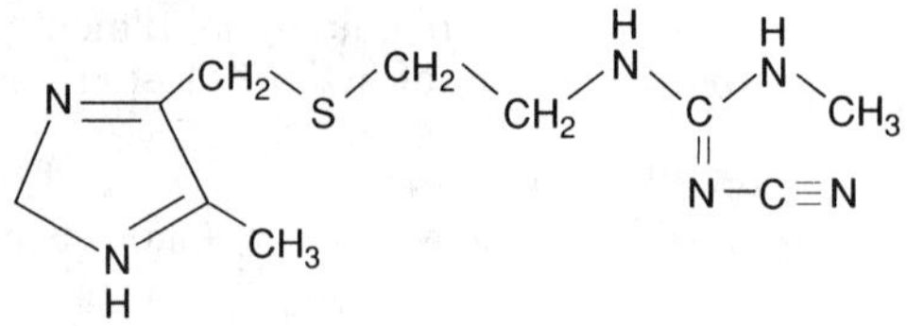

Ranitidine

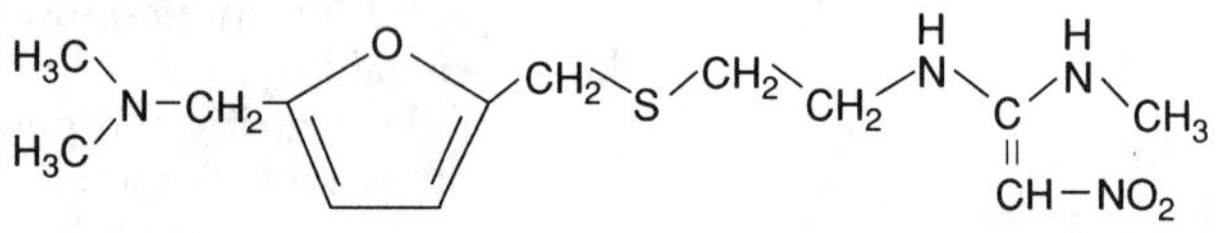

or animals with renal or hepatic disease may require dosage adjustments.

   (vi) **Drug interactions.** Cimetidine may reduce the metabolism of other drugs that undergo hepatic metabolism, thereby elevating and prolonging their concentration in the plasma.

   (b) **Ranitidine.** Many of ranitidine's actions and uses resemble those of cimetidine; however, ranitidine is three to thirteen times more potent than cimetidine.

   (i) **Mechanism of action.** Ranitidine competitively inhibits histamine at H$_2$ receptors.

   (ii) **Pharmacokinetics**

   The bioavailability of ranitidine in dogs following oral administration is 81%.

   Ranitidine is less likely than cimetidine to cause drug interactions via inhibition of the cytochrome P-450 system.

   (c) **Famotidine** and **nizatidine** are used primarily in human medicine.

   b. **Inhibitors of histamine release**

   (1) **Preparations. Cromolyn sodium** is the only drug in this class.

   (2) **Mechanism of action.** Cromolyn sodium inhibits the release of histamine and other autacoids from mast cells. It does not inhibit H$_1$ or H$_2$ receptors.

   (3) **Pharmacokinetics.** Cromolyn sodium is not well absorbed from the gut and has no clinical use when given orally.

   (4) **Therapeutic uses.** Cromolyn sodium is used prophylactically to prevent pulmonary allergic reactions.

   (5) **Administration.** In horses, cromolyn sodium can be nebulized and delivered via a face mask.

   c. **Physiologic antagonists to histamine**

   (1) **Preparations** include **epinephrine** and **ephedrine**.

   (2) **Mechanism of action.** These drugs antagonize the actions of histamine by acting on opposing physiologic systems (see Chapter 2). They either directly or indirectly activate α- and β-adrenoceptors to elevate blood pressure and relax the bronchi.

   (3) **Therapeutic uses.** Epinephrine is used to treat the immediate effects of anaphylaxis.

2. **Serotonin antagonists.** In human medicine, methysergide, cyproheptadine (also an H$_1$-receptor antagonist), and ketanserin are available. The use of serotonin antagonists in veterinary medicine is not established.

B. **Phospholipid-derived autacoid antagonists**

1. **PG antagonists.** Aspirin and other nonsteroidal anti-inflammatory agents inhibit cyclooxygenase (and, therefore, the formation of TXA_2, PGE_2, $PGF_{2\alpha}$, PGD_2, and PGI_2). There are no clinically available receptor antagonists.

2. **LT antagonists.** There are no clinically available receptor antagonists or selective inhibitors of 5-lipoxygenase.

3. **PAF antagonists.** There are no clinically available receptor antagonists or inhibitors of PAF synthesis.

C. **Polypeptide antagonists (renin–angiotensin system antagonists)**

1. **ACE inhibitors** (see also Chapter 6 I C 2)
   a. **Preparations** include **captopril, enalapril,** and **lisinopril.**
   b. **Mechanism of action.** These agents inhibit the enzymatic conversion of angiotensin I to angiotensin II. Drugs in this class do not block angiotensin II receptors.
   c. **Pharmacologic effects**
      (1) Inhibition of the sympathetic nervous system
      (2) Decreased retention of sodium and water (via reduced aldosterone secretion)
      (3) Increased levels of bradykinin, a vasodilating polypeptide that is inactivated by peptidyl dipeptidase (ACE)
      (4) Decreased blood pressure and fluid retention in animals with elevated angiotensin I blood levels

2. **β_1-Adrenoceptor antagonists.** The sympathetic nervous system promotes the release of renin from juxtaglomerular cells via β_1-adrenoceptors. Drugs such as propranolol (a β_1- and β_2-adrenoceptor antagonist) inhibit activation of β_1-adrenoceptors, thereby reducing renin release.

3. **Angiotensin-receptor antagonists**
   a. **Saralasin** is a structural analog of angiotensin. It has been used to aid in the diagnosis of angiotensin-induced hypertension, but better approaches now exist.
      (1) **At low angiotensin II concentrations,** saralasin acts as a weak partial agonist and may elevate blood pressure.
      (2) **At high angiotensin II concentrations,** its antagonist activity predominates.
   b. **Other angiotensin-receptor antagonists.** Several nonpeptide angiotensin$_1$-receptor antagonists devoid of agonist activity are under clinical evaluation.

STUDY QUESTIONS

DIRECTIONS: Each of the numbered items or incomplete statements in this section is followed by answers or by completions of the statement. Select the **one** numbered answer or completion that is **best** in each case.

1. Which of the following is a major effect of angiotensin II?

(1) Enhancement of sympathetic stimulation
(2) Vasodilation
(3) Inhibition of sodium retention and potassium loss
(4) Hypotension

2. Which one of the following statements regarding histamine H_2-receptor blockers is correct?

(1) Cimetidine may cause drug interactions by inhibiting the cytochrome P-450 enzyme system.
(2) Cimetidine is more potent than ranitidine.
(3) Ranitidine is a potent central nervous system (CNS) depressant.

(4) A side effect of ranitidine is increased gastric acid secretion.

3. Which one of the following is a function of angiotensin converting enzyme (ACE)?

(1) It converts renin to angiotensin II.
(2) It converts bradykinin to inactive metabolites.
(3) It directly promotes aldosterone secretion.
(4) It converts angiotensin II to angiotensin III.

4. Which of the following products of arachidonic acid is both an inhibitor of platelet aggregation and a vasodilator?

(1) Prostaglandin $F_{2\alpha}$ ($PGF_{2\alpha}$)
(2) Prostaglandin I_2 (PGI_2)
(3) Prostaglandin E_2 (PGE_2)
(4) Thromboxane A_2 (TXA_2)

DIRECTIONS: Each of the numbered items or incomplete statements in this section is negatively phrased, as indicated by an italicized word such as *not, least,* or *except.* Select the **one** numbered answer or completion that is **best** in each case.

5. All of the following statements concerning classic antihistaminics (H_1-receptor antagonists) are correct *except*:

(1) they block histamine receptors on the bronchi.
(2) they are the primary drugs for treating anaphylaxis.
(3) they are substituted ethylamines.
(4) sedation is a prominent side effect.

6. Which one of the following statements regarding serotonin is *incorrect*?

(1) Serotonin is a biogenic amine.

(2) Serotonin is found in platelets.
(3) Serotonin is found in enterochromaffin cells in the gastrointestinal tract.
(4) Serotonin is synthesized from tyrosine.

7. All of the following statements are correct *except*:

(1) arachidonic acid is the precursor for the synthesis of the leukotrienes (LTs).
(2) aspirin inhibits the formation of prostaglandin $F_{2\alpha}$ ($PGF_{2\alpha}$).
(3) prostaglandin E_2 (PGE_2) increases body temperature.
(4) LTs are potent relaxants of bronchiolar smooth muscle.

ANSWERS AND EXPLANATIONS

1. The answer is 1 [*IV A 3 b*].
Angiotensin II enhances sympathetic nervous system stimulation by facilitating the release of norepinephrine and by inhibiting the reuptake of released norepinephrine. Regulation of blood pressure and fluid balance are important functions of the renin–angiotensin system. As part of this function, angiotensin II produces hypertension through vasoconstriction, not vasodilation. Angiotensin II also initiates the secretion of aldosterone, which promotes sodium retention and potassium loss.

2. The answer is 1 [*V A 1 a (2)*].
Cimetidine may inhibit hepatic cytochrome P-450 metabolism of other drugs, increasing the potential for drug interactions. Ranitidine is more potent than cimetidine, but it is less likely to inhibit the cytochrome P-450 system. Ranitidine has little central nervous system (CNS) depressant activity. Ranitidine inhibits histamine-induced gastric acid secretion.

3. The answer is 2 [*V C 1 c (3)*].
Angiotensin converting enzyme (ACE, peptidyl dipeptidase) metabolizes bradykinin to biologically inactive products and converts angiotensin I to angiotensin II. Angiotensin II, not ACE, promotes aldosterone secretion, and peptidase converts angiotensin II to angiotensin III.

4. The answer is 2 [*Table 3-2*].
Prostaglandin I_2 (PGI_2, prostacyclin), which is synthesized by vascular endothelial cells, is a potent vasodilator and inhibitor of platelet aggregation. Thromboxane A_2 (TXA_2) promotes platelet aggregation. Prostaglandin $F_{2\alpha}$ (PGF_{2\alpha}) is a vasoconstrictor. Prostaglandin E_2 (PGE_2) causes bronchodilation and vasodilation, but does not inhibit platelet aggregation.

5. The answer is 2 [*V A 1 c (3)*].
Epinephrine is used to treat the immediate effects of anaphylaxis. Because they are competitive antagonists, H_1-receptor antagonists can only block the actions of histamine. Other autacoids may be involved in anaphylaxis; therefore, H_1-receptor antagonists are not generally used as first-line agents against anaphylaxis. H_1-receptor antagonists counteract the effect of histamine on the bronchi (i.e., bronchoconstriction) via H_1 receptors. Sedation is a prominent side effect of antihistamine therapy. H_1-receptor antagonists are substituted ethylamines.

6. The answer is 4 [*II B 2 a*].
Tyrosine is the precursor for catecholamine synthesis, not serotonin synthesis. Tryptophan is the precursor for serotonin, a biogenic amine that is stored in platelets. Serotonin is also synthesized and stored in the central nervous system (CNS) and in enterochromaffin cells in the gastrointestinal tract.

7. The answer is 4 [*III A 2 c (4) (a), 3 b (1) (a)*].
Leukotrienes (LTs) are potent bronchoconstrictors. Arachidonic acid is the precursor for the synthesis of the leukotrienes (LTs), as well as prostaglandins (PGs) and thromboxane (TX). Pyrogens initiate the release of interleukin-1, which promotes PGE_2 formation and leads to an increase in body temperature. Aspirin and other nonsteroidal anti-inflammatory drugs inhibit the cyclooxygenase pathway, thereby inhibiting the formation of PGs and TX.

Chapter 4

Drugs Acting on the Central Nervous System

Dean H. Riedesel

I. INTRODUCTION

A. **Function.** Drugs can alter the function of the central nervous system (CNS) to provide:

1. Anticonvulsant effects

2. Tranquilization (sedation)

3. Analgesia

4. Anesthesia

B. **Transmitter–receptor relationship.** Chemical transmitters released by a presynaptic neuron combine with receptors on the membrane of a postsynaptic neuron, altering its membrane potential.

1. **Transmitters** in the CNS include dopamine, γ-aminobutyric acid (GABA), acetylcholine (ACh), norepinephrine, epinephrine, serotonin, histamine, glutamate, glycine, and substance P.

2. **Receptors** for endogenous chemical transmitters are many times the site of action for exogenous drugs.
   a. **The transmitter–receptor complex** may directly alter the permeability of the cell membrane by opening or closing specific ion pores.
   b. **Second messengers.** The transmitter–receptor complex may initiate a sequence of chemical reactions that alter ion transport across the membrane, thereby altering the membrane potential. Specific intracellular signal molecules, or second messengers, may be generated. The second messenger system sustains and amplifies the cellular response to drug–receptor binding.

C. **Blood–brain barrier.** Circulating drugs must cross the blood–brain barrier in order to gain access to the neurons of the brain.

1. Drugs that are lipid soluble, small in molecular size, poorly bound to protein, and unionized at the pH of cerebrospinal fluid cross the blood–brain barrier most readily.

2. The blood–brain barrier tends to increase in permeability in the presence of inflammation or at the site of tumors.

3. The blood–brain barrier is poorly developed in neonates.

II. ANTICONVULSANT DRUGS

A. **General features**

1. **Preparations.** Only a few of the anticonvulsants available for human use have been proven to be clinically useful in dogs and cats.
   a. Some of the drugs are too rapidly metabolized in dogs to be effective, even at high dosages.
   b. Clinical experience and pharmacokinetic data are unavailable for many of these compounds in cats. Cats are generally assumed to metabolize drugs more slowly than dogs.

2. **Mechanism of action.** Anticonvulsants stabilize neuronal membranes.

TABLE 4-1. Commonly Used Anticonvulsants

Dogs			Cats		
Drug	**Route of Administration**	**Elimination Half-Life**	**Drug**	**Route of Administration**	**Elimination Half-Life**
Phenobarbital	Oral	32–90 hours	Phenobarbital	Oral	34–43 hours
Primidone	Oral	5–12 hours	Diazepam	Oral or intravenous	15–20 hours
Phenytoin	Oral	3–7 hours			
Diazepam	Intravenous	2–4 hours			
Potassium bromide	Oral	24–28 days			
Valproic acid	Oral	1.2–2.8 hours			

       a. Direct. They may act directly on ion channels, resulting in hyperpolarization of the membrane.

       b. Indirect. They may act indirectly by increasing the activity of GABA, an inhibitory transmitter normally present in the brain.

   3. Therapeutic uses. Anticonvulsants **reduce the incidence, severity,** or **duration of seizures.**

   4. Administration

       a. Plasma concentrations of anticonvulsant drugs should be adequate to ensure an effective concentration in the brain. Treatment for at least five half-lives must occur before stable plasma levels of these drugs are achieved and serum analyses for drug concentrations are beneficial.

          (1) Trough concentrations should be within the therapeutic range.

          (2) Peak concentrations should be below toxic levels.

       b. Drugs with long elimination **half-lives** (Table 4-1) are easier to use in veterinary medicine because owners are usually only able to administer the drug two or three times daily.

   5. Adverse effects

       a. Withdrawal symptoms, seizures, or **status epilepticus** may follow rapid cessation of administration of these drugs.

       b. A lowered seizure threshold, precipitating seizures in an otherwise well-controlled patient, may follow the administration of other drugs, such as:

          (1) Phenothiazine tranquilizers (e.g., acepromazine)

          (2) Some anthelmintics (e.g., piperazine, mebendazole)

          (3) Metoclopramide, a dopamine antagonist used to increase gastrointestinal motility

       c. Enzyme induction

          (1) Phenobarbital, primidone, and phenytoin increase the activity of metabolizing enzymes within the smooth endoplasmic reticulum of the liver. This enzyme induction may increase the biotransformation of other endogenous and exogenous chemicals.

          (2) Membrane-bound enzymes (e.g., alkaline phosphatase) can also be induced, leading to increases in serum levels that could be mistaken as an indication of liver injury.

       d. Hepatotoxicity is the most common adverse effect of anticonvulsant therapy in dogs. It develops in 6%–15% of dogs treated with primidone alone or in combination with phenytoin.

          (1) The liver should be evaluated every 6–12 months for signs of toxicity, including:

(a) Elevated serum enzyme concentrations, particularly alanine aminotransferase and glutamyl transferase activity

(b) Rising serum phenobarbital concentrations in dogs receiving a constant dosage

(c) Decreasing serum albumin concentrations

(d) Elevated postprandial serum bile acids

(2) If hepatotoxicity is detected, the dosage of primidone or phenobarbital should be decreased and potassium bromide therapy implemented.

B. Barbiturates

1. Phenobarbital

  a. Chemistry. Phenobarbital is an oxybarbiturate.

  b. Mechanism of action. The mechanism of action may depend on increasing the effect of GABA at inhibitory receptors (see II A 2 b, E 1 b, IV C 2 b). Barbiturates have also been shown to inhibit the release of ACh, norepinephrine, and glutamate.

  c. Pharmacokinetics. The oxybarbiturates are primarily metabolized in the liver. The major metabolite of phenobarbital is a parahydroxyphenyl derivative that is inactive and excreted in the urine.

  (1) Hepatic microsomal enzyme activity is increased by chronic administration of barbiturates, producing increased rates of barbiturate metabolism as well as increased metabolism of other drugs.

  (2) Hepatic microsomal enzyme activity is inhibited by certain drugs (e.g., chloramphenicol), thereby decreasing the elimination rate of barbiturates.

  d. Pharmacologic effects

  (1) Phenobarbital limits the spread of action potentials and elevates the seizure threshold.

  (2) Most barbiturates have anticonvulsant effects, but phenobarbital is unique in that it usually produces this effect at lower doses than those necessary to cause pronounced sedation.

  e. Therapeutic uses. Phenobarbital is used for **long-term control of seizures.** It is not useful for terminating an ongoing seizure because the time span from administration until the onset of effect is approximately 20 minutes.

  f. Administration

  (1) Phenobarbital is usually administered orally but can be injected intravenously or intramuscularly.

  (2) A serum drug level of 15–45 μg/ml is usually effective in controlling seizures; however, because of phenobarbital's long half-life, 14 days of therapy are required to develop a steady serum concentration.

  g. Adverse reactions

  (1) **Sedation, polydipsia, polyuria,** and **polyphagia** are common side effects. Dogs develop a tolerance to the sedative effects after 1–2 weeks, but cats may experience more pronounced sedation.

  (2) **Hepatotoxicity.** Chronic administration to dogs may result in elevated serum concentrations of hepatic enzymes and, in a small percentage of cases, actual damage.

2. Pentobarbital

  a. Chemistry. Pentobarbital is an oxybarbiturate.

  b. Pharmacokinetics. It has a rapid onset and short duration of action.

  c. Therapeutic uses. Pentobarbital will terminate seizures at a dose that produces anesthesia. This dose usually results in significant cardiopulmonary depression but may be the only way to control status epilepticus.

  d. Administration. Pentobarbital is administered intravenously.

3. Primidone

  a. Chemistry. Primidone is a deoxybarbiturate (an analog of phenobarbital).

  b. Pharmacokinetics

  (1) In dogs, primidone is rapidly metabolized by the liver to phenylethylmalonamide (PEMA) and phenobarbital.

      (a) Primidone, PEMA, and phenobarbital are all anticonvulsants, but the half-lives of the first two are too short for them to be effective.

      (b) Approximately 85% of the anticonvulsant effect of primidone is attributable to phenobarbital.

    (2) In cats, the metabolism to phenobarbital is slower and the half-life is very long; therefore, primidone is rarely used in this species.

  c. Administration. In dogs, a dose of 4–5 mg of primidone will produce a serum phenobarbital level that is equivalent to an oral dose of 1 mg of phenobarbital.

  d. Adverse effects. Prolonged use of primidone in dogs may lead to decreased serum albumin and elevated serum levels of liver enzymes. Occasionally, serious liver damage occurs.

C. Hydantoin compounds

1. Phenytoin

  a. Chemistry. Phenytoin is a hydantoin derivative.

  b. Mechanism of action. Phenytoin stabilizes neuronal membranes and limits the development and spread of seizure activity.

    (1) It reduces sodium influx during the action potential, reduces calcium influx during depolarization, and promotes sodium efflux. The resultant effect is an inhibition of the spread of seizure activity.

    (2) Potassium movement out of the cell during the action potential may be delayed, producing an increased refractory period and a decrease in repetitive depolarization.

  c. Pharmacokinetics

    (1) In dogs, phenytoin has a short half-life.

    (2) In cats, phenytoin has a very long half-life.

  d. Pharmacologic effects. The effects of phenytoin on cardiac electrophysiology are similar to those of lidocaine [see Chapter 6 II B 1 d (2) (a)].

  e. Therapeutic uses

    (1) Phenytoin is an **anticonvulsant** drug; however, because of its short half-life in dogs, use of phenytoin may be impractical.

    (2) Because of its lidocaine-like effects, phenytoin has been recommended for the treatment of **digitalis-induced ventricular arrhythmias** in dogs.

2. Mephenytoin

  a. Pharmacokinetics. Mephenytoin is rapidly metabolized to nirvanol, which has a long (27 hours in humans) half-life.

  b. Therapeutic uses. Mephenytoin may be useful in dogs as an added medication if phenobarbital and potassium bromide are not effective.

  c. Adverse reactions

    (1) In dogs, **sedation** is the only side effect reported.

    (2) In humans, dermatitis, blood dyscrasias, and hepatotoxicity have been reported.

D. Benzodiazepines (see also IV C)

1. Diazepam

  a. Chemistry. Diazepam is a water-insoluble benzodiazepine.

  b. Mechanism of action. Diazepam binds to GABA receptors and potentiates the inhibitory effect of the normal amount of endogenously released GABA.

  c. Pharmacokinetics

    (1) Absorption. Diazepam is dissolved in **propylene glycol** and **sodium benzoate** for injection.

      (a) Because of its poor water solubility, intramuscular injections of diazepam are slowly absorbed.

      (b) Diazepam is very lipid soluble and rapidly crosses the blood–brain barrier.

    (2) Distribution. It is highly (85%–99%) protein bound.

    (3) Metabolism and excretion. Metabolites are conjugated to glucuronide by the liver and excreted by the kidneys. Some of the metabolites of diazepam (e.g., desmethyldiazepam, oxazepam) are pharmacologically active. Desmethyldiazepam has a longer half-life than its parent compound.

d. Therapeutic uses and administration. Diazepam is used as an **anticonvulsant, muscle relaxant, tranquilizer,** and **appetite stimulant.**

(1) In cats, it is administered orally for seizure control. Oral therapy has been successfully used in cats for years without evidence of tolerance.

(2) In dogs, it is administered intravenously for status epilepticus and seizure control.

e. Adverse reactions. Complications related to the propylene glycol carrier include:

(1) **Venous thrombosis, transient cardiovascular depression,** and **arrhythmias** following rapid intravenous injection

(2) **Precipitation.** Mixing diazepam with most other drugs (e.g., thiobarbiturates) results in precipitation. Ketamine is an exception.

2. Midazolam

a. Chemistry. Midazolam is a water-soluble benzodiazepine.

b. Pharmacokinetics. Midazolam has a shorter half-life and duration of action than diazepam.

(1) **Distribution.** At low pH values (< 4.0), midazolam is water soluble, but at higher pH values, it is lipid soluble. Thus, in the bottle (pH = 3.5), it is water soluble, but in the body (pH = 7.4), it is lipid soluble and readily crosses the blood–brain barrier and cell membranes.

(2) **Metabolism and excretion.** The metabolites of midazolam have less pharmacologic effect than the parent compound.

c. Pharmacologic effects. Midazolam is more potent than diazepam.

d. Therapeutic uses. Midazolam is used as an anticonvulsant, muscle relaxant, tranquilizer, and appetite stimulant.

e. Administration. It is administered intramuscularly or intravenously.

3. Chlorazepate

a. Pharmacokinetics. Chlorazepate is metabolized to desmethyldiazepam.

b. Therapeutic uses. Chlorazepate may be useful in combination with phenobarbital; however, clinical studies on chlorazepate have not been reported in veterinary medicine.

c. Adverse effects. Experimental studies in dogs revealed **dependence** and **seizure activity upon abrupt withdrawal.**

E. Potassium bromide (KBr)

1. Mechanism of action

a. It is believed that competition between the bromide and chloride ions at chloride channels results in a hyperpolarized cell membrane.

b. Bromide may also enhance the inhibitory effects of GABA, which acts by increasing chloride movement into the cell. Phenobarbital, which also enhances chloride conductance, may act in synergy with potassium bromide to hyperpolarize cells, thus raising the seizure threshold.

2. Pharmacokinetics

a. Absorption. Potassium bromide is quickly absorbed from the gastrointestinal tract.

b. Metabolism. Potassium bromide is neither metabolized nor bound to serum protein. It has a long half-life, and it may take up to 4 months to achieve stable plasma levels.

c. Elimination. Potassium bromide is eliminated exclusively by the kidneys.

3. Therapeutic uses

a. Potassium bromide has been used to treat **refractory seizures** in dogs. It is not recommended for use in cats.

b. It is used **in combination with phenobarbital** to terminate **refractory generalized tonic-clinic convulsions** in dogs.

4. Adverse effects

a. Transient sedation at the beginning of therapy has been reported.

    b. Gastrointestinal effects
      (1) Stomach irritation can produce nausea and vomiting.
      (2) Vomiting, anorexia, and **constipation** are indications of toxicity.
    c. Polydipsia, polyuria, polyphagia, lethargy, irritability, and **pacing** have been reported.
    d. Pancreatitis may be precipitated by potassium bromide.

F. Valproic acid

1. **Chemistry.** Valproic acid is a derivative of carboxylic acid. It is structurally unrelated to other drugs with anticonvulsant activity.

2. **Pharmacokinetics**
    a. There is less protein binding of valproic acid in dogs than in humans.
    b. Valproic acid has a short half-life in dogs.
    c. Two of its metabolites have anticonvulsant activity.

3. **Therapeutic uses**
    a. In dogs, valproic acid is effective in **controlling seizures,** but its short half-life makes it impractical for long-term use.
    b. Its clinical usefulness in cats has not been evaluated.

III. CNS STIMULANTS (ANALEPTICS). Doxapram hydrochloride is used most frequently in veterinary medicine.

A. Therapeutic uses

1. Doxapram is used to arouse animals from **anesthetic overdosage.** At higher doses of doxapram, generalized CNS stimulation of the brain produces transient arousal from anesthesia. The depth of anesthesia is reduced, but the effect is transient, nonspecific, and not recommended.

2. Doxapram is used for **respiratory stimulation** in neonates after assisted birth or cesarean section. Low doses of doxapram increase the respiratory minute volume by stimulating the carotid bodies. Doxapram is not effective in reviving a severely depressed neonate and is not a good substitute for endotracheal intubation and ventilation.

B. Administration

1. **Intravenous administration** produces an effect for 5–10 minutes.

2. **Intramuscular administration** and **topical application** to the oral mucosa are also effective in neonates.

C. Adverse effects. High doses of doxapram may induce **seizures.**

IV. TRANQUILIZERS, ATARACTICS, NEUROLEPTICS, AND SEDATIVES. These terms are used interchangeably in veterinary medicine to refer to drugs that calm the animal and promote sleep but do not necessarily induce sleep, even at high doses. Tranquilized animals are usually calm and easy to handle, but they may be aroused by and respond to stimuli in a normal fashion (e.g., biting, scratching, kicking). When used as preanesthetic medications, these drugs enable use of less general anesthetic.

A. Phenothiazine derivatives include **acepromazine, promazine, chlorpromazine, propriopromazine,** and **triflupromazine.**

1. **Mechanism of action.** Phenothiazine derivatives affect the CNS at the basal ganglia, hypothalamus, limbic system, brain stem, and reticular activating system. They block dopamine receptors and reduce the action of serotonin (5-hydroxytryptamine, 5-HT).

2. Pharmacokinetics
   a. In general, these tranquilizers have a long duration of action (3–6 hours).
   b. Most metabolism occurs in the liver, and the kidneys excrete the metabolites over several days.

3. Pharmacologic effects
   a. Cardiovascular effects
   (1) Hypotension may develop as a result of α_1-adrenergic receptor blockade and a decrease in sympathetic nervous system tone. Animals with high sympathetic nervous system tone from hypovolemia may become profoundly hypotensive following phenothiazine administration, owing to epinephrine reversal.
      (a) Loss of α_1-receptor initiated vasoconstriction is responsible for the hypotension.
      (b) Stimulation of β_2 receptors by circulating epinephrine causes peripheral vascular dilation, compounding the problem.
   (2) Sinus bradycardia and **second-degree heart block** may occur with high doses.
   (3) Reflex sinus tachycardia may occur if hypotension develops.
   (4) Antiarrhythmic effects have been reported with phenothiazine tranquilizers. A combination of the following could be responsible.
      (a) Production of α_1-receptor blockade in the myocardium
      (b) Local anesthetic-like effect on the myocardial cells
      (c) Reduced systemic blood pressure
   (5) Inotropic effect. Myocardial contractility is either unaffected or slightly reduced.
   b. Respiratory effects
   (1) Respiratory depression
      (a) Large doses depress respiration.
      (b) In combination with an opioid to produce neuroleptanalgesia, phenothiazine tranquilizers are associated with respiratory depression.
   (2) Phenothiazines evoke a **depressed maximal response to an elevated carbon dioxide partial pressure,** although the threshold for this response remains normal.
   c. Gastrointestinal effects
   (1) Motility is depressed.
   (2) Emesis is suppressed because phenothiazines interfere with the action of dopamine on the chemoreceptor trigger zone in the medulla.
   d. Effects on blood. Packed cell volume decreases as a result of splenic sequestration of red blood cells.
   e. Metabolic effects. Body temperature tends to decrease after tranquilization because of increased heat loss from vasodilation, decreased heat production from a lack of muscular activity, and a depression of the thermoregulation center in the brain.

4. Therapeutic uses
   a. Phenothiazines are primarily used for **tranquilization.** They generally do not have analgesic effects.
   b. Most of these drugs are effective as **antiemetics.**
   c. Administration of a phenothiazine **prior to use of inhalant anesthetics** can reduce the incidence of arrhythmias caused by myocardial sensitization to catecholamines [see Chapter 5 III D 2 c (1) (c)].

5. Administration. Phenothiazines can be administered orally, intravenously, intramuscularly, or subcutaneously.

6. Adverse effects. There is no reversal agent for this class of drugs.
   a. The seizure threshold may be lowered.
   b. Accidental intracarotid administration in horses results in the immediate onset of seizure activity and, usually, death.
   c. Phenothiazine tranquilizers inhibit acetylcholinesterase (AChE) and may worsen the clinical signs of organophosphate poisoning.

    d. An antihistaminic effect makes phenothiazines an undesirable drug for sedation of animals prior to allergy testing.

    e. Paraphimosis may occur in stallions; therefore, phenothiazines should be used cautiously or avoided altogether in breeding stallions.

7. Contraindications

    a. Organophosphate poisoning

    b. Known or suspected treatment with organophosphate anthelmintics

    c. History of seizures

B. Butyrophenone derivatives

1. Preparations. Two drugs in this class are being used in veterinary medicine.

    a. Droperidol, the tranquilizer portion of Innovar-Vet

    b. Azaperone

2. Mechanism of action

    a. Like the phenothiazines, butyrophenone derivatives produce peripheral α_1-adrenergic receptor blockade.

    b. Butyrophenone tranquilizers bind to dopamine receptors in the CNS and reduce the membrane effect of normally released dopamine.

3. Pharmacokinetics

    a. Butyrophenones are metabolized in the liver.

    b. Renal excretion of the metabolites occurs primarily within the first 24 hours.

4. Pharmacologic effects

    a. Cardiovascular effects

        (1) Myocardial contractility is not altered.

        (2) The heart is protected from epinephrine-induced arrhythmias.

        (3) Azaperone produces slight α-adrenergic blockade, and the resultant vasodilation decreases blood pressure.

    b. Respiratory effects. Ventilation is minimally affected by the butyrophenones, and the response to carbon dioxide is not altered.

5. Therapeutic uses

    a. Azaperone

        (1) Azaperone, a **tranquilizer,** is often used to prevent aggressive behavior when introducing swine to the herd.

        (2) It is used as a **preanesthetic agent** in swine.

        (3) Prevention of malignant hyperthermia. Azaperone has been shown to prevent the development of porcine stress syndrome in susceptible swine, a complication of halothane anesthesia [see Chapter 5 III D 2 f (1)].

    b. Droperidol is a **long-acting tranquilizer** approved for use in dogs.

6. Adverse effects of droperidol include hypotension, transient personality changes (aggression) in dogs, and persistent head-bobbing in Doberman pinschers.

C. Benzodiazepine derivatives (see also II D)

1. Preparations. Diazepam, midazolam, and **zolazepam** are the three drugs in this group that are used in veterinary medicine.

2. Mechanism of action

    a. One portion of the GABA receptor in the brain binds the benzodiazepines, and another portion of the receptor is left available to bind to normally released GABA.

        (1) The inhibitory effect of the normal amount of GABA is enhanced by the presence of a benzodiazepine drug bound to the same receptor.

        (2) Activation of the GABA receptor results in increased chloride ion movement into the neuron, hyperpolarization of the membrane, and inhibition of cell membrane depolarization.

b. There is a synergism between benzodiazepines and barbiturates that probably involves the GABA receptor. Barbiturates bind at or near the chloride channel and, like benzodiazepines, cause membrane hyperpolarization (see II B 1 b).

3. Pharmacokinetics (see II D)

4. Pharmacologic effects
  a. Cardiovascular effects are **minimal.**
  b. Respiratory effects. Depressed ventilation may occur in an additive manner when the benzodiazepines are administered with other respiratory depressants (e.g., opioids, barbiturates).
  c. Muscular effects. Relaxation is mediated by drug effects in the spinal cord.

5. Therapeutic uses
  a. General
    (1) When used alone, benzodiazepine derivatives are not reliable tranquilizers in horses, dogs, or cats, but they provide **satisfactory tranquilization** in **sheep, goats,** and **neonatal foals.**
    (2) Benzodiazepines reduce cerebral blood flow and cerebral oxygen consumption rate, making them suitable for administration to animals with **cranial trauma.**
    (3) Benzodiazepines can be given with ketamine or tiletamine to provide **muscle relaxation.**
  b. Diazepam
    (1) Diazepam is used orally or intravenously as an **anticonvulsant** for the control of seizures and status epilepticus.
    (2) It can be used intravenously in combination with opioids (e.g., butorphanol) for **neuroleptanalgesia** or with cyclohexylamines (e.g., ketamine) or barbiturates (e.g., thiopental) for the **induction of general anesthesia.**
  c. Midazolam
    (1) Midazolam is used in combination with butorphanol and oxymorphone as a **tranquilizer** in older or debilitated dogs and cats.
    (2) It can be used as part of the drug protocol for **induction of anesthesia.** Mixed with ketamine, it provides muscle relaxation. Injected intravenously several minutes prior to thiobarbiturate administration, midazolam reduces the dose necessary for intubation in dogs and cats.
  d. Zolazepam is used exclusively with tiletamine for **anesthesia** in dogs and cats.

6. Adverse effects (see also II D 1 e)
  a. Benzodiazepines may produce **excitement** rather than tranquilization in some animals. Animals that are mentally depressed or sedated prior to the administration of a benzodiazepine are less likely to become excited.
  b. Ataxia, weakness, and **muscle fasciculations** may occur in horses.
  c. Reversal. Flumazenil is a specific competitive antagonist for benzodiazepine receptors and has minimal agonist activity.

D. α_2-**Adrenergic agonists** (see also Chapter 9 II)

1. General characteristics
  a. Preparations
    (1) Xylazine and **detomidine** are the two commercially available α_2-adrenoreceptor agonists. Both drugs also have some α-adrenoreceptor activity.
    (2) Medetomidine is not commercially available, but it is even more selective for α_2 receptors than xylazine and is thirty to forty times as potent as xylazine in dogs and cats.

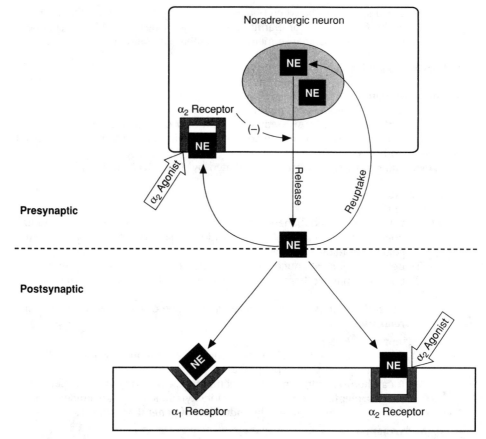

FIGURE 4-1. The effect of an α_2 agonist depends on the receptor location: presynaptic versus postsynaptic, and the tissue in which the receptor is located. Presynaptic α_2 receptors are inhibitory ($-$) to the further release of norepinephrine (*NE*) by the presynaptic neuron. Postsynaptic effects vary according to the tissue being stimulated. (Redrawn and modified with permission from Tranquilli W, Thurmon JC: Alpha adrenoreceptor pharmacology. *JAVMA* 184:1400–1402, 1984.)

    b. Mechanism of action (Figure 4-1). α_2-Adrenergic agonists stimulate central α_2 receptors. Centrally, the α_2-adrenoreceptors are located pre- and postsynaptically. Presynaptic α_2-receptor agonists reduce the release of transmitter (e.g., norepinephrine) from nerve terminals.

    c. Pharmacologic effects

      (1) Cardiovascular effects

        (a) Blood pressure

          (i) When these drugs are administered intravenously, peripheral α_2 receptors are initially stimulated, producing vasoconstriction and an **initial increase in blood pressure.** The blood pressure returns to normal or below normal in approximately 30 minutes owing to a decrease in CNS sympathetic output and, thus, norepinephrine release.

          (ii) Cardiac output initially decreases and then slowly returns to the baseline value. This decrease is the result of a decreased heart rate, an initial increase in blood pressure (increased afterload) which causes a decrease in stroke volume and a decrease in sympathetic nervous system tone. Myocardial contractility is difficult to assess, and current findings conflict.

        (b) Arrhythmia

      (i) Sinus bradycardia that is responsive to anticholinergic drugs (e.g., atropine, glycopyrrolate) and **sinus arrhythmia** are commonly associated with the administration of these drugs.

      (ii) First- and **second-degree atrioventricular (A-V) block, sinus arrest,** and **A-V dissociation** may also occur. Second-degree A-V block is common in horses and dogs following xylazine administration if anticholinergics are not administered.

    (c) Sensitivity to epinephrine. The **arrhythmic dose of epinephrine** in anesthetized or sedated animals may be altered by α_2-adrenoreceptor agonists.

      (i) Intravenous administration of high doses of drugs that have α_1 activity (e.g., xylazine) to halothane- or isoflurane-anesthetized dogs increases myocardial sensitivity to epinephrine.

      (ii) Drugs with more selective activity for α_2 receptors (e.g., medetomidine) either do not alter or increase the arrhythmic dose of epinephrine because of the resultant decreased sympathetic tone.

(2) Respiratory effects

    (a) Decreased respiratory rate and **tidal volume** decrease the arterial oxygen tension and transiently increase the arterial carbon dioxide partial pressure. In horses, these effects have been attributed to an increase in upper airway resistance.

    (b) In horses with heaves, stimulation of presynaptic α_2 receptors on cholinergic nerves within the respiratory tract reduces ACh release and causes **bronchodilation.**

(3) CNS effects. Both brain and spinal cord receptors are involved in the CNS effects of the α_2-adrenergic agonists. The brain is responsible for the sedative and analgesic effects of these agents, and the spinal cord is a site for producing analgesia and muscle relaxation.

    (a) α_2-Adrenergic agonists **potentiate the effects of opioids, barbiturates,** and **inhalant anesthetics.**

    (b) They **decrease sympathetic tone.**

    (c) The **hypnotic effect** of the drug is thought to result from its depressant action in the nucleus coeruleus (NC).

      (i) The NC is the main adrenergic nucleus of the brain and is involved in the control of sleep, analgesia, and autonomic function.

      (ii) Drugs that are agonists at receptors that mediate inhibitory transmission in the NC are anesthetics or hypnotics. The same is true of drugs that are antagonists at excitatory receptors in the NC.

(4) Gastrointestinal effects

    (a) In cats, **emesis** commonly follows intramuscular injection of xylazine. In dogs, xylazine occasionally causes emesis. The gastrointestinal tract subsequently decreases in motility.

    (b) Excessive salivation in ruminants results from decreased swallowing activity.

d. Therapeutic uses

  (1) Analgesic. Like other tranquilizers, α_2-adrenergic agonists have calming and muscle relaxing effects. In addition, they provide transient analgesia. Good **visceral analgesia** has been found in horses given α_2-adrenoreceptor agonists.

  (2) Preanesthetic agent. Administration of an α_2-receptor agonist prior to induction of anesthesia significantly reduces the required dose of general anesthetic (e.g., barbiturate, cyclohexylamine derivative, inhalant).

e. Administration. Species vary in their susceptibility to this class of tranquilizers.

  (1) Cattle require approximately one tenth the dose of xylazine required by horses for the same effect, but detomidine is used at the same dose in both species.

  (2) In swine, xylazine produces only mild sedation, even at high doses.

f. Reversal. The adverse effects of these drugs can be reversed by administering α_2-receptor antagonists (e.g., yohimbine, tolazoline, atipamezole, idazoxan).

2. Xylazine

a. Pharmacokinetics. Xylazine is metabolized to numerous metabolites that are excreted by the kidneys. Very little of the drug is excreted unchanged.

b. Therapeutic uses

(1) Xylazine produces **good sedation** in most species.

(2) Epidural administration of xylazine produces **regional analgesia** without substantial muscle weakness in horses, cows, pigs, and llamas.

c. Adverse effects

(1) In horses, **accidental intracarotid injection** of xylazine causes **immediate collapse** and **seizures.** With anticonvulsant therapy (e.g., diazepam) and support, recovery is possible.

(2) In sheep, xylazine causes the arterial oxygen tension to decrease dramatically. This **hypoxemia** is attributed to peripheral effects (e.g., airway constriction and ventilation–perfusion mismatch in the lungs).

(3) In male horses, **relaxation and extension of the penis** out of the sheath occurs. Permanent penile paralysis has not been reported in horses following the use of α_2-adrenoreceptor agonists.

(4) Decreased plasma insulin levels have been found in cats, horses, cattle, and dogs following xylazine administration. Pancreatic beta cells are effected by α_2 adrenoreceptors, resulting in decreased insulin secretion. Consequently, plasma glucose levels increase.

(5) In cattle, but not in horses, **early parturition** or **abortion** may occur if xylazine is administered in the last trimester of pregnancy, as a result of increased uterine tone.

(6) Xylazine may **increase urine output** in cattle and ponies. Normal micturition reflexes are maintained in dogs, making xylazine the preferred drug for sedation when testing this reflex.

3. Detomidine is approved for use as a sedative–analgesic in horses.

V. OPIOIDS

A. **Introduction**

1. Terminology

a. The term **"opioids"** is all-inclusive, and refers to a drug that binds to all or part of a subset of opioid receptors. An opioid may be synthetic, semisynthtic, or naturally occurring.

b. The term **"opiates"** applies to drugs derived from the poppy (opium) plant.

c. The term **"narcotics"** is commonly used to refer to opioid analgesics. In pharmacology, the term refers to drugs that induce sleep, but in the legal arena, it is used to indicate any drug that causes dependence.

2. Receptors. Opioid receptors are **naturally occurring sites in the body that respond to endogenous opiate-like substances** (i.e., enkephalins, dynorphines, endorphins).

a. The receptors are **present in numerous tissues,** including the brain, spinal cord, urinary tract, gastrointestinal tract, and vas deferens.

b. Classification. There are at least three receptor types.

(1) Mu (μ) receptors are located throughout the brain and in laminae I and II of the dorsal horn of the spinal cord.

TABLE 4-2. Effects of Opioids on Receptors

Opioid	Receptor		
	Mu	**Kappa**	**Delta**
Morphine	Ag	Ag	?
Fentanyl	Ag	Ag	?
Oxymorphone	Ag	Ag	?
Etorphine	Ag	Ag	?
Carfentanil	Ag	Ag	?
Meperidine	Ag	Ag	?
Pentazocine	Antag	Ag	Ag
Butorphanol	Antag	Ag	?
Nalbuphine	Antag	Ag	?
Nalorphine	Antag	P-Ag	?
Buprenorphine	P-Ag	Antag (?)	?
Enkephalins[†]	0	0	Ag
Endorphins[†]	Ag	Ag*	Ag
Dynorphins[†]	0	Ag	0
Naloxone	Antag	Antag	Antag
Naltrexone	Antag	Antag	Antag

Ag = agonist; Antag = antagonist; P-Ag = partial agonist; 0 = no effect; ? = unknown effect.
* For Kappa$_2$ receptor only.
[†] Endogenous opioids.

        (a) Stimulation causes supraspinal and spinal analgesia, euphoria, sedation, miosis, respiratory depression, chemical dependence, inhibition of gastrointestinal motility, and antidiuretic hormone (ADH) release.
        (b) Two receptor subtypes have been described: **Mu$_1$** and **Mu$_2$.**
    (2) Kappa (κ) receptors are found in the cerebral cortex and spinal cord.
        (a) Stimulation results in spinal analgesia, mild sedation, inhibition of vasopressin release, diuresis, and miosis.
        (b) Three subtypes have been described: **kappa$_1$, kappa$_2$,** and **kappa$_3$.**
    (3) Delta (Δ) receptors are located in the limbic system. Stimulation results in analgesia and modulation of mu receptors.
    (4) Other receptor types are described, but their existence or specificity is controversial.
        (a) Sigma (σ) receptor stimulation produces dysphoria and hallucinations. Sigma receptors bind to opioid and several nonopioid drugs (e.g., ketamine) and have no affinity for the opioid reversal agent naloxone. Consequently, sigma receptors are no longer considered opioid receptors.
        (b) Epsilon (ϵ) receptor stimulation results in analgesia, but this receptor has not been found in all species and may be the same as the kappa$_2$ receptor.
  c. Drug–receptor relationship. A drug may affect several receptors in the same way, or it may be an agonist or partial agonist on one and an antagonist on another (Table 4-2).

3. General characteristics of opioids
  a. Pharmacologic effects
    (1) Analgesic effects. Endogenous compounds (e.g., endorphins, enkephalins, dynorphins) are released by the body upon stimulation of opioid receptors. Exogenous drugs are used to stimulate these same receptors.
        (a) Opioid analgesia occurs at the level of the brain, spinal cord, and possibly the periphery.
        (b) Mu-receptor agonists produce profound analgesia.
    (2) Respiratory effects

           (a) Mu-receptor agonists are respiratory depressants; therefore, they cause an increase in the arterial carbon dioxide tension and a decrease in the arterial oxygen tension and pH. The **hypercapnia** results from a reduced sensitivity of neurons in the brain stem to carbon dioxide.

           (b) In dogs, mu-receptor agonists may cause **panting,** which may be a thermoregulatory response. The opioid resets the dog's hypothalamic temperature control point; by panting, the dog is trying to cool itself to a new set-point.

        (3) Cardiovascular effects. Opioids generally spare the cardiovascular system.

           (a) The heart rate may decrease significantly in dogs following administration of a mu-receptor agonist.

           (b) Hypotension may develop from peripheral vasodilation.

        (4) Gastrointestinal effects. Antidiarrheal effects and constipation are caused by stimulation of central (i.e., mu) receptors and peripheral (i.e., kappa and mu) receptors.

    b. Therapeutic uses. Opioids are used for:

        (1) Analgesia

        (2) Preanesthetic medication

        (3) Induction and maintenance of anesthesia. Mu agonists produce a dose-dependent decrease in the minimum alveolar concentration (MAC) of inhalant anesthetic necessary to produce anesthesia, but they will not produce anesthesia alone.

B. | **Opioid agonists** (Figure 4-2A)

    1. Morphine is the prototype opioid agonist to which all others are compared (Table 4-3).

      a. Mechanism of action. Morphine is a mu-receptor agonist.

      b. Pharmacokinetics

        (1) Morphine is metabolized in the liver by glucuronidation and excreted in the urine.

        (2) It readily crosses the placenta.

      c. Pharmacologic effects

        (1) In dogs, morphine induces **vomition** by stimulating the chemoreceptor trigger zone.

        (2) In dogs and primates, morphine causes **miosis.**

        (3) In dogs, morphine is generally considered to **inhibit gastrointestinal motility** but may initially induce defecation.

      d. Therapeutic uses

        (1) Morphine is used for the **treatment of acute pain** in dogs, cats, and horses.

           (a) In cats, low doses of morphine can be safely used for pain relief.

           (b) In horses, the addition of tranquilizers (e.g., xylazine) reduces pacing activity and results in good analgesia for standing procedures.

        (2) Morphine may be used as an **anesthetic premedication** in dogs.

        (3) The venodilation that results from morphine administration has been used in **canine heart failure therapy** as a means of reducing cardiac preload.

        (4) Antitussive effects in dogs are significant.

      e. Adverse effects

        (1) Hyperexcitability may occur in cats, pigs, cattle, and horses following mu-receptor agonist administration. Low doses, concurrent administration of a tranquilizer, or both will eliminate this side effect.

        (2) Hypotension. Intravenous morphine causes histamine release, which may induce hypotension as a result of the vasodilation.

        (3) Cerebral hemorrhage and edema. Opioids should be used with caution in dogs with head injuries because if respiration is depressed and arterial carbon dioxide values increase, the resultant increased cerebral blood flow may contribute to further cerebral hemorrhage and edema.

        (4) Reduced urine formation. High doses may stimulate the release of ADH and reduce urine formation.

A. Agonist

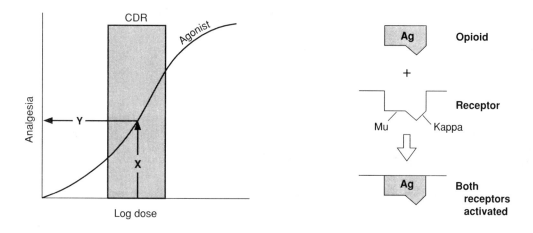

B. Antagonist

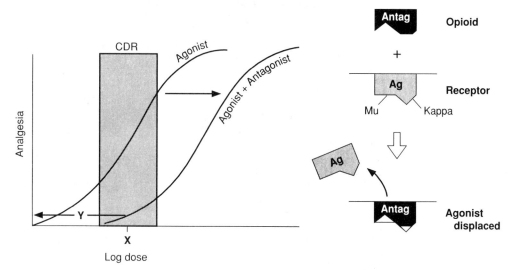

FIGURE 4-2. (*A*) An opioid agonist (*Ag*) binds to the mu and kappa receptors, producing a dose-related analgesia. The steep portion of the dose–response curve is within the clinical dose range (*CDR*). When an opioid agonist is administered within the CDR (*X*), analgesia results (*Y*). (*B*) An opioid antagonist (*Antag*) binds to the mu and kappa receptors but does not stimulate them. The antagonist causes the dose–response curve to shift to the right. Consequently, the analgesia (*Y*) produced by an opioid agonist (*Ag*) previously or subsequently administered within the CDR (*X*) will be reduced (reversed).

TABLE 4-3. Relative Opioid Potencies

Drug	Analgesic Potency	Histamine Release
Meperidine	0.1–0.2	Yes
Pentazocine	0.25–0.5	
Nalbuphine	0.5–1.0	
Morphine	1	Yes
Butorphanol	4.0–7.0	
Oxymorphone	10	
Alfentanil	7.5–25	
Buprenorphine	30	
Fentanyl	75–125	
Sufentanil	375–1,250	
Etorphine	1,000–10,000	
Carfentanil	10,000	

2. **Oxymorphone**
   a. **Chemistry.** Oxymorphone is a dihydroxy derivative of morphine.
   b. **Pharmacologic effects**
      (1) **Analgesic effects.** The analgesic potency of oxymorphone is approximately ten times that of morphine.
      (2) **Gastrointestinal effects.** It occasionally causes vomition.
      (3) **Cardiovascular effects.** When administered intravenously to normovolemic dogs, the cardiac output transiently decreases, while mean arterial pressure, systemic vascular resistance, and arterial carbon dioxide tension increase.
   c. **Therapeutic uses**
      (1) **Analgesia.** Oxymorphone is used as an analgesic in dogs and cats. In cats, it should be used at a low dose or in combination with a tranquilizer.
      (2) **Preanesthetic medication.** In dogs, oxymorphone is used as a preanesthetic medication.
      (3) **Neuroleptanalgesia** is a state of sedation and analgesia without unconsciousness, produced by administering a tranquilizer and an opioid. Oxymorphone combined with acepromazine is one example of a neuroleptanalgesic combination that is frequently used in dogs.
      (4) **Anesthetic.** In swine, it has been used in combination with xylazine and ketamine for intravenous anesthesia.
   d. **Adverse effects** are reversible with naloxone and some of the agonist–antagonist opioids (see V D).
      (1) **Panting** and **bradycardia** are common in dogs.
      (2) **Dose-dependent excitement** may occur in cats.
      (3) **Cerebral hemorrhage** or **edema** may be exacerbated in animals with head trauma.

3. **Fentanyl**
   a. **Chemistry.** Fentanyl is a synthetic opioid.
   b. **Pharmacokinetics**
      (1) Fentanyl has a more rapid onset than morphine after intravenous administration because it is more lipid soluble.
      (2) It has a shorter duration of action than morphine.
      (3) It is approximately 75–125 times more potent than morphine.
   c. **Therapeutic uses.** Fentanyl may be used in dogs as part of an **anesthetic induction** regimen or as a continuous infusion to provide **analgesia.**
      (1) It is difficult to induce anesthesia with fentanyl alone without the addition of another drug (e.g., droperidol, midazolam, thiopental, isoflurane).
      (2) Neuroleptanalgesia can be achieved in dogs using **Innovar-Vet,** a combination of 0.4 mg/ml of fentanyl and 2 mg/ml of droperidol.
   d. **Adverse effects**

(1) Auditory stimuli may evoke a **motor response** from the animal.

(2) **Panting, defecation,** and **flatulence** are common.

(3) **Bradycardia** and **salivation** may warrant treatment with anticholinergic drugs (e.g., glycopyrrolate).

4. Meperidine

  a. Chemistry. Meperidine is a synthetic opioid agonist. The structure of meperidine is very similar to that of atropine.

  b. Pharmacokinetics. Meperidine has approximately 10%–20% the potency of morphine.

  c. Pharmacologic effects resemble those of morphine because meperidine is primarily a mu-receptor agonist. It produces a slight atropine-like effect.

  d. Therapeutic uses. Meperidine is used to relieve **moderate to severe pain** and as a **preanesthetic.**

  e. Adverse effects. Meperidine should not be administered intravenously to dogs because of the resultant histamine release, tachycardia, and reduced myocardial contractility.

5. Carfentanil

  a. Pharmacokinetics

   (1) Carfentanil is approximately 10,000 times more potent than morphine.

   (2) The half-life of carfentanil is quite variable and may be long (2–24 hours). Thus, short-acting opioid reversal agents (e.g., naloxone) are metabolized faster than the carfentanil and their effects will not last as long.

  b. Therapeutic uses

   (1) Carfentanil is an opioid **used to immobilize large exotic animals,** mostly nondomestic ungulates (e.g., elk, giraffe, zebra).

   (2) It has been used with xylazine **to immobilize wild horses,** but its effects in domestic horses (e.g., muscle rigidity, paddling, tachycardia, and hypertension) are unacceptable.

C. **Opioid antagonists** (Figure 4-2B) bind to mu, kappa, and delta receptors but do not stimulate the receptors. They are pure antagonists with no agonist activity.

1. Naloxone

  a. Mechanism of action. Naloxone has a high affinity for mu and, to a lesser extent, delta and kappa receptors, which allows it to displace opioid agonists from these receptors. Mu-receptor agonists are the easiest to reverse because their receptor affinity is low.

  b. Pharmacokinetics

   (1) Naloxone has a duration of action many times shorter than that of the agonists for which it is administered to reverse. Consequently, repeat administration may be necessary to maintain opioid reversal.

   (2) It is metabolized in the liver and excreted in the urine after the metabolite is conjugated to glucuronide.

  c. Therapeutic uses

   (1) **Reversal of respiratory depression**

     (a) Naloxone is used **postoperatively** to reverse the respiratory depression caused by mu-receptor opioids. However, the analgesic effects will also disappear. The resultant pain may initiate undesirable behavioral and physiologic responses (e.g., excitement, tachycardia, hypertension) that are difficult to reverse because of the strong affinity that antagonists have for the receptors.

     (b) Naloxone is used to reverse opioid-induced ventilatory depression **in neonates.**

   (2) **Treatment of shock.** High doses have been beneficial in the treatment of septic, hypovolemic, and cardiogenic shock.

  d. Administration is intravenous or intramuscular. Oral administration is not very effective.

2. Naltrexone
   a. Mechanism of action. Naltrexone is a long-acting mu-, delta-, and kappa-receptor antagonist.
   b. Pharmacokinetics. It is metabolized in the liver, and the primary metabolite (6-beta-naltrexol) has opioid-receptor blocking activity.
   c. Therapeutic uses. It has been used to treat **behavioral problems in dogs** (e.g., continuous licking).
   d. Administration is oral.

3. Nalmefene is a long-lasting injectable opioid antagonist recently approved for use in humans. In humans, its half-life is 8–10 hours.

D. Opioid agonist–antagonist drugs

1. General information
   a. Classification. Opioid agonist–antagonists bind to several receptors (usually mu and kappa) and affect each receptor in a different way. They are subdivided into two types.
      (1) One type (e.g., butorphanol, nalbuphine, pentazocine) has a high affinity for mu receptors but induces no activity (Figure 4-3A). These drugs also have high affinity for, and moderate activity at, kappa receptors.
      (2) The other type (e.g., buprenorphine) has a high affinity for mu receptors but is only a partial agonist (Figure 4-3B).
   b. Therapeutic uses
      (1) Analgesia. Agonist–antagonist drugs are used to produce analgesia through stimulation of the mu or kappa receptors.
      (2) Reversal of respiratory and CNS depression. Agonist–antagonist drugs can also be used to reverse the respiratory and CNS depression of a pure mu-receptor agonist. These agents have the advantage of eliminating most of the ventilatory depression without totally eliminating the analgesia.
   c. Disadvantages. Agonist–antagonist opioids are more difficult to reverse than agonists because of their high receptor affinity.

2. Pentazocine is an agonist at the kappa and delta receptors and a weak antagonist at the mu receptor. It has about 25%–50% the potency of morphine.

3. Butorphanol tartrate resembles pentazocine but has an analgesic potency four to seven times that of morphine.
   a. Mechanism of action
      (1) Butorphanol has a moderate affinity for mu receptors but no activity (i.e., it is a mu-receptor antagonist).
      (2) It has a high affinity for kappa receptors and moderate activity.
      (3) It has moderate affinity for sigma receptors and moderate activity.
   b. Pharmacokinetics. Butorphanol is metabolized in the liver, and the inactive metabolites are excreted in the urine.
   c. Pharmacologic effects
      (1) Analgesia is produced until a certain point is reached. Increasing the dose does not produce further analgesia (see Figure 4-3A).
      (2) Increasing doses does not progressively depress respiration in a dose-dependent fashion.
   d. Therapeutic uses
      (1) Opioid reversal. Butorphanol can be used to reverse the mu effects of other opioids (e.g., morphine, oxymorphone). It allows reversal of sedation and respiratory depression while maintaining some analgesia (kappa effect).
      (2) Analgesic. Butorphanol is used as an analgesic.
      (3) Antitussive. In dogs, butorphanol doses lower than those necessary to produce analgesia have antitussive effects.
   e. Reversal. Butorphanol's agonist activity can be antagonized with naloxone.

4. Buprenorphine has thirty times the analgesic potency of morphine.
   a. Chemistry. Buprenorphine is derived from opium.

A. Agonist – antagonist

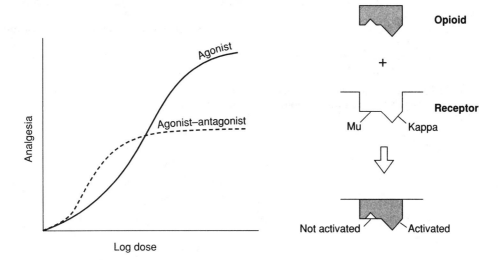

B. Partial agonist

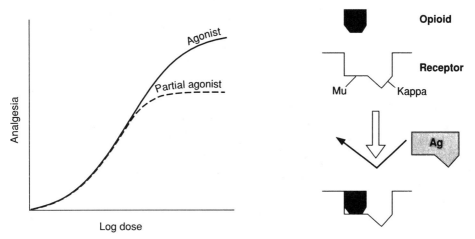

FIGURE 4-3. (*A*) An opioid agonist–antagonist (e.g., butorphanol) binds to the mu and kappa receptors, but only the kappa receptor is stimulated. The mu receptor site is occupied but unstimulated. The peak level of analgesia on the dose–response curve is less than what can be achieved with a pure agonist (ceiling effect). (*B*) A partial agonist (e.g., buprenorphine) binds to the mu receptor, producing dose-related analgesia. The peak level of analgesia is less that that possible with a pure agonist. Because buprenorphine has a high affinity for mu receptors, once it binds to the mu receptor, it prevents binding of the pure agonist (*Ag*).

    b. Mechanism of action. Buprenorphine has a strong affinity for mu receptors, fifty times that of morphine. It is a partial agonist at the mu receptor.

       (1) Buprenorphine can have antagonistic effects by displacing pure mu receptor agonists.

       (2) It is resistant to antagonism by naloxone because of its strong affinity for mu receptors.

    c. Pharmacokinetics. Buprenorphine has a longer duration of action than other opioids (up to 8 hours).

5. Nalbuphine is an agonist–antagonist with a potency equal to that of morphine. It is an antagonist at the mu receptor and an agonist at the kappa receptor.

STUDY QUESTIONS

DIRECTIONS: Each of the numbered items or incomplete statements in this section is followed by answers or by completions of the statement. Select the **one** numbered answer or completion that is **best** in each case.

1. Which one of the following drugs will reverse the respiratory depression caused by previous oxymorphone administration but still leave the dog with some analgesia?

(1) Carfentanil
(2) Fentanyl
(3) Naloxone
(4) Morphine
(5) Butorphanol

2. Which one of the following statements concerning buprenorphine is true?

(1) It is an agonist–antagonist opioid with antagonist activity at the mu receptor and agonist activity at the kappa receptor.
(2) It is an agonist–antagonist opioid with partial agonist activity at the mu receptor.
(3) It is a very potent mu agonist used to immobilize nondomestic ungulates.
(4) It is an antagonist at mu, kappa, and delta receptors.
(5) It is an α_2-adrenoreceptor agonist in the central and peripheral nervous system.

3. Immediately after an intravenous injection of xylazine to a healthy animal, what would be the expected cardiovascular response?

(1) Decreased arterial blood pressure, cardiac output, and heart rate
(2) Increased arterial blood pressure but a decreased cardiac output and heart rate
(3) Increased arterial blood pressure, cardiac output, and heart rate
(4) Increased arterial blood pressure and cardiac output but a decreased heart rate
(5) Decreased arterial blood pressure but an increased cardiac output and heart rate

4. Which one of the following drugs is an antagonist at the mu, kappa, and delta receptors?

(1) Naloxone
(2) Morphine
(3) Oxymorphone
(4) Pentazocine
(5) Butorphanol

5. Compared to morphine, which one of the following drugs is the most potent (in terms of analgesic effect)?

(1) Oxymorphone
(2) Meperidine
(3) Butorphanol
(4) Fentanyl
(5) Naloxone

6. A common side effect of oxymorphone administration in the dog is:

(1) panting.
(2) vomition.
(3) defecation.
(4) hypotension.
(5) tachycardia.

7. Which one of the following opioid receptors is correctly matched with its function?

(1) Mu—supraspinal analgesia
(2) Mu—respiratory stimulation
(3) Delta—respiratory depression
(4) Kappa—antidiuresis
(5) Kappa—respiratory depression

8. Phenobarbital can be used as an oral anticonvulsant. What other anticonvulsant drug is metabolized in the liver and produces phenobarbital as a metabolite?

(1) Primidone
(2) Phenytoin
(3) Diazepam
(4) Pentobarbital
(5) Potassium bromide

9. A horse to be tranquilized is given an intravenous injection of xylazine. The horse immediately falls to the ground and goes into violent seizures. What is the probable cause?

(1) The horse was prone to seizures, and xylazine lowered the threshold enough for a seizure to occur.
(2) The injection was given into the carotid artery instead of the jugular vein.
(3) Extreme hypotension from epinephrine reversal led to cerebral hypoxia and seizures.
(4) α_2-Adrenoreceptor stimulation decreased activity at the γ-aminobutyric acid (GABA) receptors.
(5) Increased insulin release by the pancreas secondary to α_2 adrenoreceptor stimulation caused acute hypoglycemia.

10. Which one of the following drugs will reverse the effects of diazepam?

(1) Butorphanol
(2) Naloxone
(3) Flumazenil
(4) Yohimbine
(5) Zolazepam

ANSWERS AND EXPLANATIONS

1. The answer is 5 [V D 1 a (1), b (2)].
The agonist–antagonist opioid butorphanol will reverse the effects of oxymorphone at the mu receptor while still providing analgesia via stimulation of the kappa receptor. Fentanyl, morphine, and carfentanil are mu agonists, like oxymorphone. Naloxone is an antagonist at all opioid receptors and would reverse the analgesia as well as the respiratory depression.

2. The answer is 2 [V D 1 a (2)].
Buprenorphine is an agonist–antagonist opioid with partial agonist activity at the mu receptor. Butorphanol is an agonist–antagonist with antagonist activity at the mu receptor and agonist activity at the kappa receptor. Carfentanil is the very potent mu agonist used to immobilize nondomestic ungulates. Naloxone and naltrexone are antagonists at mu, kappa, and delta receptors. Xylazine, detomidine, and medetomidine are α_2-adrenoreceptor agonists in the central and peripheral nervous systems.

3. The answer is 2 [IV D 1 c (1)].
α_2 Agonists (e.g., xylazine) initially cause peripheral vasoconstriction via stimulation of α_2 receptors in the arterioles. Xylazine has some α_1 receptor activity, which also produces vasoconstriction. The vasoconstriction leads to an increased arterial blood pressure. The heart rate decreases because of a decrease in sympathetic nervous system tone and an increase in parasympathetic tone. These changes in autonomic nervous system tone are central nervous system (CNS) effects of the drug and are secondary to the baroreceptor response to the increased arterial blood pressure. The baroreceptor response to an acute increase in arterial blood pressure is to slow the heart rate by increasing tone in the vagus nerve. The cardiac output decreases because of the decreased heart rate and a decrease in stroke volume secondary to the increased afterload (blood pressure) on the left ventricle.

4. The answer is 1 [V C 1 a].
Naloxone, nalmefene, and naltrexone are pure antagonists at all three opioid receptors (mu, kappa, and delta). Morphine and oxymorphone are agonists at mu and kappa recep-

tors. Pentazocine and butorphanol are antagonists at the mu receptor but agonists at the kappa receptor.

5. The answer is 4 [Table 4-3].
Fentanyl is 75 to 125 times more potent than morphine. Meperidine, which is 0.1 to 0.2 times as potent as morphine, is the least potent opioid analgesic. Butorphanol is four to seven times as potent as morphine, and oxymorphone is 10 times as potent as morphine. Naloxone is a mu-receptor antagonist and therefore has no analgesic activity.

6. The answer is 1 [V B 2 d (1)].
Administration of oxymorphone to dogs commonly causes panting and bradycardia. Occasionally, dogs will vomit. The fentanyl–droperidol combination (Innovar-Vet) commonly causes defecation, panting, and flatulence. Morphine and meperidine may cause hypotension because of associated histamine release and vasodilation.

7. The answer is 1 [V A 2 b].
Mu receptor stimulation causes supraspinal and spinal analgesia, euphoria, respiratory depression, and sedation. Kappa receptor stimulation causes spinal analgesia, mild sedation, diuresis, and miosis. Delta receptor stimulation causes analgesia.

8. The answer is 1 [II B 3].
Primidone is a deoxybarbiturate that is metabolized by the liver to produce phenylethylmalonamide (PEMA) and phenobarbital. Primidone and its two active metabolites have anticonvulsant activity. Phenytoin, diazepam, pentobarbital, and potassium bromide are all anticonvulsants, but none of them is metabolized by the liver to form phenobarbital.

9. The answer is 2 [IV D 2 c (1)].
Accidental intracarotid injection of xylazine is very uncommon, but it can occur in horses because of the anatomical proximity of the carotid artery and the jugular vein. The high concentration of xylazine delivered by the carotid artery to the brain results in convulsions and immediate collapse of the horse. Most horses survive with supportive therapy. Ace-

promazine gives a similar initial response when injected in the carotid artery, but many horses do not survive. Xylazine given by the intravenous route is not normally associated with seizure activity and has no direct effect on γ-aminobutyric acid (GABA) receptors. Blood pressure is not decreased initially. Xylazine inhibits insulin release in horses, leading to hyperglycemia, not hypoglycemia.

10. The answer is 3 *[IV C 6 c]*.
Flumazenil, a specific benzodiazepine-receptor–blocking drug, will reverse the effects of diazepam. It has high affinity for the drug receptor, great specificity, and very little intrinsic activity. Flumazenil is a competitive antagonist and will not displace an agonist, but it will occupy the receptor when the agonist dissociates from the receptor. Naloxone is an opioid antagonist. Yohimbine is an α_2-receptor antagonist. Butorphanol is an agonist–antagonist opioid. Zolazepam is a benzodiazepine-receptor agonist (like diazepam).

Chapter 5

Anesthetics

Dean H. Riedesel

I. INTRODUCTION

A. **Local anesthetics** interfere with nerve impulse conduction and **render an area or region of the body insensitive to painful stimuli.** These agents do not induce unconsciousness. Local anesthetics may be administered:

1. **Topically**

2. **By injection**
   a. **Into the tissues that are to be anesthetized** (i.e., **infiltration**)
   b. **Around nerves** to desensitize the tissues they innervate
   c. **Into the epidural or subarachnoid space** to desensitize a large region of the body bilaterally
   d. **Into joint spaces**

B. **General anesthetics** render the patient **unconscious** and **hyporeflexic** as well as **analgesic.** General anesthesia can be administered by **inhalation** of the drug as a vapor or by parenteral **injection.**

II. LOCAL ANESTHETICS

A. **Introduction**

1. **Action potentials** are changes in the resting membrane potential that convey information within the nervous system. Action potentials result from differences in the intracellular and extracellular **concentrations of certain ions** (mainly sodium and potassium) and the **permeability of the cell membrane** to these ions. This concentration difference is maintained by an ion pump within the cell membrane that is fueled by adenosine triphosphate (ATP). This pump, the **Na^+-K^+-ATPase pump,** transports three sodium ions out of the cell for every two potassium ions transported into the cell.

   a. **Phases of the action potential**
      (1) **Threshold.** The **resting membrane potential** must reach a specific threshold value before an action potential results.
         (a) Small decreases in the membrane potential (toward zero potential) that do not reach the threshold value do not lead to the propagation of an action potential.
         (b) Action potentials are an **all-or-none response** to a stimulus (i.e., they do not reflect the strength of the stimulus).
      (2) **Depolarization** results from a **rapid change** in the cell's permeability to **sodium.** Positively charged sodium ions rapidly **stream into the cell,** altering the membrane potential.
      (3) **Repolarization.** The channels that allow the sodium to move into the cell close at the peak of the action potential. **Potassium** then rapidly **diffuses out** of the cell, returning the membrane potential to its resting level.
         (a) **Absolute refractory period.** The nerve is **refractory** to stimulation during repolarization. This phenomenon limits the number of impulses that can be conducted along a nerve fiber per unit of time.
         (b) **Relative refractory period.** A period of **relative refractoriness** occurs toward the end of repolarization. During the relative refractory period, the

cell will respond only to stimuli of greater intensity than those necessary to invoke a response when the cell is at a resting membrane potential.

    (4) Return to resting potential. After repolarization, the Na^+-K^+-ATPase pump reestablishes the normal concentration difference of sodium and potassium across the membrane of the cell, readying it to fire again.

  b. Propagation of action potentials. Action potentials **self-perpetuate** along the length of the nerve fiber.

    (1) Unmyelinated nerves develop a flow of current from the depolarized region into the resting segment. The current flow reduces the membrane potential of the resting segment to a value that exceeds threshold and the action potential is propagated.

    (2) Myelinated nerves. In myelinated nerves, action potentials are generated only at the nodes of Ranvier. Action potentials appear to "jump" from node to node. Nerve impulse conduction velocity is much faster in myelinated nerves, as compared with unmyelinated nerves.

  2. Classification of nerves. Nerves are classified according to their size, myelination, and function.

    a. Nonmyelinated fibers are easier to block with local anesthetics than myelinated fibers.

    b. Small fibers are easier to block with local anesthetics than large fibers.

B. **Mechanism of action**

  1. Local anesthetics decrease the rate and degree of depolarization by elevating the threshold value and decreasing membrane permeability to sodium.

  2. The exact site of action of local anesthetics is thought to be one of the following:

    a. The external surface of the sodium channel

    b. The internal surface (axoplasmic side) of the sodium channel

    c. Within the nerve cell membrane, where the anesthetic produces lateral pressure and constriction of the sodium channels

    d. The axoplasmic side of the sodium channel and within the cell membrane

C. **Chemistry**

  1. Structure. Local anesthetics have three structural components: an **aromatic group,** an **intermediate bond,** and a **tertiary amine** (Figure 5-1).

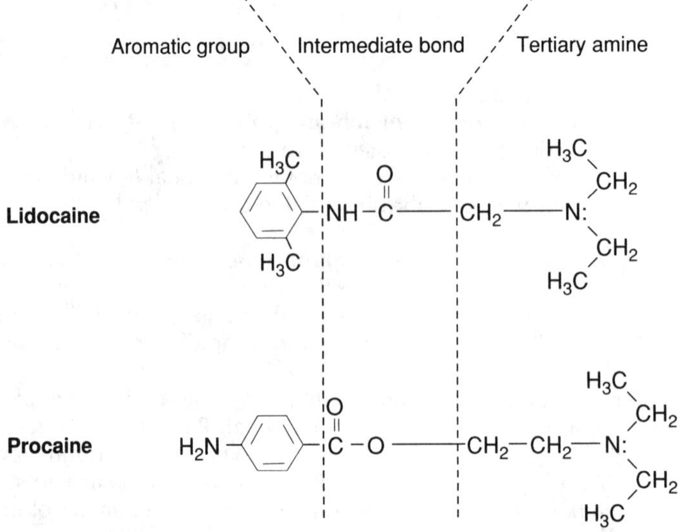

FIGURE 5-1. Lidocaine, an amide-linked local anesthetic, and procaine, an ester-linked local anesthetic.

    a. The **intermediate bond** is a connecting hydrocarbon chain that is either an **ester** or an **amide.**

    b. The **addition of carbon atoms** to the **aromatic region** or the **amine end** of the molecule **increases its lipid solubility** and, therefore, its potency.

2. Characteristics

    a. Local anesthetic drugs are **weak bases;** therefore, they are usually **water insoluble.** Commercial products are usually prepared as hydrochloride salt solutions, which are acidic. The acidity increases the stability and water solubility of the local anesthetic solution.

    b. Local anesthetics **exist in solution as uncharged** and **charged molecules.**

$$B + H^+ <\!\!-\!\!> BH^+, \text{ where}$$

$$B = \text{the basic uncharged form of the local anesthetic}$$

$$BH^+ = \text{the positively charged cation form}$$

$$H^+ = \text{hydrogen ion}$$

    (1) The relative proportions of uncharged and charged molecules depend on the pH of the solution and the dissociation constant (pK_a) of the drug.

       (a) If the local anesthetic is injected into an acidic environment, the $[H^+]$ increases, producing more ionized drug (BH^+) and decreasing the effectiveness of the local anesthetic.

       (b) Conversely, if the local anesthetic is injected into an alkaline environment, which has a low $[H^+]$, then greater amounts of the drug will exist in the base form, increasing the effectiveness of the local anesthetic.

    (2) The uncharged molecule (B) diffuses more rapidly across the nerve sheath than the ionized or charged molecule (BH^+). The charged molecule is thought to be the active form of the drug in the axoplasm.

D. **Pharmacokinetics**

1. Absorption and speed of onset (Table 5-1)

    a. **Lipid solubility** is directly proportional to **potency** and **duration of action.** The higher the lipid solubility, the more potent the agent and the longer its duration of action.

    b. The **pK_a correlates with the speed of onset.**

    (1) Drugs with a pK_a closest to the body's pH of 7.4 (e.g., 7.6–7.9) have a rapid onset of action.

    (2) Drugs with a high pK_a (e.g., 8.1–8.9) have a slower rate of onset.

2. Distribution

    a. **Protein binding** correlates with the **duration of action.** The binding site for the local anesthetic within the sodium channel is thought to be a protein.

    b. Epinephrine is added to some local anesthetics (e.g., lidocaine) to prolong the duration of action. The local vasoconstriction induced by the epinephrine limits sys-

TABLE 5-1. Characteristics of Local Anesthetics

Intermediate Group	Drug	Liquid Solubility	Potency	pK_a	Duration
Ester	Procaine	1	Low	8.9	Short
	Chloroprocaine	8	Intermediate	9.1	Short
	Tetracaine	58	High	8.4	Long
Amide	Lidocaine	3.7	Intermediate	7.8	Intermediate
	Mepivacaine	1.3	Intermediate	7.7	Intermediate
	Bupivacaine	34	High	8.1	Long

temic absorption of the drug, maintaining the local concentration. When epinephrine is combined with drugs that already have a long duration of action (e.g., bupivacaine), the effect is less dramatic.

3. Metabolism
  a. Ester-linked local anesthetics undergo hydrolysis by cholinesterase in the plasma and, to a lesser extent, in the liver.
  b. Amide-linked local anesthetics are metabolized by microsomal enzymes, primarily in the liver.

E. **Therapeutic uses**

1. Anesthesia
  a. Topical anesthesia. Local anesthetics are used to desensitize the mucous membranes of the eye, nose, and larynx.
    (1) Lidocaine is commonly used to desensitize the larynx in cats prior to endotracheal intubation.
    (2) Proparacaine is used to desensitize the cornea.
  b. Infiltrative anesthesia. Local anesthetics are used to numb tissues in a limited area (e.g., in order to debride and suture a laceration).
  c. Peripheral nerve blocks are used to desensitize larger areas. For example, a paravertebral nerve block would be used to desensitize the paralumbar fossa of a cow prior to a laparotomy.
  d. Spinal anesthesia. Epidural injection of a local anesthetic anesthetizes the spinal cord or cauda equina and is useful for procedures such as caudal abdominal, pelvic limb, or perineal surgery.
  e. Neurolytic anesthesia. Ethyl alcohol, which is neurolytic, has been used in veterinary medicine to produce prolonged nerve blockade in animals. Loss of nerve function can last as long as 1 year (i.e., as long as it takes the nerve to regenerate).

2. Control of arrhythmias. Lidocaine infused or injected intravenously is used to control premature ventricular contractions.

3. Facilitation of general anesthesia. Intravenous injections of lidocaine are used to decrease the dose of thiobarbiturate needed to induce anesthesia and prevent ventricular arrhythmias associated with thiobarbiturate use in dogs. Alternate injections of lidocaine and thiopental are given until an endotracheal tube can be inserted, and then inhalant anesthesia is continued.

F. **Adverse effects** can occur if the plasma concentration of the local anesthetic reaches certain threshold values. The relative toxicity of the local anesthetics closely follows their anesthetic potency. For example, bupivacaine is toxic at a lower plasma concentration than lidocaine.

1. Central nervous system (CNS). Skeletal muscle twitches are the first sign of toxicity, but **tonic-clonic seizures** are imminent and often the first clinical sign.

2. Cardiovascular system. Signs of toxicity usually occur at higher plasma concentrations than those associated with CNS signs. Plasma concentrations of lidocaine that produce cardiovascular toxicity may be lower for cats than in other species.
  a. Prolongation of the PR and QRS intervals may result from slowed impulse conduction.
  b. Hypotension and **decreased myocardial strength** (i.e., a negative inotropic effect) may occur.

3. Methemoglobinemia may occur following use of prilocaine or benzocaine in cats and rabbits.

III. **INHALANT ANESTHETICS.** The primary site of action of these agents is the brain and spinal cord. Analgesia and unconsciousness are produced when the concentration of the anesthetic reaches a specific level in the CNS.

A. **Mechanism of action.** Because the physiologic mechanism of consciousness is unknown, it is not surprising that the mechanism of action of inhalant anesthetics is also unknown.

1. **Single mechanism.** The observation that anesthesia has been produced using the gaseous phase of a wide variety of chemically unrelated compounds has led to the **unitary hypothesis,** which holds that all general anesthetics act through one basic mechanism.

   a. The fact that increasing the atmospheric pressure reverses the anesthetic effect of all inhalant anesthetics tested seems to support a single mechanism of action.

   b. In 1908, Meyer and Overton observed that anesthetic potency is correlated with the solubility of the drug in olive oil. This observation has been cited as support for a common mechanism of action.

2. **Multiple mechanisms.** Each anesthetic may have a unique mechanism of action.

B. **Pharmacokinetics.** Through ventilation of the lungs, an anesthetic partial pressure is established within the alveoli. Increasing either the inspired concentration of anesthetic or alveolar ventilation will increase the partial pressure in the alveolus. The drug diffuses from the alveoli into the blood and is circulated to all parts of the body. Anesthetic molecules move from areas of high partial pressure to areas of low partial pressure. Removal of anesthetic from the alveolus is affected by the solubility of the anesthetic in blood (i.e., the blood:gas partition coefficient), cardiac output, and the difference in partial pressure between the alveolus and the venous blood entering the lung.

1. **Minimum alveolar concentration (MAC).** The MAC of an inhalant anesthetic is the alveolar concentration that prevents gross purposeful movement in 50% of patients in response to a standardized painful stimulus. The MAC is used as a measure of **potency.** MAC values for the most frequently used inhalant anesthetics are listed in Table 5-2.

   a. **Correlation of MAC values and doses**

      (1) The anesthetic dose required to anesthetize 95% of animals is approximately 1.2 to 1.4 times the MAC. Surgical anesthesia levels are achieved by obtaining alveolar concentrations equal to 1.4 to 1.8 times the MAC.

      (2) If two anesthetics are administered simultaneously, the MAC multiples are additive.

   b. **Factors affecting MAC values**

      (1) Hypothermia, severe hypotension, advanced age, pregnancy, severe hypoxemia, severe anemia or the concurrent administration of certain drugs (e.g., opioids, tranquilizers) may decrease the MAC value for a particular patient.

      (2) Hyperthermia or hyperthyroidism may increase the MAC value for a particular patient.

      (3) The duration of anesthesia, patient gender, acid–base balance, and hypertension have no effect on the MAC value.

   c. **Relationship to lipid solubility.** The **Meyer-Overton observation** states that the oil:gas partition coefficient correlates inversely with anesthetic potency. The more lipid soluble the anesthetic, the lower the MAC and the higher the potency.

TABLE 5-2. Minimum Alveolar Concentration (MAC) Values in Dogs, Cats, and Horses

Anesthetic	Canine MAC (%)	Feline MAC (%)	Equine MAC (%)
Methoxyflurane	0.29	0.23	0.22
Halothane	0.87–0.92	0.81–1.14	0.88
Enflurane	2.20	2.37	2.12
Isoflurane	1.28	1.63	1.31
Nitrous oxide	188–222	255	190
Sevoflurane	2.16–2.36	2.58	2.31
Desflurane	7.2	9.79	—

TABLE 5-3. Inhalent Anesthetics in Decreasing Order of Lipid Solubility

Inhalant Anesthetic	Oil/Gas Partition Coefficient	Potentcy Ranking	(MAC)
Methoxyflurane	970	1	(0.29%)
Halothane	224	2	(0.87%)
Enflurane	96	4	(2.20%)
Isoflurane	91	3	(1.28%)
Sevoflurane	53.4	5	(2.36%)
Desflurane	18.7	6	(7.20%)
Nitrous oxide	1.4	7	(188%)

MAC = minimal alveolar concentration.

Conversely, the lower the lipid solubility, the higher the MAC and the lower the potency (Table 5-3).

2. **Blood:gas partition coefficient.** The **solubility** of an agent is most commonly expressed in terms of a blood:gas partition coefficient. Solubility of the agent in blood **correlates with the speed of induction and recovery.** Table 5-4 contains the blood:gas partition coefficients for the inhalant anesthetics.

   a. A high blood:gas partition coefficient indicates that the blood can hold a large amount of the anesthetic. Therefore, it will take longer to raise the alveolar partial pressure because the blood will keep absorbing the anesthetic as it is brought by ventilation to the alveolus.

   b. In addition, it takes a long time before the blood is saturated with enough drug to cause diffusion of adequate amounts into the tissues. Therefore, induction and recovery are slow.

3. A plot of the ratio of concentration of anesthetic concentration in the alveolus (F_A) to the concentration inspired (F_I) provides information about the various inhalant anesthetics (Figure 5-2).

C. **Administration**

1. By controlling the anesthetic concentration in the alveolus, the anesthetist is controlling the anesthetic concentration in the brain. Because the inhalant anesthetics move in the body by diffusion, it is necessary to administer high concentrations to the lungs initially in order to establish the necessary partial pressure in the brain.

2. Most inhalant anesthetics are liquid at room temperature and require a vaporizer to form a safe and accurate vapor concentration to be inhaled by the patient.

   a. The **boiling point** indicates what physical state the drug will be in at room temperature. If the boiling point is below room temperature (20°C), then the drug exists

TABLE 5-4. Blood:Gas Partition Coefficients for the Inhalant Anesthetics in Humans

Agent	Blood:Gas Partition Coefficient
Methoxyflurane	13.0–15.0
Halothane	2.3–2.5
Enflurane	2.0
Isoflurane	1.4
Sevoflurane	0.6
Nitrous oxide	0.5
Desflurane	0.42

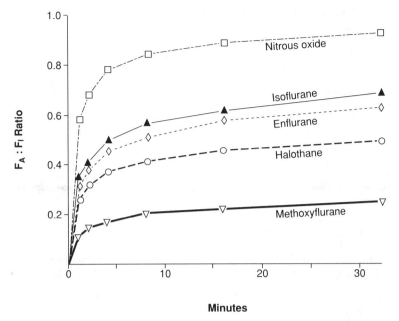

Minutes

FIGURE 5-2. A plot of the ratio of concentration of anesthetic in the alveolus (F_A) to that inhaled (F_I) over time provides information about the various inhalant anesthetics. The ratio begins at 0 and over time approaches the inspired concentration. When the body becomes saturated with the anesthetic and no longer removes a significant quantity from the alveolus, the ratio will equal 1. Anesthetics that are very soluble in blood (e.g., methoxyflurane) have F_A:F_I plots that rise very slowly. The alveolar concentration is much lower than the concentration inhaled because the blood rapidly absorbs a large quantity. Anesthetics that are poorly soluble in blood (e.g., nitrous oxide) have F_A:F_I plots that rise toward 1.0 quickly, indicating that the blood is rapidly becoming saturated and that the concentration in the alveolus is similar to what is being inhaled. After approximately 20 minutes, the F_A:F_I for methoxyflurane is about 0.2, which means that the alveolar concentration is only 20% of the inspired concentration. If the desired alveolar concentration is the MAC (in this case, 0.23%) then the inhaled concentration will have to be about five times the MAC, or 1.15% (0.23 / 0.2 = 1.15%). After about 20 minutes, the F_A:F_I for isoflurane is about 0.6, which means that the alveolar concentration is approximately 60% of the inspired concentration. If the desired alveolar concentration is the MAC (1.28%), then the inspired concentration should be 2.13% (1.28 / 0.6 = 2.13%).

    as a gas at room temperature. Table 5-5 contains the boiling points for the inhalant anesthetics.

  b. The **vapor pressure** of a liquid compound indicates how volatile it is and the maximum concentration that can be achieved (see Table 5-5).

    (1) The higher the vapor pressure, the easier it is to vaporize the compound.

    (2) The maximum concentration that can be achieved is calculated by dividing

TABLE 5-5. Physical-Chemical Properties of the Inhalant Anesthetics

Agent	Boiling Point (°C)	Vapor Pressure (mm Hg)	Maximum Concentration (%)
Methoxyflurane	105	24	3
Halothane	50	244	32
Enflurane	57	172	23
Isoflurane	48	240	32
Nitrous oxide	−89	760	100
Desflurane	23.5	664	87
Sevoflurane	58.5	160	21

TABLE 5-6. Inhalant Anesthetics: Physical-Chemical Properties of the Liquid Phase and Gas Volume after Vaporization

Inhalant	Gram Molecular Weight (g/mole)	Specific Gravity at Room Temperature (g/ml)	Volume at Room Temperature (ml)
Halothane	197.4	1.8680	228
Methoxyflurane	165.0	1.420	207
Isoflurane	184.5	1.5019	196
Enflurane	184.5	1.5230	198
Desflurane	168.0	1.4651	210
Sevoflurane	200.0	1.5203	183

the vapor pressure by the atmospheric pressure (760 mm Hg at sea level) and multiplying by 100.

(3) To determine the volume of gaseous anesthetic that will result from the vaporization of a liquid anesthetic, the following formula can be used:

$$\frac{(X)\ (SG)}{GMW} \times 22{,}400 = V_1, \text{ where}$$

$$X = \text{volume of liquid anesthetic (ml)}$$
$$SG = \text{specific gravity (g/ml)}$$
$$GMW = \text{gram molecular weight (g/mole)}$$
$$V_1 = \text{volume of anesthetic gas produced (ml)}$$

The resultant volume (V_1) assumes standard conditions of 1 atm of pressure (760 mm Hg) and 0°C. To convert the volume to room temperature (20°C) requires Charles' law, which states that if pressure is held constant, volume and temperature will vary directly.

$$\frac{V_1}{T_1} = \frac{V_2}{T_2}, \text{ where}$$

$$V_1 = \text{volume of gas at 0°C (273°K)}$$

$$T_1 = 273°K$$

$$V_2 = \text{volume at room temperature}$$

$$T_2 = \text{room temperature (293°K, 20°C)}$$

Table 5-6 contains the specific gravity, gram molecular weight, and volume at room temperature for some of the common inhalant anesthetics.

D. **Preparations.** Table 5-7 is a comparative summary of some of the more common inhalant anesthetics. Physical examination and clinical test results, as well as the underlying condition necessitating anesthesia, are factors that must be considered when selecting an anesthetic agent.

1. **Nitrous oxide**
   a. **Chemistry** (Figure 5-3). Nitrous oxide is an odorless, nonflammable, inorganic gas at room temperature. It will support combustion by dissociating into nitrogen and oxygen.
   b. **Pharmacokinetics**
      (1) **Induction and recovery from anesthesia** are rapid because of nitrous oxide's extremely low solubility—the body quickly becomes saturated with the inhaled concentration.
      (2) **Second gas effect.** The physical movement of nitrous oxide out of the alveolus into the blood stream tends to concentrate the other components of the alveolus, enhancing their absorption.

TABLE 5-7. A Comparative Summary of the Characteristics of Enflurane, Halothane, Isoflurane, and Methoxyflurane

Characteristic	Comparison Among Anesthetics
Chemical stability	[I] = [E] > M > H
Blood solubility	M > H > E > [I]
MAC	E > I > H > [M]
Dysrhythmia with catecholamines	H > M = E > [I]
Respiratory depresssion	E > I > M > [H]
Muscle relaxation	[I] ≥ [E] > M > H
Metabolism	M > H > E > [I]
Seizure activity	E > M ≥ [I] = [H]
Reduction in cardiac output	E > H ≥ M > [I]
Vasodilation	[I] > E > H ≥ M
Hypotension	E > [I] ≥ [H] ≥ [M]

Data compiled from Haskins, SC: Inhalational anesthetics. *Vet Clin North Am Small Anim Pract* 22: 297–307, 1992 and Steffey EP: Inhalation anesthetics and gases. In *Equine Anesthesia.* Edited by Muir WW, Hubbell JAE. St Louis, Mosby-Yearbook, 1991, pp 279–352.
    E = enflurane; H = halothane; I = isoflurane; M = methoxyflurane; MAC = minimal alveolar concentration.
    Brackets ([ ]) indicate most ideal manifestation of the characteristic.

    (a) The second gas effect can be **advantageous during mask induction,** decreasing the length of time that the animal may struggle before unconsciousness and relaxation occur.
    (b) It may be a **liability during recovery** when the nitrous oxide in the blood quickly moves from the blood into the alveolus. This physical movement of gas dilutes the other components of the alveolus (e.g., oxygen) and may lead to **diffusion hypoxia.** To prevent hypoxemia, 100% oxygen should be administered to all patients for at least 5 minutes after nitrous oxide is discontinued.
  c. Pharmacologic effects
    (1) The **cardiopulmonary effects** of nitrous oxide are **minimal.**
      (a) Nitrous oxide directly depresses myocardial function. However, because

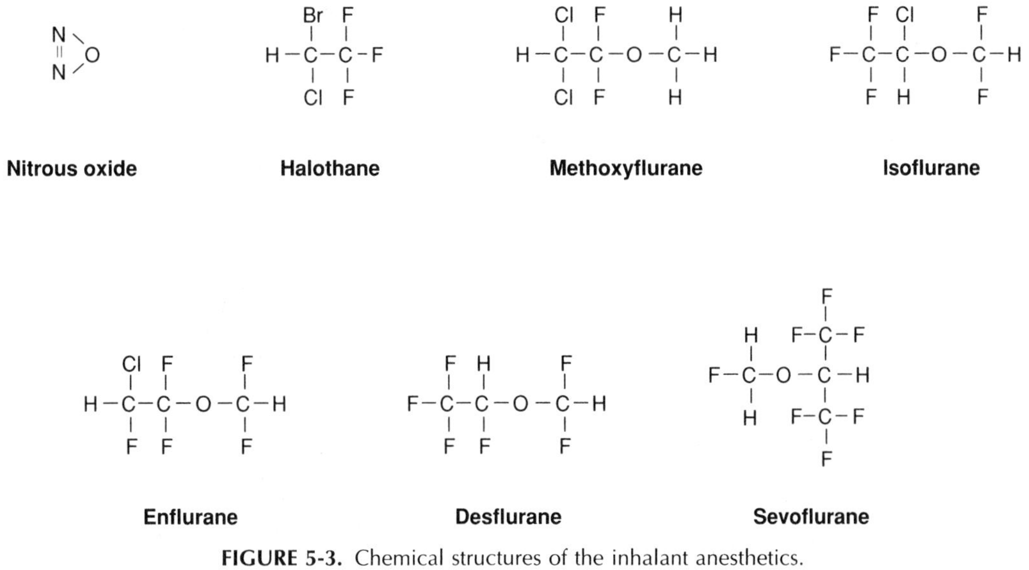

FIGURE 5-3. Chemical structures of the inhalant anesthetics.

nitrous oxide also directly stimulates the sympathetic nervous system, depression of myocardial function is minimal.

(b) Nitrous oxide does not sensitize the myocardium to epinephrine.

(2) **Hepatic and renal effects.** Liver and kidney function are unaffected by nitrous oxide.

(3) **Effects during pregnancy and delivery.** Nitrous oxide readily crosses the placenta; hypoxemia may develop if a neonate is allowed to breath room air immediately after cesarean delivery.

d. **Therapeutic uses.** Nitrous oxide is not a very potent anesthetic; surgical anesthesia is not obtainable in animals with nitrous oxide alone. Concentrations of 50%–66% are commonly used and the remainder of the anesthetic dose is provided by some other inhalant drug (e.g., halothane). The analgesic effect of nitrous oxide allows the anesthetist to administer lower concentrations of more potent anesthetics, minimizing the cardiopulmonary effects of these agents.

e. **Administration.** Nitrous oxide is administered quantitatively using flowmeters. A mixture of oxygen and nitrous oxide is determined by the respective flowmeters so that the desired percent of nitrous oxide is delivered to the anesthetic circuit. For example, if the ratio of oxygen to nitrous oxide is 1:1, then the mixture consists of 50% nitrous oxide and 50% oxygen.

f. **Adverse effects**

(1) **Hypoxemia** in anesthetized animals is frequently the result of ventilation–perfusion ($\dot{V}/\dot{Q}$) mismatch in the lung. A high percentage of inhaled oxygen usually prevents the arterial oxygen from becoming dangerously low, whereas a low percentage predisposes animals to hypoxemia.

(a) Large domestic animals frequently develop $\dot{V}/\dot{Q}$ mismatch during anesthesia–recumbency, and reducing the inhaled oxygen percentage with typical concentrations of nitrous oxide further predisposes them to hypoxemia. Therefore, nitrous oxide is seldom used in adult horses and cattle because it may increase the incidence and severity of hypoxemia.

(b) Administration of nitrous oxide at concentrations greater than 70% is discouraged because it places any anesthetized animal at risk of developing hypoxemia.

(2) **Distention of gas-filled spaces.** The blood solubility of nitrous oxide is thirty-five times greater than that of nitrogen. Because room air is 79% nitrogen, nitrous oxide will accumulate in and distend closed, gas-filled spaces (such as those that occur with pneumothorax or intestinal blockage). Nitrous oxide is contraindicated in animals with pockets of trapped gas.

(3) **Pernicious anemia** and **neurologic dysfunction** have been reported in humans following chronic exposure to nitrous oxide, which inhibits the activity of vitamin B_{12}-dependent enzymes in the body.

2. **Halothane,** a very potent inhalant anesthetic, has been widely used in veterinary medicine since its introduction in 1956.

a. **Chemistry.** Halothane, a halogenated hydrocarbon (see Figure 5-3), is a colorless, nonflammable liquid with a characteristic odor. Halothane is sold in brown bottles to prevent exposure to light and contains thymol as a preservative.

b. **Pharmacokinetics**

(1) **Induction and recovery** are faster with halothane than with methoxyflurane, but slightly slower than with isoflurane.

(2) **Elimination.** Most of the absorbed anesthetic is eliminated by the lungs, but it has been estimated that as much as 20%–25% is converted to trifluoroacetic acid, chloride, fluoride, and bromide by the liver. The chloride, fluoride, and bromide are excreted by the kidneys.

c. **Pharmacologic effects**

(1) **Cardiovascular effects**

(a) Halothane causes a **dose-related depression of the cardiovascular system.** Myocardial contractility is reduced, causing a progressive **decrease in cardiac output, stroke volume,** and **arterial blood pressure.** Cardiac function improves over time (i.e., in about 4 hours).

(b) **Vasodilation** may occur in the peripheral vasculature.

(c) **Myocardial sensitization.** Halothane is notorious for sensitizing the myocardium to catecholamines (e.g., epinephrine, dopamine, norepinephrine, ephedrine). Very low doses of these agents can lead to the development of **arrhythmias** (most commonly premature ventricular contractions, but ventricular tachycardia or fibrillation may occur as well). If it is deemed necessary to use a catecholamine in a halothane-anesthetized animal, the dosage should be reduced.

(d) **Heart rate may slow** and **second-degree atrioventricular block** may occur. These effects can be reversed with anticholinergics.

(e) Light levels of halothane anesthesia may **increase cardiac automaticity,** resulting in spontaneous premature ventricular contractions. The overall incidence of spontaneous arrhythmias with halothane anesthesia is low.

(f) Cats may develop **atrioventricular dissociation** as a result of junctional tachycardia. This is usually not a serious development and can be treated with anticholinergics if the ventricular rate becomes too slow.

(2) **Respiratory effects.** Halothane is nonirritating to the respiratory tract, but respiratory function is impaired.

(a) The tidal volume and breathing rate are decreased, reducing the minute volume and placing the animal at risk of developing **respiratory acidosis.** The respiratory function of horses and cattle is particularly affected by halothane.

(b) In dogs, **respiratory arrest** occurs at 2.9 MAC. Bronchodilation results in an increased anatomical dead space.

(3) **CNS effects**

(a) **CNS depression** occurs.

(b) **Thermal regulation** is depressed and body temperature usually decreases unless a supplemental heat source is provided.

(c) **Cerebral vessels dilate,** causing cerebral blood flow to increase. At the same time, cerebral **oxygen consumption decreases** in a dose-dependent manner. Therefore, animals with increased intracranial pressure should not receive halothane unless hypocapnia can be simultaneously induced by alveolar hyperventilation. Inducing hypocapnia reduces the effect of halothane on intracranial blood flow and pressure.

(4) **Muscular effects.** Muscle relaxation is good with surgical levels of halothane. The neuromuscular junction is sensitized to nondepolarizing neuromuscular blocking drugs (e.g., muscle relaxants such as atracurium).

(5) **Renal effects.** Halothane is not toxic to the kidneys of animals; however, it does reduce renal blood flow and the glomerular filtration rate. Consequently, **urine production is reduced.**

(6) **Effects during pregnancy and delivery.** Halothane crosses the placenta and will depress the fetus. Neonates delivered by cesarean section from dams anesthetized with halothane will quickly arouse when they start to breathe.

(7) **Analgesic effects.** Halothane is not analgesic at subanesthetic concentrations. Therefore, the animal will feel pain as soon as it emerges from anesthesia.

d. Therapeutic uses

(1) **Anesthetic maintenance.** Halothane is often used for maintaining anesthesia in dogs, cats, and horses. It has also been safely used in birds, laboratory animals, and exotics.

(2) **Muscle relaxation** is usually adequate at surgical levels of anesthesia. Methoxyflurane may provide better muscle relaxation, especially at light levels of anesthesia.

e. Administration

(1) Periodic cleaning of the vaporizer is required to remove accumulated thymol.

(2) Halothane reacts with metals, causing them to deteriorate. Halothane is soluble in rubber and some plastics and also leads to their deterioration. Generally speaking, plastic breathing hoses will last longer than rubber hoses.

f. Adverse effects

(1) Halothane is a trigger for **malignant hyperthermia** in pigs (i.e., **porcine stress**

syndrome). Malignant hyperthermia has also been reported in horses, dogs, and cats anesthetized with halothane.

  (2) The question of **hepatotoxicity** is complex and unresolved.

    (a) Halothane is not a classic hepatotoxin (i.e., it does not invariably result in hepatic damage). However, there have been reports of centrolobular hepatic necrosis and icterus developing in goats during the postanesthetic period. Concurrent drug administration and hypoxemia are probably significant contributing factors in the development of this condition.

    (b) It is also known that certain human patients are immunologically sensitive to the drug and develop hepatic necrosis after minimal exposure. The halothane metabolite trifluoroacetic acid has been implicated as the initiating factor.

3. Methoxyflurane has been used in veterinary medicine since about 1960.

  a. Chemistry

    (1) Structure. Methoxyflurane is a halogenated ether (see Figure 5-3).

    (2) Characteristics

      (a) Methoxyflurane has a very low vapor pressure and is very potent.

      (b) It is a clear, light-sensitive liquid.

      (c) It is nonexplosive and nonflammable.

      (d) It has a distinctive, "fruity" odor that is not objectionable to animals.

  b. Pharmacokinetics

    (1) Inductions and recoveries are slow as a result of methoxyflurane's high blood solubility. Its solubility in rubber is also very high, which may reduce the initial inhaled concentration during induction and increase the inhaled concentration during recovery.

    (2) Elimination. It has been estimated that as much as 50% of the inhaled methoxyflurane is metabolized by the liver and kidneys; excretion via the lungs also takes place. The metabolites are potentially toxic (see III D 3 f).

  c. Pharmacologic effects

    (1) Cardiovascular effects

      (a) Myocardial contractility is reduced and the peripheral vasculature dilates, leading to a **dose-dependent decrease in cardiac output and arterial blood pressure.**

      (b) Methoxyflurane **directly depresses the myocardium.**

      (c) It **sensitizes the myocardium** to catecholamines. The catecholamine sensitization associated with methoxyflurane is less than that seen with halothane.

    (2) Respiratory effects. Methoxyflurane is nonirritating to the respiratory tract, but **respiratory function is depressed.**

      (a) In dogs, the respiratory depression caused by methoxyflurane is at least as great as that associated with halothane.

      (b) The respiratory rate and tidal volume are decreased, leading to an **increase in the arterial carbon dioxide partial pressure.**

        (i) In spontaneously breathing anesthetized dogs, the elevated arterial carbon dioxide partial pressure stimulates the sympathetic nervous system, alleviating some of the cardiovascular depression seen with methoxyflurane.

        (ii) In mechanically ventilated dogs with a normal arterial carbon dioxide partial pressure, the cardiovascular depression is equivalent to that seen with halothane.

    (3) CNS effects

      (a) Methoxyflurane causes a **dose-dependent CNS depression,** but the exact mechanism is unknown.

      (b) Cerebral blood vessels dilate and blood flow increases with methoxyflurane. Animals with suspected increases in intracranial pressure should not be anesthetized with methoxyflurane.

      (c) Body temperature usually decreases unless a supplemental heat source is provided.

    (4) **Hepatic effects.** Liver function is reversibly depressed by methoxyflurane.

    (5) **Renal effects.** Renal blood flow, glomerular filtration rate, and urine flow are all reduced by methoxyflurane.

    (6) **Effects during pregnancy and delivery.** Methoxyflurane rapidly crosses the placenta and will depress the fetus. Neonates delivered by cesarean section from dams anesthetized with methoxyflurane will slowly arouse as they exhale the anesthetic.

    (7) **Analgesic effects.** Methoxyflurane is analgesic in subanesthetic doses. Animals recovering from anesthesia may benefit from this effect.

  d. Therapeutic uses. Methoxyflurane is widely used in dogs and cats, but its slow induction and recovery times have discouraged usage in horses. Because of its low vapor pressure and high solubility, methoxyflurane is not very useful for mask induction of anesthesia. However, it functions well as a **maintenance agent** after induction with another drug (e.g., a thiobarbiturate).

  e. Administration. Methoxyflurane contains an antioxidant [butylated hydroxytoluene (BHT)] that is not readily vaporized and slowly accumulates in the vaporizer, causing a yellow-brown discoloration of the anesthetic. When this occurs, the vaporizer should be cleaned and the discolored liquid discarded.

  f. Adverse effects. Hepatic necrosis and renal failure have been associated with methoxyflurane anesthesia in dogs. It may be best to avoid using methoxyflurane in animals receiving other potentially nephrotoxic drugs or with known hepatic or renal disease.

    (1) The free fluoride ion and oxalic acid that are produced by metabolism of this compound can be nephrotoxic.

    (2) Hepatotoxicity from metabolites has been suspected in rare cases of postanesthetic hepatic necrosis.

4. Isoflurane is the newest inhalant anesthetic cleared for veterinary use.

  a. Chemistry

    (1) **Structure.** Isoflurane is a halogenated ether (see Figure 5-3).

    (2) **Characteristics**

      (a) Isoflurane is a colorless liquid with a characteristic, pungent odor. It is a stable compound that does not require additives to maintain shelf-life; however, it is supplied in brown bottles.

      (b) The specific gravity and the vapor pressure are similar to those of halothane.

  b. Pharmacokinetics

    (1) **Induction and recovery.** Because of its low blood:gas partition coefficient, isoflurane rapidly induces anesthesia, patients change levels of anesthesia quickly, and recovery is rapid.

    (2) **Elimination.** Metabolism of isoflurane is very low (approximately 0.17% is metabolized); consequently, it has not been associated with organ toxicity. Thus, isoflurane can be considered for anesthesia in animals with hepatic or renal disease.

  c. Pharmacologic effects

    (1) **Cardiovascular effects**

      (a) Isoflurane depresses cardiovascular function and decreases arterial blood pressure in a dose-related manner. However, isoflurane-anesthetized animals maintain a higher cardiac output at deeper levels of anesthesia than halothane-anesthetized animals because the decrease in stroke volume is counteracted by an increase in heart rate.

      (b) Heart rhythm remains relatively normal.

      (c) Catecholamine sensitization occurs with isoflurane, but to a lesser extent than with other inhalant anesthetics.

    (2) **Respiratory effects.** In most species, the respiratory rate and tidal volume are decreased, leading to an increase in the arterial carbon dioxide partial pressure.

      (a) In horses, isoflurane causes more respiratory depression than halothane, but in dogs, the respiratory effects are similar to those produced by halothane.

      (b) Apnea occurs in most species at around 2.5 MAC.

(3) CNS effects
  (a) Isoflurane is a dose-dependent CNS depressant that produces general anesthesia by an unknown mechanism.
  (b) Body temperature usually decreases unless a supplemental heat source is provided.
  (c) Cerebral blood flow is unchanged at doses of less than 1.2 MAC. Cerebral blood flow increases at high multiples of MAC, but the vessels are still responsive to carbon dioxide. Thus, controlled ventilation to decrease the arterial carbon dioxide partial pressure will counteract the cerebral vasodilation of deep levels of isoflurane anesthesia.
(4) Muscular effects. Isoflurane potentiates the nondepolarizing muscle relaxant drugs (e.g., atracurium) more than halothane.
(5) Hepatic effects. Hepatic function is **reversibly depressed.** No cases of hepatic necrosis resulting from the use of isoflurane have been reported.
(6) Renal effects. Renal function is reversibly depressed, causing a **decrease in renal blood flow, glomerular filtration rate,** and **urine production.**
  d. Therapeutic uses. Isoflurane is widely used in dogs, cats, birds, and horses and is not contraindicated in any species. It is the current **agent of choice for animals with suspected increases in intracranial pressure.**
  e. Adverse effects. Because of its inertness, isoflurane has not been associated with any organ toxicities.

5. **Enflurane** (see Figure 5-3) is widely used in human medicine, but not in veterinary medicine. It has few advantages over other, less expensive inhalants (e.g., halothane).
  a. Pharmacokinetics. The blood:gas partition coefficient is low; therefore, rapid changes in the anesthetic depth are possible and mask induction is feasible. Metabolism is minimal.
  b. Pharmacologic effects
    (1) Cardiovascular effects. Cardiovascular function is depressed in a dose-dependent manner.
      (a) The **arterial blood pressure** and **cardiac output decrease** more than what is seen with halothane at comparable anesthetic depth.
      (b) Catecholamine sensitization is not as severe as that seen with halothane.
    (2) Respiratory effects. Enflurane decreases the respiratory rate and tidal volume. The degree of **hypoventilation** is dose-dependent and is greater than that produced by halothane, methoxyflurane, or isoflurane.
    (3) Central nervous system effects
      (a) Most volatile anesthetics cause a progressive slowing of the electroencephalogram (EEG) waves as the depth of anesthesia increases to the point of electrical silence. Enflurane is different, however, in that at moderate to deep levels of anesthesia, the typical slow wave activity is interrupted by high voltage, high-frequency patterns. These bursts of activity are accompanied by **skeletal muscle twitches** or **tonic-clonic seizures.** Consequently, enflurane is not recommended for anesthesia in animals suffering from seizure disorders.
      (b) Enflurane **dilates cerebral blood vessels** and **increases cerebral blood flow.** Like halothane and methoxyflurane, enflurane is not recommended for use in animals that may have increased intracranial pressure.
      (c) Body **temperature decreases.**
    (4) Hepatic effects. Hepatic blood flow and function are transiently reduced by enflurane.
    (5) Renal effects. Renal blood flow, glomerular filtration rate, and urine production are reduced by enflurane.
  c. Adverse effects. The free fluoride ion produced by enflurane metabolism is potentially nephrotoxic. Although the percent of metabolism is very small, enflurane should be used cautiously in animals with renal disease.

6. **Desflurane** is a new inhalant anesthetic agent that is approved for use in humans. Its use in veterinary medicine has been very limited.

a. **Chemistry** (see Figure 5-3). Desflurane's structure is similar to that of isoflurane.

b. **Pharmacokinetics.** Induction and recovery are rapid with desflurane, which has a blood:gas partition coefficient similar to that of nitrous oxide. Compared with other inhalants that are currently in use, desflurane's potency is low.

c. **Pharmacologic effects.** Cardiovascular effects are similar to those produced by isoflurane.

d. **Administration.** The vapor pressure of desflurane is high; therefore, a sophisticated vaporizer is necessary in order to accurately control the vaporization.

7. **Sevoflurane** has been approved for human, but not veterinary, use.

a. **Chemistry.** Sevoflurane is a polyfluorinated methyl isopropyl ether inhalant anesthetic (see Figure 5-3).

b. **Pharmacokinetics**

(1) **Induction and recovery.** Sevoflurane has a low blood:gas partition coefficient; therefore, induction and recovery are rapid.

(2) **Elimination.** Sevoflurane is metabolized by the liver to fluoride ion and hexafluoroisopropanol. It is degraded by carbon dioxide absorbents (i.e., soda lime) but the resulting compound (olefin, or compound A) has not been shown to be nephrotoxic in human clinical studies.

IV. INJECTABLE ANESTHETICS

A. Barbiturates and barbituric acid derivatives

1. **General information**

a. **Chemistry.** Barbituric acid is formed by combining urea and malonic acid.

(1) **Substitutions** at the various carbon and nitrogen atoms produce drugs with varying characteristics (Table 5-8, Figure 5-4).

(a) **Oxybarbiturates** have an oxygen molecule bound to C2.

(b) **Thiobarbiturates** have a sulfur molecule bound to C2. Thiobarbiturates are generally more lipid soluble and more highly protein bound than the oxybarbiturates.

(2) The resulting **weak acids** are **supplied as sodium salts.** Solutions consisting of barbiturate salts dissolved in water are very alkaline (pH 10–11.5).

b. **Mechanism of action**

TABLE 5-8. Barbiturates Commonly Used in Veterinary Medicine

Drug	X	R_1	R_2	R_3	Duration of Action
Pentobarbital	O	Ethyl	1-Methylbutyl	H	Short
Phenobarbital	O	Ethyl	Phenyl	H	Long
Methohexital	O	Allyl	1-Methyl-2-pentynyl	CH_3	Ultrashort
Thiopental	S	Ethyl	1-Methylbutyl	H	Ultrashort
Thiamylal	S	Allyl	1-Methylbutyl	H	Ultrashort

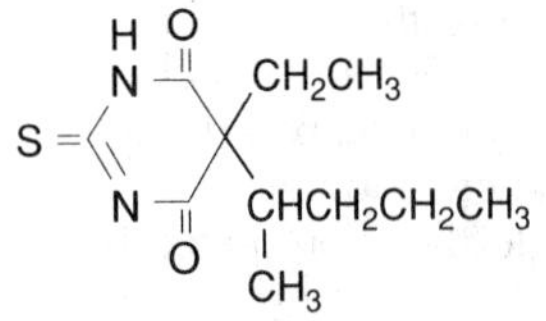

Thiopental

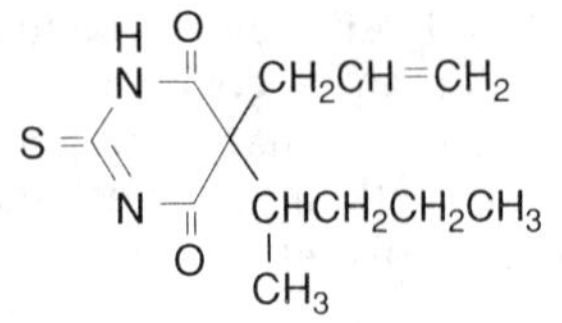

Thiamylal

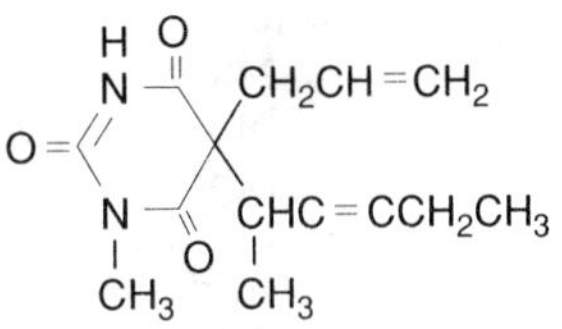

Methohexital

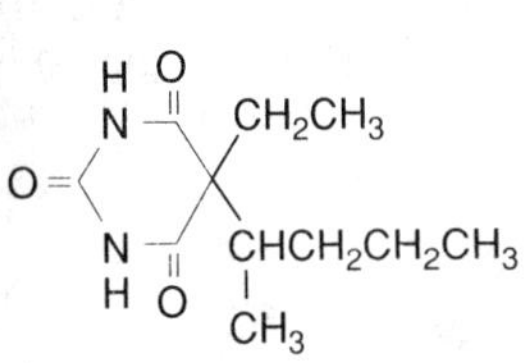

Pentobarbital

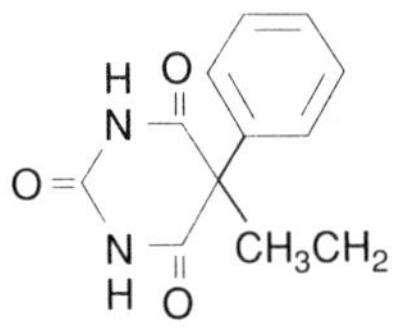

Phenobarbital

FIGURE 5-4. Chemical structures of the injectable anesthetics.

(1) Barbiturates bind to γ-aminobutyric acid (GABA) receptors, decreasing the rate of dissociation of the inhibitory neurotransmitter from the receptor.

(2) Barbiturates decrease the excitatory effects of the neurotransmitter glutamate.

(3) They alter synaptic transmission by inhibiting sodium and calcium channels and potentiating potassium channels.

c. Pharmacokinetics

(1) **Distribution** depends on the lipid solubility of the agent, protein binding, and ionization. Only non–protein-bound and nonionized molecules cross the blood–brain barrier.

    (a) Lipid solubility

        (i) Oxybarbiturates are less lipid soluble and slower to enter the brain than thiobarbiturates, but their duration of action is longer.

        (ii) Thiobarbiturates are rapid in onset because of their high lipid solubility and ultrashort in duration because they redistribute in the body to muscle tissue (Figure 5-5).

    (b) Protein binding parallels lipid solubility. Barbiturates bind to plasma proteins. Decreased protein binding (e.g., as a result of uremia or hypoalbuminemia) will increase the clinical effect of a dose of a thiobarbiturate.

    (c) Ionization. The degree of ionization in the blood stream depends on the pK_a of the particular drug and the pH of the blood. The nonionized form of the drug has greater lipid solubility and will penetrate the CNS quickly.

(2) **Metabolism and redistribution** (see Figure 5-5) are important in determining early recovery from anesthesia with these drugs.

    (a) Initially, metabolism is quite high when plasma levels are elevated and delivery of the drug to the liver is high, but after plasma levels decrease, the metabolism of these drugs is quite slow.

    (b) The fat compartment of the body slowly accumulates these drugs because of their high lipid solubility; however, blood flow to fat is low and rapid redistribution to this compartment does not occur (see Figure 5-5).

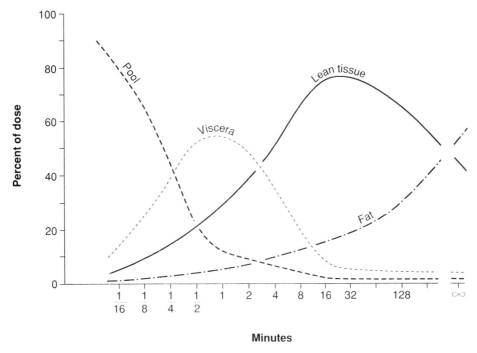

FIGURE 5-5. Distribution of a thiopental dose following intravenous injection. Initially, the drug is primarily in the central blood pool, but it rapidly redistributes to the viscera, lean tissue (muscle), and adipose tissue. At the time of recovery (approximately 10–15 minutes postinjection), most of the drug is in the lean tissue compartment. (Redrawn with permission from Price HL et al: The uptake of thiopental by body tissues and its relation to the duration of narcosis. *Clin Pharmacol Ther* 1:16, 1960.)

Repeat doses of thiobarbiturates may result in high drug concentrations in the fat compartment. When drug administration is stopped, the accumulated stores may return to the blood stream, resulting in prolonged elevation of plasma drug levels and prolonged recovery from anesthesia.

  d. Pharmacologic effects

  (1) Cardiovascular effects. Intravenous injection in the normovolemic patient causes **transient hypotension** and an **increase in heart rate.**

  (2) Respiratory effects. Transient apnea following the intravenous injection of these compounds occurs fairly commonly as a result of depression of the respiratory centers in the brain stem.

  (3) CNS effects

   (a) Barbiturates cause a dose-dependent depression of CNS function.

   (i) Low doses may cause sedation or excitement.

   (ii) Moderate doses cause general anesthesia.

   (iii) High doses lead to profound CNS depression.

   (iv) Overdoses cause apnea and, eventually, cardiovascular depression and death.

   (b) Barbiturates decrease cerebral blood flow, cerebral blood volume, and intracranial pressure.

  (4) Effects during pregnancy and delivery. Placental transfer of barbiturates is rapid after intravenous injection.

  (5) Analgesic effects. Barbiturates are not analgesic in subanesthetic doses. There is evidence that some barbiturates are hyperalgesic at subanesthetic doses.

 2. Preparations and therapeutic uses

  a. Ultrashort-acting barbiturates are very lipid soluble; therefore, their onset of action is rapid and their duration of action is short (10–30 minutes).

(1) Thiopental and thiamylal. Thiamylal is slightly more potent than thiopental. In large domestic animals (e.g., horses, cattle) the thiobarbiturates are commonly administered with guaifenesin, a central acting muscle relaxant (see V D).

    (a) Therapeutic uses

        (i) Thiobarbiturates are considered one of the **drugs of choice for induction of anesthesia in animals with suspected increased intracranial pressure.**

        (ii) These agents can be used for **maintenance of anesthesia;** however, repeat doses may lead to slow recovery because of saturation of the redistribution sites.

        (iii) Thiobarbiturates are safe for induction of anesthesia for **cesarean section** because these drugs redistribute rapidly in the dam and fetus. By the time the fetus is delivered, the fetal blood levels are quite low.

    (b) Adverse effects

        (i) Prolonged recovery. Plasma clearance of these drugs is prolonged in greyhounds. Therefore, they experience a long duration of effect and slow recovery. Use of thiobarbiturates in greyhounds and other sight hounds is not recommended.

        (ii) Cardiac arrhythmias may occur if a large intravenous dose of a thiobarbiturate is administered rapidly. Premature ventricular contractions are most common. The ventricular arrhythmia is usually short in duration but potentially detrimental to the patient.

        (iii) Allergic reactions to these drugs have been reported but are extremely rare.

        (iv) Local irritation. Perivascular injection may lead to necrosis and sloughing of substantial amounts of tissue. Use of dilute solutions, injection of saline into the area, or injection of lidocaine to dilute the drug and alter the pH may help prevent tissue irritation.

(2) Methohexital is more rapidly metabolized than the thiobarbiturates and the other oxybarbiturates because of its higher lipid solubility, which results from the addition of a methyl group. It is more potent than thiopental.

    (a) Therapeutic uses

        (i) Like the thiobarbiturates, methohexital is safe for use during **cesarean section.**

        (ii) It is **safe for use in greyhounds** and other sight hounds. Because of methohexital's rapid redistribution and metabolism by the liver, recovery is quick.

    (b) Adverse effects. Methohexital is more likely than the thiobarbiturates to cause a period of excitement during induction and recovery.

b. Short-acting barbiturates (e.g., **pentobarbital**) are less lipid soluble and have a longer duration of action (approximately 30–60 minutes) than the ultrashort-acting agents.

    (1) Therapeutic uses

        (a) Pentobarbital, which has a very low margin of safety, is the primary ingredient of **euthanasia** agents.

        (b) Pentobarbital is **occasionally used for intravenous anesthesia** in dogs, cats, pigs, and small ruminants.

    (2) Adverse effects

        (a) Low doses administered intravenously may cause an excitement phase characterized by whining, paddling, and incoordination.

        (b) Recovery is slow and characterized by paddling of the limbs and incoordination. Sedation, physical assistance, or both may be required to ensure a smooth recovery.

c. Long-acting barbiturates (e.g., **phenobarbital**) are the least lipid soluble and the slowest in their onset of action, but they have a long duration of action (6–12 hours). Phenobarbital is used primarily as an **anticonvulsant** at subanesthetic doses, not as a general anesthetic (see Chapter 4 II B 1).

B. Cyclohexylamines

1. **Dissociative anesthesia,** which is characterized by analgesia and superficial sleep, is a term used to describe the CNS state produced by these drugs. Different levels of the CNS seem to become dissociated from one another—the EEG reveals depression of the thalamoneocortical portion of the brain and enhanced activity in the limbic system.
   a. **Many reflexes** (e.g., palpebral, laryngeal, pharyngeal) **are maintained** and the skeletal muscles of the eyelid are contracted, opening the orbit.
   b. **Somatic analgesia is good, but visceral analgesia is poor.**
   c. **Muscle relaxation is poor.** Animals are described as **cataleptic,** a state characterized by rigidity and partial extension of the limbs.

2. **Pharmacologic effects**
   a. **Cardiovascular effects.** Cyclohexylamines directly depress cardiovascular function; however, in healthy animals, they increase sympathetic tone, masking the direct effect and resulting in overall stimulation of cardiovascular function.
      (1) The heart rate is maintained or increased.
      (2) The blood pressure and cardiac output are increased.
   b. **Respiratory effects.** Respiration is depressed, causing the arterial oxygen tension to decrease and arterial carbon dioxide tension to increase. Cats and many other species develop an **apneustic breathing pattern,** characterized by an inspiratory hold with a very short expiratory pause.
   c. **CNS effects**
      (1) Cerebral blood flow and intracranial pressure are increased by these anesthetic drugs.
      (2) Dilation of pupils occurs.
   d. **Effects during pregnancy and delivery.** These drugs rapidly cross the placenta and affect the fetus.

3. **Preparations** include **phencyclidine, ketamine,** and **tiletamine.**
   a. **Phencyclidine,** introduced in the 1960s, was the first cyclohexylamine used to produce anesthesia. It is no longer available for veterinary use.
   b. **Ketamine** is approved by the Food and Drug Administration (FDA) for use in cats, but numerous other species have been safely anesthetized with ketamine.
      (1) **Chemistry.** Ketamine is commercially available as an aqueous solution with a pH of 3.5. The solution contains a racemic mixture of the two isomers of ketamine.
      (2) **Mechanism of action**
         (a) Ketamine inhibits the polysynaptic actions of the excitatory neurotransmitters acetylcholine (ACh) and L-glutamate in the spinal cord and N-methyl-D-aspartate (NMDA) in the brain. It is a potent noncompetitive antagonist at the NMDA receptor complex.
         (b) It stimulates receptors that may be the same as or closely related to the sigma receptor [see Chapter 4 V A 2 b (4) (a)].
      (3) **Pharmacokinetics.** Ketamine is metabolized by the liver, and some of the metabolites have anesthetic activity. The metabolites are excreted in the urine. The older literature indicates that in cats, the majority of ketamine is excreted unchanged by the kidney. More recent studies, however, indicate that the majority of ketamine administered to cats is metabolized in the liver and only a small amount is renally excreted.
      (4) **Administration**
         (a) Ketamine can be **administered intramuscularly** or **intravenously** to cats, dogs, small ruminants, and swine. In adult horses and cattle, it is only administered intravenously.
         (b) **Ketamine combinations.** Animals usually receive a tranquilizer (e.g, acepromazine, xylazine, diazepam) along with ketamine in order to provide muscle relaxation.
            (i) Xylazine, guaifenesin, or both are frequently administered to horses

prior to administration of ketamine. Both xylazine and guaifenesin provide muscle relaxation.

(ii) Diazepam, midazolam, or xylazine are frequently used with ketamine in dogs and cats in order to prevent seizures and provide muscle relaxation.

(iii) Guaifenesin, diazepam, or xylazine may be used in combination with ketamine in pigs, cattle, sheep, and goats.

(5) Adverse effects

(a) **Seizures** are common in horses and dogs following administration of ketamine alone.

(b) **Profuse salivation** may occur in cats. Laryngeal and pharyngeal reflexes are present, but they are not active enough to prevent life-threatening **airway obstruction.** Anticholinergic drugs administered before or along with ketamine will prevent excessive salivation.

(c) **Corneal ulceration.** Because the eyes remain open during anesthesia, the cornea may dry out and ulcerate if not protected by an ophthalmic ointment.

c. **Telazol** contains equal amounts of tiletamine, a cyclohexylamine, and zolazepam, a benzodiazepine tranquilizer.

(1) Therapeutic uses

(a) Telazol is used for **anesthesia of short duration in dogs and cats.** It is very useful in **feral cats** or **uncooperative dogs** because it can be administered intramuscularly, has a rapid onset of action, and the dose is small.

(b) Telazol is used in many other domestic and exotic species.

(i) It has been used for short-term anesthesia in horses following administration of xylazine and butorphanol.

(ii) It is combined with xylazine and ketamine for use in pigs.

(iii) It may be used alone or in combination with xylazine in small ruminants.

(2) Administration. Telazol can be administered intramuscularly, subcutaneously, or intravenously.

(3) Adverse effects

(a) Recoveries are slow and smooth in cats, but in dogs, recoveries are sometimes accompanied by muscle tremors, paddling, and whining. Rough recoveries may occur in dogs because they metabolize the zolazepam more rapidly than the tiletamine.

(b) Hyperthermia may result from the increased muscle activity.

(c) Tachycardia may occur in dogs.

4. Contraindications

a. Cyclohexylamines may increase intraocular pressure by inducing contraction of the extraocular muscles; therefore, they are contraindicated in animals with **corneal ulcers** or **lacerations.**

b. They are contraindicated in animals with **head trauma** or a **space-occupying mass** in the brain.

C. **Propofol**

1. Chemistry. Propofol, a substituted isopropylphenol, is an alkylphenol derivative that is unrelated to any other anesthetic drug currently in use. It is formulated in a 1% aqueous emulsion containing 10% soybean oil, 1.2% egg lecithin, and 2.25% glycerol.

2. Pharmacokinetics

a. **Induction.** The onset of action is rapid and induction is smooth. Repeat doses in dogs do not accumulate.

b. **Distribution.** Propofol is highly protein bound.

c. **Metabolism**

(1) The duration of anesthesia following a single intravenous injection is very short (2–10 minutes) because propofol is rapidly metabolized by glucuronide synthetase in the liver. Cats have less glucuronide synthetase with which to

metabolize propofol; therefore, prolonged infusions or consecutive day injections may not be tolerated.

(2) The lungs have been shown to remove a significant amount of propofol from the circulating blood and may participate in drug metabolism as well.

3. **Therapeutic uses**
   a. The milky white emulsion is used primarily in dogs and cats for intravenous induction of anesthesia for **short procedures** or **prior to inhalant anesthesia.**
   b. Rapid redistribution and metabolism result in quick recovery of psychomotor function; therefore, propofol is **ideal for outpatient cases.**
   c. Propofol decreases cerebral blood flow and cerebral oxygen consumption; therefore, it is safe for use in animals with **head trauma** or **increased intracranial pressure.**

4. **Adverse effects**
   a. **Myoclonic twitching** and **limb paddling** are sometimes seen in dogs following propofol administration.
   b. **Direct myocardial depression, peripheral vasodilation,** and **venodilation** occur, causing blood pressure and cardiac output to decrease. Propofol must be used cautiously in traumatized animals and those with hypovolemia or impaired left ventricular function.
   c. **Apnea** following a rapid, intravenous bolus dose is common in dogs and cats.
   d. **Heinz body formation.** Phenolic compounds may cause oxidative damage to erythrocytes in cats. Daily infusions resulted in the formation of Heinz bodies, anorexia, and malaise.
   e. **Septicemia.** Propofol's vehicle (soybean oil, egg lecithin, and glycerol) is supportive of bacterial growth; therefore, great care must be taken to avoid contamination of the drug prior to injection or septicemia may result.

D. **Etomidate** is a sedative hypnotic nonbarbiturate drug of ultrashort duration. It has a wide margin of safety, with a therapeutic index of 16 (as compared with thiopental, which has a therapeutic index of 4–7).

1. **Pharmacokinetics.** Etomidate undergoes rapid hepatic hydrolysis and does not accumulate, even following repeated doses.

2. **Pharmacologic effects**
   a. Etomidate causes **minimal depression of cardiovascular and respiratory function.**
   b. It decreases cerebral blood flow, metabolic rate, and oxygen consumption.
   c. Etomidate inhibits adrenal steroidogenesis, reducing the normal increase in plasma cortisol levels associated with anesthesia and surgery. The clinical importance of this inhibition is unknown.

3. **Therapeutic uses.** Etomidate is administered intravenously to dogs and cats for induction of anesthesia for **short procedures** or **prior to inhalant anesthesia.**

3. **Adverse effects. Myoclonus** and **excitement** can occur either on induction or recovery. These effects can be prevented by adequate preinduction sedation with a tranquilizer or opioid drug.

V. **PREANESTHETIC MEDICATIONS** facilitate anesthesia and surgery by improving the rapidity and smoothness of induction, reducing anxiety, providing analgesia and amnesia, and compensating for some of the side effects of anesthesia (e.g., salivation, bradycardia).

A. **Opioids** (see Chapter 4 V) are administered to provide analgesia.

B. **Tranquilizers** (see Chapter 4 IV) provide preoperative sedation and amnesia and help to prevent or counteract the CNS stimulation caused by some anesthetics.

C. **Anticholinergic agents** (see Chapter 2 VI) prevent profuse salivation and bradycardia.

D. **Muscle relaxants. Guaifenesin** is a central acting muscle relaxant that is used intravenously with thiobarbiturates and ketamine for induction of anesthesia in horses, cattle, and swine.

1. **Chemistry.** Guaifenesin is a white powder that is dissolved in water, 0.9% saline, or 5% dextrose to produce a final drug concentration of 5%–10%.

2. **Mechanism of action.** Guaifenesin is a centrally acting muscle relaxant that blocks polysynaptic reflexes and depresses impulse transmission by internuncial neurons in the spinal cord.

3. **Pharmacokinetics.** Guaifenesin is metabolized by the liver, and the conjugated metabolites are excreted by the kidney. The plasma half-life is approximately 60–80 minutes.

4. **Pharmacologic effects**
   a. **Cardiovascular effects.** Guaifenesin decreases arterial blood pressure in horses but has minimal effects on cardiac output or heart rate.
   b. **Respiratory effects.** Diaphragmatic function and respiration are minimally depressed.
   c. **Analgesic effects.** Sedation accompanies the muscle relaxation, but analgesia is minimal.
   d. **Effects during pregnancy and delivery.** It readily crosses the placenta but does not adversely affect the fetus.

5. **Administration.** Guaifenesin is usually mixed with either a thiobarbiturate or ketamine. This combination is then rapidly infused into the jugular vein of a tranquilized horse to induce anesthesia.

6. **Adverse effects**
   a. Perivascular injection causes **acute inflammation, necrosis,** and **sloughing at the injection site.**
   b. Prolonged infusions will lead to drug accumulation in the body and **extremely long recovery times.**
   c. **Urticaria** is occasionally seen in horses following guaifenesin administration. This effect is thought to be a drug-induced allergic reaction.
   d. Overdoses can cause **bradycardia, hypotension, extensor rigidity, apneustic breathing,** and **cardiac arrest.**
   e. Concentrations exceeding 10% in cattle or 12.5% in horses are associated with **intravascular hemolysis** and **hemoglobinuria.**

STUDY QUESTIONS

DIRECTIONS: Each of the numbered items or incomplete statements in this section is followed by answers or by completions of the statement. Select the **one** numbered answer or completion that is **best** in each case.

1. What is the first indicator of local anesthetic toxicity?

(1) Skeletal muscle twitching
(2) Tonic-clonic convulsions
(3) Hypotension
(4) Cardiac arrhythmias
(5) Vomiting

2. Which inhalant anesthetic has a vapor pressure almost identical to that of halothane?

(1) Methoxyflurane
(2) Enflurane
(3) Isoflurane
(4) Desflurane
(5) Sevoflurane

3. If several dogs are breathing 50% nitrous oxide, they would probably all be responsive to a painful stimuli. If the minimum alveolar concentration (MAC) of nitrous oxide is approximately 200%, how much halothane would have to be administered to render 50% of these dogs unresponsive to a painful stimulus?

(1) 1.00 MAC halothane
(2) 0.75 MAC halothane
(3) 0.67 MAC halothane
(4) 0.50 MAC halothane
(5) 0.25 MAC halothane

4. Inhalant anesthetics vary in how quickly the alveolar concentration (blood concentration) will approximate the inspired concentration. Which one of the following anesthetics has the fastest rate of rise in alveolar concentration?

(1) Halothane
(2) Enflurane
(3) Methoxyflurane
(4) Isoflurane
(5) Nitrogen

5. Which inhalant anesthetic would enhance the nephrotoxic effect of other drugs (e.g., flunixin meglumine)?

(1) Methoxyflurane
(2) Halothane
(3) Enflurane
(4) Isoflurane
(5) Nitrous oxide

6. A dog with myocardial disease needs to be anesthetized. Which inhalant anesthetic maintains the highest cardiac output at deep levels of anesthesia?

(1) Halothane
(2) Methoxyflurane
(3) Enflurane
(4) Thiopental
(5) Isoflurane

7. Which injectable anesthetic is best suited for use in a small animal requiring an outpatient procedure?

(1) Propofol
(2) Pentobarbital
(3) Thiopental
(4) Telazol
(5) Guaifenesin

8. Which of the following drugs is a highly lipid-soluble oxybarbiturate with an ultrashort duration of action?

(1) Methohexital
(2) Pentobarbital
(3) Thiopental
(4) Thiamylal
(5) Phenobarbital

9. Which inhalant anesthetic has a high boiling point (above that of water) and is delivered to the patient at its maximum concentration during the initial phase of anesthesia?

(1) Halothane
(2) Nitrous oxide
(3) Enflurane
(4) Isoflurane
(5) Methoxyflurane

ANSWERS AND EXPLANATIONS

1. The answer is 1 [*II F 1*].
Skeletal muscle twitching is the first recognizable sign of local anesthetic toxicity. Twitching of the skeletal muscles may rapidly progress to tonic-clonic convulsions. Cardiovascular toxicity (as manifested by hypotension and arrhythmias) usually occurs at a higher dose than that necessary to produce neurologic toxicity. Gastrointestinal signs (e.g., vomiting) are not usually associated with local anesthetic toxicity.

2. The answer is 3 [*III D 4 a (2) (b); Table 5-5*].
Halothane and isoflurane have almost equivalent and fairly high vapor pressures (244 mm Hg and 240 mm Hg, respectively), which can produce a maximum concentration of 32%. Such a high concentration would be rapidly fatal; therefore, fairly sophisticated vaporizers have been developed to accurately control the vapor concentration delivered to the patient. The maximum concentration that can be achieved can be calculated by dividing the vapor pressure by the atmospheric pressure and multiplying by 100. Desflurane is very volatile at room temperature and develops a concentration of 87% because its vapor pressure is 664 mm Hg. Enflurane and sevoflurane are slightly less volatile than isoflurane and halothane, with vapor pressures of 172 mm Hg and 160 mm Hg, respectively. Methoxyflurane, which has a low vapor pressure (24 mm Hg), can only develop a 3% maximum concentration.

3. The answer is 2 [*III B 1 a (2); Table 5-2*].
The minimum alveolar concentration (MAC) of nitrous oxide is approximately 200%. Thus, animals breathing 50% nitrous oxide will be receiving 0.25 MAC (50% / 200% = 25%). Simultaneously inhaled anesthetics are additive; therefore, another 0.75 MAC would be required to reach a level that would be equivalent to 1.0 MAC. By definition, this is the MAC that would render 50% of the animals unresponsive to painful stimuli.

4. The answer is 4 [*III D 4 b (1); Figure 5-2*].
Isoflurane and nitrous oxide are the least soluble gases in current veterinary use; therefore,

the alveolar concentration quickly approaches the inspired concentration. In other words, the ratio of the concentration of anesthetic in the alveolus to that inhaled (F_A:F_I) approaches 1.0 quickly. Methoxyflurane is the most soluble inhalant anesthetic; therefore, it is the slowest to achieve its effective alveolar concentration. Nitrogen is the primary gas component of room air and is not an inhalant anesthetic.

5. The answer is 1 [*III D 3 f*].
Methoxyflurane is metabolized in the body to produce free fluoride ion and other compounds. The fluoride ion itself may be nephrotoxic if present in a high enough concentration, and it will add to the nephrotoxic effect of other drugs like tetracyclines, aminoglycosides, and flunixin meglumine. Dogs and cats seem to be resistant to methoxyflurane nephrotoxicity, except when other nephrotoxic drugs are used concurrently.

6. The answer is 5 [*III D 4 c (1) (a); Table 5-7*].
All inhalant anesthetics are myocardial depressants and reduce cardiac output. However, isoflurane causes the least depression of the inhalants listed. Thiopental is an injectable thiobarbiturate anesthetic that is also a myocardial depressant.

7. The answer is 1 [*IV C 3 b*].
Propofol is rapidly redistributed and metabolized in the body; therefore, the recovery times for the return of normal activity and behavior is very short. Even though thiopental is classified as an ultrashort-acting barbiturate, there is a longer time period necessary for return of normal activity and behavior. Pentobarbital and Telazol are longer-acting drugs. Guaifenesin is primarily a muscle relaxant used for the induction of anesthesia in horses and cattle.

8. The answer is 1 [*IV A 2 a (2)*].
Most oxybarbiturates, with the exception of methohexital, are less lipid soluble than thiobarbiturates. A methyl side chain increases methohexital's lipid solubility and results in

an ultrashort duration of action. Pentobarbital and phenobarbital are long-acting oxybarbiturates. Thiopental and thiamylal are ultrashort-acting thiobarbiturates.

9. The answer is 5 [*III D 3; Table 5-5*]. Methoxyflurane has a boiling point of 105°C, which exceeds that of water (100°C). It is administered at its maximum concentration (3%) during the initial phase of anesthesia. Halothane, nitrous oxide, enflurane, and isoflurane have lower boiling points and must be administered at much lower than maximum concentration or they would cause severe cardiopulmonary depression and death.

Chapter 6

Drugs Acting on the Cardiovascular System

Wendy A. Ware

I. DRUGS USED IN THE TREATMENT OF CONGESTIVE HEART FAILURE

A. Introduction

1. **Definitions.** Heart failure occurs when abnormal cardiac function results in inadequate blood delivery to the tissues or provides adequate delivery only with elevated cardiac filling pressures. Several types of pathophysiologic abnormalities can lead to heart failure.
   a. **Right ventricular congestive failure** results in:
      (1) Systemic venous hypertension
      (2) Congestion of the liver and other abdominal viscera
      (3) Pleural effusion
   b. **Left ventricular congestive failure** results in pulmonary venous congestion and edema. Chronic pulmonary congestion can lead to development of right ventricular failure if pulmonary arterial pressure rises as a result of severe pulmonary venous hypertension.
   c. **Low-output failure** of either ventricle can coexist with congestive failure and can cause weakness, syncope, and prerenal azotemia.

2. **Pathophysiology of heart failure**
   a. **Pathophysiologic mechanisms.** As an aid to choosing optimal therapy, the causes of heart failure can be categorized according to the underlying pathophysiologic mechanism (Table 6-1).
      (1) **Myocardial dysfunction (systolic** or **pump failure).** Poor myocardial function may be a secondary complication in heart failure as well as the primary cause.
      (2) **Volume–flow overload**
      (3) **Pressure overload**
      (4) **Restricted diastolic filling (diastolic failure)**
      (5) **Persistent arrhythmias**
   b. **Cardiac compensatory mechanisms**
      (1) **Frank-Starling mechanism.** Increases in heart filling cause stronger contraction to help normalize output. Examples include:
         (a) Valvular insufficiency
         (b) Arterial hypertension
         (c) Ventricular outflow obstruction
      (2) **Myocardial hypertrophy** helps normalize wall stress and oxygen consumption, which increases with volume and, especially, pressure overloads. Hypertrophy can interfere with diastolic function by making the ventricle less compliant.
         (a) **Systolic pressure loads** mainly cause **concentric hypertrophy** and myocardial fiber thickening.
         (b) **Volume loads** mainly cause **eccentric hypertrophy,** with myocardial fiber elongation and chamber enlargement.
   c. **Neurohormonal compensatory mechanisms**
      (1) Neurohormonal compensatory mechanisms include:
         (a) **Increased sympathetic nervous tone**
         (b) **Activation of the renin-angiotensin-aldosterone system**
         (c) Release of **antidiuretic hormone (ADH, vasopressin)**
      (2) Working independently or together, these systems cause **volume retention** and **vasoconstriction.**

TABLE 6-1. Therapeutic Approaches to Heart Failure

Type of Problem	Common Causes	Therapeutic Goals*	Means of Achieving Therapeutic Goals
Myocardial dysfunction	Idiopathic dilated cardiomyopathy; infective myocarditis; drug toxicities (e.g., from doxorubicin); myocardial ischemia or infarction	Improve ventricular contractility	Positive inotropic drugs
		Control edema and effusions	Diet, diuretics, vasodilators
		Improve cardiac output	Positive inotropic drugs, vasodilators
		Reduce cardiac workload	Rest, vasodilators, diuretics
Volume–flow overload	Valvular insufficiency (mitral, tricuspid, or aortic); ventricular septal defect; patent ductus arteriosus; chronic anemia; thyrotoxicosis	Control edema and effusions	Diet, diuretics, vasodilators
		Reduce valvular regurgitation, if present	Arterial vasodilators
		Improve forward cardiac output	Arterial vasodilators; positive inotropic drugs may help in severe failure
		Reduce cardiac workload	Rest, vasodilators, diuretics
Pressure overload	Ventricular outflow obstruction (subaortic or aortic stenosis, pulmonic stenosis); systemic hypertension; heartworm disease	Reduce cardiac workload	Rest, diuretics, β-blockers or antihypertensives (depending on the cause)
		Control edema and effusions	Diet, diuretics, possibly vasodilators (depending on the cause)
		Support cardiac function	Positive inotropic drugs may help in severe failure
Restricted ventricular filling	Hypertrophic cardiomyopathy; restrictive cardiomyopathy	Enhance myocardial relaxation and filling by slowing heart rate	β-blockers or calcium channel blockers
		Control edema and effusions	Diet, diuretics
		Reduce cardiac workload	Rest
	Cardiac tamponade; constrictive pericardial disease	Relieve impediment to ventricular expansion	Pericardiocentesis; partial pericardiectomy may be necessary

* Cardiac arrhythmias frequently occur with all manifestations of heart failure. It should be noted that, generally, pharmacologic treatment of congestive heart failure focuses on relieving symptoms, not treating the underlying cause. If the cause of heart failure is known and treatable, specific therapy should be undertaken.

   (a) They may be life-saving with acutely low cardiac output (e.g., in cases of hemorrhage), but **in heart failure, continued neurohormonal activation exacerbates congestive signs,** increases systolic demands on the heart, and increases morbidity and mortality rates.

   (b) In general, as heart failure worsens, the degree of neurohormonal activation increases.

   3. Therapeutic approaches (see Table 6-1). Treatment of heart failure usually includes dietary salt reduction and moderate exercise restriction in addition to drug therapy.

B. **Diuretics** are used to counteract the sodium and volume retention caused by the activation of neurohormonal compensatory mechanisms. Diuretics are discussed in more detail in Chapter 7.

1. **High-ceiling (loop) diuretics. Furosemide** is used almost exclusively to reduce edema associated with congestive heart failure. Adverse effects are usually related to excessive fluid losses, electrolyte losses, or both.

2. **Thiazide diuretics** (e.g., **chlorothiazide, hydrochlorothiazide**) are occasionally used in early congestive heart failure. Thiazides decrease renal blood flow and should not be used in the presence of azotemia.

3. **Potassium (K$^+$)-sparing diuretics** (e.g., **spironolactone, triamterene**)
   a. **Therapeutic uses.** K$^+$-sparing diuretics are rarely used alone in heart failure. In conjunction with furosemide, K$^+$-sparing diuretics reduce potassium wasting. They are useful in the presence of hypokalemia or when high doses of furosemide do not sufficiently control fluid accumulation.
   b. **Contraindications.** The K$^+$-sparing diuretics are generally contraindicated in patients receiving potassium supplementation or an angiotensin converting enzyme (ACE) inhibitor.

C. Vasodilators

1. **Introduction**
   a. Vasodilators can **improve cardiac output** and **reduce edema and effusions** resulting from heart failure. They affect arterioles, venous capacitance vessels, or both (balanced vasodilators).
      (1) **Arteriolar dilators** decrease systemic vascular resistance, arterial blood pressure, and afterload on the heart by relaxing arteriolar smooth muscle; thus, the heart can eject more blood. When mitral regurgitation is present, arteriolar dilators decrease the systolic pressure gradient across the mitral valve, reduce regurgitant flow, and enhance forward flow out of the aorta. Reduction of regurgitant flow decreases left atrial pressure and pulmonary congestion.
      (2) **Venodilators** relax systemic veins, increase venous capacitance, decrease cardiac filling pressures (i.e., the preload), and reduce pulmonary congestion.
   b. Treatment with an arteriolar or balanced vasodilator should be initiated cautiously to avoid hypotension and reflex tachycardia.

2. **ACE inhibitors**
   a. **Preparations.** The following ACE inhibitors have been used in animals. Enacard is the only ACE inhibitor licensed for veterinary use.
      (1) **Captopril** (Capoten)
      (2) **Enalapril maleate** (Enacard, Vasotec)
      (3) **Lisinopril** (Prinivil, Zestril)
      (4) **Benazepril** (Lotensin)
   b. **Mechanism of action** (Figure 6-1). ACE inhibitors interfere with the conversion of angiotensin I to angiotensin II. Angiotensin II has a variety of effects, which lead to volume retention and vasoconstriction.
   c. **Pharmacokinetics**
      (1) **Captopril** is a weak organic acid with an active sulfhydryl group (lacking in the other ACE inhibitors).
         (a) **Absorption.** Approximately 75% is rapidly absorbed following oral administration. Administration with food reduces absorption.
         (b) **Fate** (in dogs)
            (i) Captopril is approximately **40% protein bound.**
            (ii) The acute hemodynamic effects last for less than 4 hours, necessitating oral **administration 2–3 times daily.**
            (iii) Total body clearance (Cl$_T$) is approximately 10 ml/min/kg, with a volume of distribution (V$_d$) of 2.5 L/kg and an elimination half-life (t$_{1/2}$) of approximately 2.8 hours.
         (c) **Elimination.** Captopril is eliminated by the kidneys.
      (2) **Enalapril maleate**
         (a) **Absorption.** Administration with food does not decrease bioavailability.
         (b) **Fate**

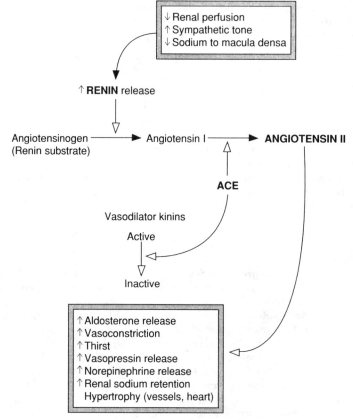

FIGURE 6-1. The renin-angiotensin cascade and effects of angiotensin II. Angiotensin converting enzyme *(ACE)* catalyzes the conversion of angiotensin I to angiotensin II and degrades vasodilator kinins (e.g., brad-ykinin). *Open arrows* = enzymatic reaction.

    (i) Enalapril has a slower onset (the peak plasma concentration is reached within 4–6 hours) but longer duration of action than capto-pril. It is **administered** orally **1–2 times daily.**
    (ii) Enalapril is transformed in the liver to the active metabolite **enala-prilat.**
   (c) Elimination. Both enalapril and enalaprilat are excreted unchanged in the urine.
  (3) Lisinopril is a lysine analog of enalaprilat. It is **administered once daily.**
  (4) Benazepril
   (a) Absorption. Approximately 40% is absorbed following oral administra-tion. Administration with food does not affect absorption.
   (b) Fate. Benazepril, which is administered **once daily,** is converted to **bena-zeprilat** in the liver.
   (c) Elimination is approximately 50% biliary and 50% renal.
 d. Pharmacologic effects
  (1) Arteriolar and venous dilation
   (a) Inhibition of locally produced ACE within vascular walls may cause a local vasodilating effect, even in the absence of high circulating renin levels.
   (b) The vasodilating effects of ACE inhibitors may be enhanced by vasodila-tor kinins normally degraded by ACE.
  (2) Reduced sodium and water retention. Inhibition of angiotensin II production decreases the secretion of aldosterone, a hormone that promotes renal so-dium retention.

e. Therapeutic uses. Because of their multiple effects in moderating excessive neurohumoral compensatory responses, ACE inhibitors have significant advantages over hydralazine and other arteriolar dilators in heart failure; however, in dogs and cats with hypertension, these drugs have variable effectiveness.

(1) The addition of ACE inhibitors to standard therapy (i.e., diuretics and digoxin) lowers morbidity and mortality rates in humans (and most likely, other species) with heart failure caused by myocardial dysfunction.

(2) ACE inhibitors are also useful for treating heart failure caused by valvular insufficiency and other volume overloads.

(3) Cats with right-sided congestive failure secondary to chronic hypertrophic or restrictive cardiomyopathy also may benefit from ACE inhibitor use.

f. Adverse effects

(1) **Hypotension** can occur.

(2) **Gastrointestinal upset** (especially with captopril) may persist even with dose reduction and may necessitate drug withdrawal.

(3) **Renal failure or worsening of renal function** has occurred. Decreasing diuretic or ACE inhibitor dosage may help restore renal function.

(4) In humans, rash, pruritus, impairment of taste, proteinuria, and neutropenia have also been noted.

(5) ACE inhibitors may cause **hyperkalemia** when used with K^+-sparing diuretics or potassium supplements. Animals with renal insufficiency may also experience hyperkalemia following administration of ACE inhibitors.

3. Hydralazine (Apresoline)

a. Mechanism of action. Hydralazine directly relaxes arteriolar smooth muscle but has little effect on the venous system. Intact vascular endothelium is necessary.

b. Pharmacokinetics

(1) **Absorption.** Administration with food decreases bioavailability by more than 60%.

(2) **Fate**

(a) Hydralazine is subject to extensive first-pass hepatic metabolism. In dogs, large doses saturate the first-pass metabolism mechanism, increasing bioavailability.

(b) Total body clearance is approximately 70 ml/min/kg, and the volume of distribution is 9 L/kg.

c. Pharmacologic effects. Hydralazine decreases mean arterial pressure and vascular resistance, increasing cardiac output. The cerebral, coronary, splanchnic, and renal circulations are most affected.

d. Therapeutic uses

(1) **Mitral valve insufficiency**

(a) Hydralazine in combination with furosemide is especially useful for dogs with mitral valve insufficiency and severe pulmonary edema.

(b) It rapidly reduces arterial resistance (afterload), which reduces regurgitant volume and pulmonary venous pressure and increases cardiac output.

(2) **Myocardial failure**

(3) **Hypertension**

e. Adverse effects

(1) **Hypotension** is the most common adverse effect.

(2) **Reflex tachycardia** may occur in some animals, in which case the dosage should be reduced. Addition of digoxin or a β-blocker to the therapeutic regimen may be necessary.

(3) Hydralazine may enhance the neurohumoral response to heart failure and increase **sodium and water retention.**

(4) **Gastrointestinal upset** may occur, especially in cats.

4. Nitrates

a. Preparations

(1) **Sodium nitroprusside** (Nipride)

(2) **Nitroglycerine ointment**

(3) **Isosorbide dinitrate** (Isordil)

b. Mechanisms of action

  (1) Sodium nitroprusside, which is administered intravenously, directly dilates both arteriolar and venous smooth muscle.

  (2) Nitroglycerine and isosorbide dinitrate, which are administered orally or transcutaneously, dilate venous smooth muscle, possibly by stimulating production of cyclic guanosine 3′,5′-monophosphate (cGMP).

c. Pharmacokinetics. Nitroglycerine undergoes extensive first-pass hepatic metabolism after oral administration.

d. Pharmacologic effects

  (1) Sodium nitroprusside is a potent arterial and venous dilator.

  (2) Other nitrates primarily increase venous capacitance and reduce cardiac filling pressures.

e. Therapeutic uses

  (1) Sodium nitroprusside is sometimes used for **fulminant congestive heart failure** in dogs. Hemodynamic monitoring is necessary because severe hypotension may result.

  (2) Nitroglycerine and isosorbide dinitrate help relieve **acute cardiogenic pulmonary edema.** One or the other is sometimes used as **long-term therapy for** animals that have **persistent pulmonary edema** despite diuretic therapy. Hydralazine may be added to the therapeutic regimen for a more balanced vasodilating effect; however, ACE inhibitor therapy may be more advantageous than nitrate–hydralazine therapy.

f. Administration

  (1) Sodium nitroprusside must be administered by intravenous infusion because of its short duration of action.

    (a) The dosage should be titrated to maintain mean arterial pressure above 70 mm Hg.

    (b) Tolerance develops rapidly, further necessitating careful monitoring and dosage adjustments.

  (2) Nitroglycerine

    (a) Transcutaneous. The transcutaneous route is the most commonly used route in animals.

      (i) Nitroglycerine ointment is applied to the animal's skin (usually the groin, axillary area, or ear pinna) every 4–6 hours. Application papers or gloves should be used.

      (ii) Dosage and absorption are variable. Tolerance has developed in humans following long-term administration of high doses and frequent application of long-acting formulations.

      (iii) The self-adhesive, sustained-release preparations may be useful but have not been sufficiently evaluated in small animals.

    (b) Sublingual nitroglycerine is also well-absorbed.

g. Adverse effects

  (1) Hypotension is the major side effect of sodium nitroprusside and can be profound. Hypotension may result from excessive or inappropriate use of other nitrates as well.

  (2) Cyanide toxicity can result from excessive or prolonged used of sodium nitroprusside.

5. Prazosin (Minipress)

  a. Mechanism of action. Prazosin selectively blocks α_1 receptors. These postsynaptic receptors mediate arterial and venous vasoconstriction.

  b. Therapeutic uses. Initial therapy may result in hemodynamic improvement, but drug tolerance develops over time. The drug is not commonly used because of tolerance and inconvenient capsule sizes for small animals. No controlled clinical animal studies are available.

D. **Positive inotropic drugs**

1. Digitalis glycosides. This discussion focuses on **digoxin** because **digitoxin** is rarely, if ever, used clinically at this time.

a. **Mechanisms of action**
  (1) **Positive inotropic effect.** Digitalis glycosides increase the availability of calcium to contractile proteins by competitively binding to and inhibiting the Na^+-K^+-ATPase pump at the myocardial cell membrane. The intracellular accumulation of sodium promotes calcium entry via the Na^+-Ca^{2+} exchanger.
  (2) **Antiarrhythmic effects**
      (a) The antiarrhythmic effects of digoxin are mediated mostly by increased parasympathetic tone to the sinoatrial (S-A) and atrioventricular (A-V) nodes and the atria.
      (b) Digoxin also has some direct effects that prolong the conduction time and the refractory period of the A-V node.
  (3) Digoxin improves arterial baroreceptor sensitivity in heart failure, helping to counteract excessive neurohormonal activation.
b. **Pharmacokinetics**
  (1) **Digoxin**
      (a) **Absorption** is approximately 60% for the tablet form and 75% for the elixir. In horses, the oral bioavailability is approximately 20%. Absorption is decreased by the presence of food, kaolin-pectin compounds, antacids, or malabsorption syndromes.
      (b) **Fate**
          (i) Approximately 27% of the drug in serum is protein bound.
          (ii) There is minimal hepatic metabolism.
          (iii) Differences among species in the metabolism and excretion of digoxin are summarized in Table 6-2.
  (2) **Digitoxin**
      (a) **Absorption.** Digitoxin is well absorbed orally. It is nonpolar and highly fat-soluble.
      (b) **Fate**
          (i) Digitoxin is approximately **90% protein bound** in serum.
          (ii) The half-life is only 8–12 hours in dogs, but **in cats, digitoxin** has an extremely long half-life (over 100 hours), and **should not be used.**

TABLE 6-2. Pharmacokinetics of Digoxin: Differences Among Species

Species	Half-life	Therapeutic Serum Concentrations	Steady State	Elimination
Dogs	23–39 hours	1.0–2.4 ng/ml; achieved within 2–4.5 days (with oral administration every 12 hours)	Achieved in approximately 7 days	Primarily by glomerular filtration and renal secretion; approximately 15% is metabolized by the liver
Cats	25–78+ hours (increases with prolonged oral administration)	1.0–2.0 ng/ml; achieved with low doses every 48 hours*	Achieved in approximately 10 days	Renal and hepatic elimination equally important
Horses	13–23 hours	0.5–2.0 ng/ml; achieved within 1–2 hours†	Achieved in approximately 3–5 days	Primarily renal elimination

* Serum concentrations are approximately 50% higher with the alcohol-based elixer than with tablets; however, the elixer is less palatable. Administration of tablets with food results in serum concentrations 50% lower than when administered on an empty stomach.
† Significant enterohepatic recycling may produce a second peak serum concentration in horses.

(iii) Serum digitoxin concentration is measured 6–8 hours after the previous dose. The **therapeutic serum concentration** is 15–35 ng/ml.

(c) Elimination. Digitoxin is cleared by the liver, although it appears to be tolerated in the presence of liver disease as well as renal failure.

c. Pharmacologic effects

(1) The digitalis glycosides increase the contractility of cardiac muscle, but are relatively weak positive inotropic agents.

(2) The digitalis glycosides reduce the sinus rate, prolong atrioventricular conduction time, and suppress atrial premature depolarizations and supraventricular tachycardia.

d. Therapeutic uses

(1) Digoxin is generally used in the treatment of heart failure associated with myocardial dysfunction. In these patients, digoxin increases cardiac output, decreases cardiac filling pressures, decreases heart size, and decreases venous and capillary pressures.

(2) Digoxin is also used for its antiarrhythmic effect against supraventricular arrhythmias. It is only moderately effective in slowing the ventricular response in atrial fibrillation, and it does not cause conversion to sinus rhythm.

e. Administration. Fatal myocardial toxicity [see I D 1 f (1)] may occur, especially in patients with myocardial failure; therefore, dosage guidelines should be based on the attainment of therapeutic serum concentrations and clinical improvement, and not on the appearance of PR interval prolongation or signs of gastrointestinal toxicity.

(1) Initial dosage

(a) Generally, oral maintenance doses of digoxin should be used to initiate therapy, because loading doses often cause toxic serum concentrations.

(b) Slow intravenous administration (over at least 15 minutes) can be used in an emergency (e.g., supraventricular tachycardia).

(i) Rapid injection causes peripheral vasoconstriction.

(ii) Ideally, the calculated dose is divided and given slowly over several hours.

(iii) Other intravenous positive inotropic drugs are safer and more effective than digoxin for immediate support of myocardial contractility.

(2) Maintenance dosage

(a) After 1 week of initial therapy or dosage alteration, the serum concentration can be measured. Blood is taken 8–10 hours after dosing.

(i) The therapeutic serum concentration range is considered to be 1.0–2.4 ng/ml.

(ii) If the serum level is less than 0.8 ng/ml, the digoxin dose can be increased by no more than 30%. The serum concentration should be rechecked the following week.

(b) If the serum concentration cannot be measured and toxicity is suspected, the drug should be discontinued for 1–2 days, then reinstituted at half of the original dose.

(3) Factors affecting dosage

(a) Renal disease. Serum digoxin concentrations are increased in cats and dogs with renal failure because of reduced total body clearance and volume of distribution, thereby increasing the risk of toxicity.

(i) There appears to be no correlation between the degree of azotemia and the serum digoxin concentration in dogs, rendering extrapolations from human formulas invalid. (Similar data for cats is unavailable.)

(ii) Reduced dosage and close monitoring of serum digoxin concentration are recommended in animals with renal disease.

(b) Heart disease. There is only a weak correlation between digoxin dosage and serum concentration in dogs with heart failure, indicating that other factors are important in determining the serum concentrations of this drug.

(c) Weight

(i) **Cachexia.** Because much of the drug is bound to skeletal muscle, animals with reduced muscle mass or cachexia, as well as those with compromised renal function, can easily achieve toxic levels of the drug at the usual calculated dosages.

(ii) **Obesity.** Because digoxin has poor lipid solubility, the dosage should be based on the calculated lean body weight, especially in obese animals.

(d) **Liver disease. A prolonged Bromsulphalein retention** of over 5% at 30 minutes has been associated with digoxin toxicity in cats.

f. Adverse effects

(1) **Myocardial toxicity** can cause almost any cardiac rhythm disturbance, including ventricular tachyarrhythmias, supraventricular premature complexes and tachycardia, sinus arrest, Mobitz type I second degree A-V block, and junctional rhythms.

(a) **Causes**

(i) **Calcium overload.** Diastolic sequestration and systolic release of calcium may be impaired in diseased myocardial cells. The use of digoxin can lead to cellular calcium overload and electrical instability.

(ii) **Toxic levels of digoxin** increase sympathetic tone to the heart, causing increased automaticity. In addition, the parasympathetic effects of a prolonged conduction time and altered refractory period facilitate the occurrence of re-entrant arrhythmias.

(iii) Digoxin also can stimulate spontaneous automaticity of myocardial cells by inducing and potentiating **late after-depolarizations.** This effect is enhanced by cellular stretch, calcium overload, and hypokalemia.

(b) **Predisposing factors**

(i) **Hypokalemia** can cause myocardial toxicity by leaving more available binding sites on membrane Na^+-K^+-ATPase pumps for the digitalis glycosides.

(ii) **Hypercalcemia** and **hypernatremia** potentiate both the inotropic and toxic effects of the drug.

(iii) **Abnormal thyroid hormone levels** can lead to digitalis glycoside toxicity. Hyperthyroidism increases the drug's myocardial effects, and hypothyroidism reduces its total body clearance.

(iv) **Hypoxia** sensitizes the myocardium to the toxic effects of the digitalis glycosides.

(v) **Certain drugs** increase the serum concentration of the various digitalis glycosides (see I D 1 h).

(c) **Therapy**

(i) Atrioventricular conduction abnormalities usually resolve with **drug withdrawal,** although sometimes an anticholinergic agent is needed.

(ii) Ventricular tachycardia induced in dogs by the digitalis glycosides is treated with **lidocaine** or **phenytoin** (diphenylhydantoin).

(iii) **Cholestyramine**

Digoxin. Oral administration of cholestyramine, a steroid-binding resin, is only useful very soon after accidental overdosage of digoxin, because digoxin undergoes minimal enterohepatic circulation.

Digitoxin. Much greater enterohepatic circulation occurs with digitoxin, which allows for increased binding to cholestyramine within the intestines.

(iv) Other therapies include **intravenous potassium supplementation** (if serum potassium is less than 4.0 mEq/L), **intravenous fluids** to correct dehydration and maximize renal function, and **propranolol** to help control ventricular tachyarrhythmias (as long as no conduction blocks are present).

(v) **Digoxin immune Fab** (Digibind) is a preparation of digoxin-specific antigen-binding fragments derived from ovine antidigoxin antibodies.

It has been used to treat digoxin and digitoxin overdose in humans.

   (2) Gastrointestinal upset

     (a) Gastrointestinal signs (e.g., anorexia, vomiting, borborygmus, diarrhea) may appear before signs of myocardial toxicity, especially in patients without myocardial failure.

     (b) Some gastrointestinal signs may be caused by direct effects of the digitalis glycosides on chemoreceptors in the area postrema of the medulla.

     (c) Gastrointestinal signs usually respond to drug withdrawal and correction of fluid or electrolyte disturbances.

g. Relative contraindications

  (1) Hypertrophic cardiomyopathy. Digoxin may worsen existing ventricular outflow obstruction, although it has been used when clinical signs of right ventricular failure develop.

  (2) Pericardial disease. Digoxin is generally not useful in the treatment of pericardial disease.

  (3) Sinus or A-V nodal disease

  (4) Ventricular tachyarrhythmias. Digoxin may exacerbate ventricular arrhythmias.

h. Drug interactions

  (1) Digoxin

    (a) Digoxin concentration is increased by:

      (i) Quinidine, which displaces the drug from skeletal muscle binding sites and reduces its renal clearance

      (ii) Verapamil and amiodarone

      (iii) Possibly diltiazem, prazosin, spironolactone, and triamterene

    (b) Digoxin metabolism may be altered by drugs that affect hepatic microsomal enzymes.

    (c) Digoxin bioavailability is decreased by neomycin and sulfasalazine.

    (d) Digoxin toxicity may be potentiated by thyroid and electrolyte disturbances (especially hypokalemia).

  (2) Digitoxin clearance is increased by phenylbutazone, primidone, and phenobarbital. It is decreased by chloramphenicol, quinidine, and tetracycline.

2. Sympathomimetic agents (catecholamines) [see also Chapter 2]

a. Preparations

  (1) Dopamine (Intropin)

  (2) Dobutamine (Dobutrex), a synthetic analog of dopamine

b. Mechanism of action. Sympathomimetic agents stimulate cardiac β_1-adrenergic receptors, activating adenyl cyclase, which converts adenosine triphosphate (ATP) into cyclic adenosine monophosphate (cAMP). cAMP stimulates a protein kinase system, which, via phosphorylation of certain membrane proteins, leads to increased calcium influx and greater contractility.

c. Pharmacokinetics

  (1) Dopamine and dobutamine have very short half-lives (less than 2 minutes).

  (2) They undergo extensive hepatic metabolism.

  (3) Clinically, they are suitable only for intravenous administration, usually by constant infusion.

d. Pharmacologic effects. Catecholamines increase heart rate and contractility, especially at high doses.

  (1) Dopamine

    (a) At low doses (less than 2–5 μg/kg/min), dopamine stimulates **vasodilator** dopaminergic receptors in the renal, mesenteric, coronary, and cerebral circulations.

    (b) At higher doses, it stimulates β and α receptors. Peripheral vasoconstriction occurs at 10–15 μg/kg/min.

  (2) Dobutamine increases contractility, with minimal effects on heart rate and blood pressure at lower infusion rates (3–7 μg/kg/min).

        (a) Dobutamine stimulates β_1 receptors but has only weak action on β_2 and α receptors.

        (b) It does not stimulate dopaminergic receptors.

    e. Therapeutic uses

        (1) Myocardial failure (dilated cardiomyopathy). Dopamine and dobutamine are used in conjunction with other therapy for short-term inotropic support in dogs and cats. Use of catecholamines for heart failure is limited by the development of β receptor down-regulation (i.e., decreased number of receptors, affinity for receptors, or both). Generally these drugs are given for no more than 3 days.

        (2) Hypotension that is not responsive to fluid loading

        (3) Acute oliguric renal failure. Dopamine is also used to increase renal blood flow.

    f. Adverse effects

        (1) At high doses, dopamine and dobutamine may cause:

            (a) Increased heart rate

            (b) Increased myocardial oxygen demand

            (c) Arrhythmias (ventricular tachyarrhythmias, sinus tachycardia)

                (i) Development of tachyarrhythmias should prompt a decrease in infusion rate.

                (ii) Dobutamine is less arrhythmogenic than other catecholamines, but it may precipitate supraventricular and ventricular arrhythmias at higher infusion rates (10–20 μg/kg/min).

        (2) Cats are more sensitive to dobutamine than dogs and may exhibit seizures or other adverse effects at relatively low dosages.

    g. Drug interactions. By increasing renal blood flow, dopamine may enhance the renal clearance of other drugs.

  3. Amrinone

    a. Preparations

        (1) Inocor

        (2) Milrinone, a more potent relative of amrinone, has undergone testing in humans and dogs but has not been marketed.

    b. Mechanism of action. Amrinone and milrinone inhibit phosphodiesterase III, an intracellular enzyme that degrades cAMP. Increased cAMP levels within cardiac myocytes increase calcium influx and, thus, increase myocardial contractility.

    c. Pharmacokinetics

        (1) The effects of amrinone are short-lived (less than 30 minutes) in normal dogs after intravenous injection; thus, constant infusions are required for sustained effect.

        (2) Peak effects in dogs are seen after 45 minutes of constant-rate infusion.

    d. Pharmacologic effects

        (1) Contractility improvements of 40%–200% have been reported in dogs with experimentally induced myocardial failure.

        (2) Vasodilation also occurs because increased cAMP reduces calcium uptake in vascular smooth muscle and promotes relaxation.

            (a) Much of the clinical benefit of amrinone may be the result of this vasodilating effect.

            (b) Higher dosages result in greater vasodilation with reduced blood pressure and increased heart rate.

    e. Therapeutic use. Amrinone is used for **acute inotropic support** in dogs and cats with **severe myocardial failure.**

    f. Adverse effects. Amrinone has a relatively wide margin of safety. It may, however, **exacerbate ventricular** arrhythmias.

E. | β**-blockers and calcium channel blockers.** Heart disease causing diastolic dysfunction (e.g., hypertrophic cardiomyopathy) responds to drugs that slow the heart rate (thereby increasing filling time and reducing ischemia), facilitate cardiac relaxation, or both.

1. β-Blockers (II B 2; see also Chapter 2). Propranolol and atenolol are commonly used to slow the heart rate and reduce myocardial oxygen consumption. Many other β-blockers are also available.

2. Calcium channel blockers, as a group, cause coronary and systemic vasodilation, enhanced myocardial relaxation, and, sometimes, reduced cardiac contractility. Diltiazem is used in cats with hypertrophic cardiomyopathy (see II B 4).

II. ANTIARRHYTHMIC DRUGS

A. Introduction

1. The **sinus node** normally controls the heart rate and rhythm.

2. **Causes of abnormal heart rhythms** include:
   a. Disturbances in sinus node function
   b. Altered automaticity of other cardiac fibers
   c. Abnormal conduction anywhere in the heart
   d. Combinations of these factors

B. Drugs used for tachyarrhythmias (Table 6-3)

1. **Class I agents** are local anesthetics.
   a. **Preparations**

TABLE 6-3. Classification of Antiarrhythmic Drugs

Class	Agents	Mechanism of Action	ECG Effects
I		Decrease fast inward Na^+ current; stabilize membrane by decreasing conductivity, excitability, and automaticity	
A	Quinidine Procainamide Disopyramide	Moderately decrease conductivity, increase action potential duration	Prolonged QRS and QT intervals
B	Lidocaine Phenytoin Tocainide Mexiletine	Decrease action potential duration with little change in conductivity	Unchanged QRS and QT intervals
C	Flecainide Encainide Propafenone	Markedly decrease conductivity without changing action potential duration	
II	Propranolol Atenolol Esmolol Metoprolol Nadolol Pindolol	β-Adrenergic blockade (reduce sympathetic stimulation with no direct effects on myocardium at clinical dosages)	
III	Bretylium Amiodarone Sotalol	Selectively prolong action potential duration and refractory period; antiadrenergic effects	Prolonged QT intervals
IV	Verapamil Diltiazem	Decrease slow inward Ca^{2+} current (greatest effects on S-A and A-V nodes)	

A-V = atrioventricular; Ca^{2+} = calcium; ECG = electrocardiogram; Na^+ = sodium; S-A = sinoatrial.

      (1) **Class IA** drugs include quinidine, procainamide, and disopyramide.

      (2) **Class IB** drugs include lidocaine, phenytoin (Dilantin), tocainide, and mexiletine.

      (3) **Class IC** drugs include flecainide, encainide, and propafenone.

  b. Mechanisms of action

      (1) Class I agents have **local anesthetic effects,** which alter the automaticity, excitability, conduction, and refractoriness of the cardiac membranes.

      (2) Some Class I agents (e.g., quinidine, procainamide) also have **indirect autonomic effects.**

      (3) Most Class I agents are dependent on extracellular potassium concentration for their effects.

  c. Pharmacokinetics

      (1) Class IA drugs

        (a) Procainamide

          (i) Absorption. Procainamide is well absorbed orally.

          (ii) Fate (Table 6-4). Procainamide is thought to be 20% protein bound in the dog. The metabolite N-acetylprocainamide is found in horses but is not present to any significant degree in dogs and cats.

          (iii) Elimination is by hepatic metabolism as well as renal excretion in proportion to the creatinine clearance.

        (b) Quinidine

          (i) Absorption. Quinidine is well absorbed orally with little first-pass hepatic elimination.

          (ii) Fate (see Table 6-4). The extensive hepatic metabolism of quinidine is not greatly dependent on liver blood flow. Quinidine is highly protein bound in dogs and cats.

TABLE 6-4. Pharmacokinetics of Classes IA and IB Antiarrhythmic Agents

Class	Agent	Half-life	Therapeutic Plasma Range	Total Body Clearance	Volume of Distribution
IA	Procainamide				
	Dogs	2.5–4 hours 3–6 hours (sustained release)	4–10 μg/ml	Not specifically known	1.4–2.1 L/kg
	Horses	3–7 hours	Not specifically known	3.9 ml/min/kg	2.4 L/kg
	Quinidine				
	Dogs	6 hours	2.5–5.0 μg/ml	6 ml/min/kg	2.9 L/kg
	Cats	2 hours	Not specifically known	14.8 ml/min/kg	2.2 L/kg
	Horses	4–7 hours	2–4 μg/ml	6–16 ml/min/kg	2.9–6.3 L/kg
IB	Lidocaine				
	Dogs	1–1.5 hours	2–6 μg/ml	62 ml/min/kg	5.7 L/kg
	Horses	3.1 hours	Not specifically known	64/4 ml/min/kg	1.7 L/kg
	Tocainide				
	Dogs	8–12 hours	Not specifically known	4.2 ml/min/kg	1.7 L/kg
	Phenytoin				
	Dogs	3 hours	10–16 μg/ml	4 ml/min/kg	1.2 L/kg
	Cats	>24 hours*	Not specifically known		

* Phenytoin should not be used in cats because of its extended half-life in this species.

(iii) **Elimination.** Quinidine is metabolized in the liver and excreted in the urine.

(2) Class IB drugs

(a) Lidocaine

(i) **Fate** (see Table 6-4). Lidocaine undergoes rapid hepatic metabolism. Some metabolites may contribute to lidocaine's antiarrhythmic effects, as well as its toxic ones.

(ii) **Elimination.** Lidocaine has almost complete first-pass hepatic elimination; therefore, it is administered intravenously, usually as slow boluses followed by constant-rate infusion. Constant-rate infusion without a loading dose results in steady state levels in 4–6 hours.

(b) Tocainide

(i) **Absorption.** Tocainide is well absorbed orally and does not undergo extensive first-pass metabolism.

(ii) **Fate** (see Table 6-4)

(iii) **Elimination.** Tocainide is eliminated by both the kidneys and the liver. Its clearance is not significantly influenced by changes in liver blood flow.

(c) Phenytoin

(i) **Absorption.** Phenytoin is usually given slowly intravenously because oral bioavailability is poor.

(ii) **Fate** (see Table 6-4). The drug is metabolized in the liver.

(iii) **Elimination.** By stimulating hepatic microsomal enzymes, phenytoin may speed its own elimination.

(d) Mexiletine

(i) **Absorption.** Mexiletine appears to have good oral absorption.

(ii) **Fate.** Mexiletine undergoes liver metabolism, which is influenced by liver blood flow. The half-life in dogs is 4.5–7 hours, depending on the urine pH.

(iii) **Elimination.** Approximately 10% of the drug is excreted unchanged in the urine. Alkaline urine prolongs elimination.

d. Pharmacologic effects

(1) Class IA drugs

(a) Procainamide and **quinidine** depress automaticity and conduction velocity and prolong the effective refractory period. These effects result from both the electrophysiologic (direct) and vagolytic (indirect) actions of the drugs. At low doses, quinidine's vagolytic effects may cause increases in the sinus rate or the ventricular response rate to atrial fibrillation by antagonizing the drug's direct effects.

(b) Disopyramide is similar to quinidine and procainamide electrophysiologically but has significant depressive effects on the canine myocardium. It also has a half-life of less than 2 hours in dogs; thus, it is not used clinically.

(2) Class IB drugs

(a) Lidocaine

(i) Lidocaine suppresses automaticity in both normal Purkinje fibers and diseased myocardial tissue, slows conduction, and reduces the supernormal period. Its effects are enhanced in diseased or hypoxic cardiac cells.

(ii) Lidocaine produces minimal hemodynamic effects and little to no depression of contractility at therapeutic doses when given slowly intravenously; however, hypotension has been associated with toxic levels.

(iii) Lidocaine has little effect on sinus rate, A-V conduction rate, and refractoriness.

(b) Tocainide is similar to lidocaine in its electrophysiologic and hemodynamic properties.

(c) Phenytoin is similar to lidocaine; however, it also has some slow calcium channel inhibitory and central nervous system (CNS) effects that may con-

tribute to its effectiveness against arrhythmias induced by the digitalis glycosides.

(d) **Mexiletine** is similar to lidocaine in its electrophysiologic, hemodynamic,
and antiarrhythmic properties.

(3) **Class IC drugs. Flecainide** and **encainide** markedly reduce cardiac conduction velocity and may depress automaticity in the sinus node and specialized
conducting tissues at high dosages.

e. **Therapeutic use.** Class I antiarrhythmic agents are used primarily for frequent ventricular premature contractions and ventricular tachycardia.

(1) **Class IA drugs. Procainamide** and **quinidine** may also be effective for atrial
premature depolarizations and tachycardias.

(a) Quinidine may cause conversion to sinus rhythm in horses, cattle, and
large dogs with recent onset of atrial fibrillation and clinically normal ventricular function.

(b) Procainamide is less effective than quinidine for atrial arrhythmias, and it
is not effective in converting chronic atrial fibrillation to sinus rhythm.

(2) **Class IB drugs**

(a) **Lidocaine** is usually the intravenous ventricular antiarrhythmic agent of
choice in the dog, but it is generally ineffective for supraventricular arrhythmias.

(b) **Phenytoin** is used only in dogs for the therapy of digitalis glycoside-in-
duced ventricular arrhythmias that are not responsive to lidocaine. **Phenytoin is not used in cats or horses.**

(3) **Class IC drugs. Flecainide** and **encainide** have been associated with an increased mortality rate in humans; thus, they are used only with caution and
for life-threatening ventricular arrhythmias refractory to more conventional
therapy.

f. **Administration**

(1) **Class IA drugs**

(a) **Procainamide**

(i) **Oral** and **intramuscular administration** of procainamide are not associated with marked hemodynamic effects.

(ii) **Constant intravenous infusion** may be used, but rapid intravenous injection can cause significant hypotension and cardiac depression.
With constant infusion, steady state is achieved in 12–22 hours.

(b) **Quinidine**

(i) **Oral** and **intramuscular administration.** Slow-release sulfate, gluconate, and polygalacturonate salts prolong quinidine's absorption and
elimination.

Slow-release preparations should be administered every 8 hours in
dogs; standard quinidine sulfate should be administered every 6
hours. Therapeutic blood levels are usually achieved within 12–24
hours.

The sulfate salt is more rapidly absorbed than the gluconate salt.
Adverse hemodynamic effects are not common but may occur in
patients with underlying cardiac disease.

(ii) **Intravenous administration** can cause vasodilation (via nonspecific
α-adrenergic receptor blockade), cardiac depression, and hypotension.

(iii) **Nasogastric intubation** is the preferred method of administration in
the horse. Quinidine is usually administered every 2 hours for up to
six doses to convert atrial fibrillation.

(2) **Class IB drugs**

(a) **Lidocaine** is administered by slow intravenous boluses, followed (if effective) by constant rate infusion.

(b) **Phenytoin**

(i) Rapid intravenous injection of phenytoin is avoided because the propylene glycol vehicle can depress myocardial contractility and cause vasodilation, hypotension, exacerbation of arrhythmias, and respiratory arrest.

(ii) **Slow intravenous infusion** and **oral administration of phenytoin** do not cause significant hemodynamic disturbances.

(3) **Class IC drugs** are administered orally. Intravenous administration of **flecainide** and **encainide** can cause significant hypotension and myocardial depression.

g. **Adverse effects.** All antiarrhythmic drugs, but especially the class IC agents, may exacerbate arrhythmias (i.e., they have a proarrhythmic effect).

(1) **Class IA drugs**

(a) **Procainamide**

(i) The most serious toxic effects of procainamide include hypotension, depressed A-V conduction, and worsening of arrhythmias, which may result in syncope or ventricular fibrillation.

(ii) Some of procainamide's toxic effects are similar to those of quinidine [see II B 1 g (1) (b)], but they are usually more mild.

(iii) The ventricular response rate to atrial fibrillation may increase when procainamide is used without digoxin, a β-blocker, or a calcium channel blocker.

(b) **Quinidine.** Toxicity occurs as an extension of the drug's electrophysiologic and hemodynamic actions. Because of quinidine's extensive protein binding, severe hypoalbuminemia can predispose to toxicity.

(i) Prolongation of electrocardiographic (ECG) intervals occurs as plasma concentration increases. Toxicity is indicated by marked QT interval prolongation, development of bundle branch block, QRS widening greater than 25%, and all degrees of A-V block and ventricular tachyarrhythmias.

(ii) Lethargy, weakness, and congestive heart failure can result from quinidine's negative inotropic and vasodilating effects. Cardiotoxicity and hypotension may be partially reversed by sodium bicarbonate therapy, which temporarily decreases serum potassium and enhances the binding of quinidine to albumin.

(iii) Gastrointestinal signs (nausea, vomiting, and diarrhea) commonly occur with oral quinidine therapy.

(iv) In horses, apprehension, depression, diarrhea, and anorexia are common.

(v) In humans (and possibly in dogs and cats), reversible thrombocytopenia has occurred.

(2) **Class IB drugs**

(a) **Lidocaine.** CNS excitation is the most common toxic effect. Signs include agitation, disorientation, muscle twitches, nystagmus, generalized seizures, and, less frequently, nausea.

(i) Cats are particularly sensitive to lidocaine toxicity and may suffer respiratory arrest along with seizures.

(ii) Horses are also very sensitive to lidocaine. QRS widening can occur.

(b) **Tocainide** is similar to lidocaine in its toxic effects.

(i) Gastrointestinal side effects (anorexia and vomiting) may be common.

(ii) Occasionally, neurotoxic signs (ataxia, disorientation, and twitching) are observed.

(c) **Phenytoin**

(i) Intravenous administration has been associated with bradycardia, A-V blocks, ventricular tachycardia, and cardiac arrest.

(ii) Signs of neurotoxicity include depression, nystagmus, disorientation, and ataxia.

(d) **Mexiletine.** Toxic effects are similar to those of lidocaine. Vomiting and disorientation have been reported in dogs.

(3) **Class IC drugs. Flecainide** and especially **encainide** can worsen ventricular arrhythmias. Bradycardia, intraventricular conduction disturbance, and consis-

tent (although transient) hypotension have occurred in dogs. Nausea, vomiting, and anorexia have also been reported.
  h. **Contraindications**
    (1) All Class I agents are contraindicated in the presence of complete heart block.
    (2) Class I agents should be used cautiously in patients with sinus bradycardia, sick sinus syndrome, and first- or second-degree A-V nodal block.
  i. **Drug interactions**
    (1) Positive interactions. Concurrent use of a class I drug and a drug of another class (or even subclass) may increase antiarrhythmic efficacy in cases refractory to a single agent.
    (2) Negative interactions
      (a) Class IA drugs
        (i) Cimetidine blocks renal tubular secretion of **procainamide** and predisposes the patient to quinidine toxicity by slowing elimination of **quinidine.**
        (ii) Quinidine can precipitate **digoxin** toxicity when both drugs are used together, because it displaces digoxin from skeletal muscle binding sites and decreases digoxin's renal clearance.
        (iii) Anticonvulsants and **other drugs** that induce hepatic microsomal enzymes can speed the metabolism of **quinidine** so that an increased dosage may be needed.
      (b) Class IB drugs
        (i) Propranolol, cimetidine, and **other drugs that decrease liver blood flow** slow the metabolism of **lidocaine.** Reduced hepatic blood flow associated with heart failure can also predispose the patient to toxicity.
        (ii) Cimetidine, chloramphenicol, and **other drugs that inhibit microsomal enzymes** can result in toxic serum concentrations of **phenytoin.**

2. **Class II agents** are β-blockers (see also Chapter 2).
  a. **Preparations** (see Table 6-3). **Propranolol** (Inderal) has been used most widely in veterinary medicine. Atenolol and other β-blockers are also used now.
  b. **Mechanism of action.** β-Adrenergic antagonists act by inhibiting catecholamine effects on the heart.
  c. **Pharmacokinetics**
    (1) Absorption. Food delays the rate of oral absorption of propranolol and increases the clearance of an intravenous dose (by increasing hepatic blood flow).
    (2) Fate. Propranolol undergoes extensive first-pass hepatic metabolism; however, long-term administration and higher doses cause hepatic enzyme saturation and increased bioavailability.
      (a) In dogs, the half-life of propranolol is less than 1.5 hours, but active metabolites exist. A volume of distribution of 3.3–6.5 L/kg and a total body clearance of 34–70 ml/min/kg have been reported.
      (b) In cats, the half-life ranges from 0.5 to more than 4.2 hours.
      (c) In horses, the half-life is 1.2–1.7 hours, the volume of distribution is 2.3 L/kg, and the total body clearance is 12–21 ml/min/kg. Bioavailability is low.
    (3) Elimination. Propranolol lowers hepatic blood flow, thereby prolonging its own elimination and that of other drugs dependent on liver blood flow for their metabolism.
  d. **Pharmacologic effects.** Class II agents slow the heart rate and A-V conduction velocity and reduce contractility, myocardial oxygen consumption, and systemic vascular resistance.
    (1) Class II agents block sympathetic effects; therefore, pharmacologic effects are proportional to existing sympathetic tone.
    (2) Although β-blockers have a minimal negative inotropic effect in normal ani-

mals, in those with severe underlying myocardial disease that depend on increased sympathetic drive to maintain cardiac output, they can depress cardiac contractility, conduction, and heart rate.

e. Therapeutic uses
   (1) β-Blockers are indicated for the treatment of **supraventricular tachyarrhythmias,** such as paroxysmal atrial tachycardia and frequent atrial premature complexes. They may also be helpful for some ventricular tachyarrhythmias.
   (a) In cats, β-blockers are the drug of choice for both supraventricular and ventricular tachyarrhythmias.
   (b) Esmolol, a newer agent with β_1 selectivity and a half-life of less than 10 minutes, is potentially useful for short-term treatment of acute tachyarrhythmias and hypertrophic obstructive cardiomyopathy.
   (2) β-blockers slow the ventricular response rate in **atrial fibrillation.** They are often used in combination with digoxin.
   (3) β-Blockers are also used to decrease heart rate and myocardial oxygen demand in hypertension, **hypertrophic cardiomyopathy,** and other causes of myocardial hypertrophy.

f. Administration. In dogs, the combination of propranolol (or another β-blocker) with a class I agent often provides better arrhythmia suppression than either agent alone.
   (1) Oral administration every 8 hours appears to be adequate in both dogs and cats. Because the drug's effects are dependent on the level of sympathetic activation, individual response is quite variable; therefore, initial doses should be low and titrated upward as needed.
   (2) Intravenous administration is used mainly in the treatment of refractory ventricular tachycardia (in conjunction with a class I drug) and in the emergency management of atrial or junctional tachycardia.

g. Adverse effects
   (1) Toxicity is usually related to excessive β blockade, resulting in bradycardia, heart failure, and hypotension. Bronchospasm or increased vascular resistance can occur with nonselective β-blockers (e.g., propranolol).
   (2) Propranolol and other lipophilic β-blockers can cause depression and disorientation.
   (3) Abrupt discontinuation of therapy can result in serious cardiac arrhythmias because of the possibility of β receptor up-regulation (i.e., an increased number of receptors, affinity for receptors, or both) during chronic β blockade.
   (4) β-Blockers may prevent the appearance of early signs of acute hypoglycemia (e.g., tachycardia, blood pressure changes) in diabetic animals. These drugs also reduce the release of insulin in response to hyperglycemia.

h. Drug interactions
   (1) β-Blockers enhance the depression of A-V conduction produced by the digitalis glycosides, class I antiarrhythmic drugs, and calcium channel blockers. The simultaneous use of a β-blocker and a calcium channel blocker is not recommended and can lead to marked decreases in heart rate and myocardial contractility.
   (2) β-Blockers may decrease liver blood flow, leading to reduced elimination of drugs that are highly dependent on liver blood flow for clearance (e.g., lidocaine and phenytoin).

3. Class III agents prolong action potentials.
   a. Preparations
      (1) Bretylium tosylate
      (2) Amiodarone
      (3) Sotalol
   b. Mechanism of action. Class III agents prolong the cardiac action potential duration and the effective refractory period without decreasing conduction velocity.
   c. Pharmacokinetics
      (1) Absorption. Extremely poor oral absorption of bretylium limits its use to the

intramuscular or intravenous routes. Amiodarone and sotalol can be administered orally.

(2) Fate.

(a) The half-life of bretylium is approximately 10.4 hours.

(b) Bretylium tissue concentrations rise slowly, peaking in 1.5–6.0 hours. The tissue concentration is more closely related to the drug's antifibrillatory effects than the plasma concentration.

(c) The pharmacokinetics of amiodarone are complex. The time to achieve steady state and myocardial concentrations is prolonged, and chronic oral administration leads to the accumulation of an active metabolite.

(3) Elimination. Bretylium is eliminated through the kidneys.

d. Pharmacologic effects

(1) Bretylium causes an initial catecholamine release, followed by a longer period where norepinephrine release is inhibited. Intravenous administration produces a transient increase, followed by a prolonged decrease, in sinus rate, A-V conduction velocity, vascular resistance, and arterial blood pressure. The antifibrillatory effects of bretylium may be delayed 4–6 hours after administration.

(2) Amiodarone in therapeutic dosages slows the sinus rate, decreases the A-V conduction velocity, and causes minimal depression of myocardial contractility and blood pressure.

(3) Sotalol is a nonselective β-blocker with primarily class III activity; thus it prolongs repolarization time and refractoriness.

e. Therapeutic uses

(1) Class III agents are most effective for **suppressing re-entrant arrhythmias** and **preventing ventricular fibrillation.**

(2) Bretylium, amiodarone, and d-sotalol may be indicated for the treatment of life-threatening ventricular arrhythmias that are not responsive to conventional therapy and for other patients at risk for developing ventricular fibrillation. They are **not indicated for initial therapy of ventricular arrhythmias.**

f. Adverse effects

(1) Bretylium

(a) Rapid intravenous injection may cause ataxia, nausea, and vomiting.

(b) Significant hypotension may occur, but is rare.

(c) Aggravation of arrhythmias and tachycardia may occur during the early stages of treatment.

(2) Amiodarone. Long-term therapy in humans is associated with significant side effects, including bluish skin discoloration, corneal microdeposits, abnormalities in thyroid function, liver disease, and fatal pulmonary fibrosis.

g. Contraindications include extreme bradycardia or hypotension.

h. Drug interactions. Amiodarone increases the serum concentration of digoxin, quinidine, procainamide, phenytoin, and theophylline.

4. Class IV agents are calcium channel blockers.

a. Preparations

(1) Diltiazem (Cardizem)

(2) Verapamil (Calan, Isoptin)

b. Mechanisms of action. Class IV drugs reduce calcium influx by blocking the slow inward calcium current. Tissues dependent on the slow inward calcium current (e.g., the sinus and A-V nodes) are most affected.

c. Pharmacokinetics

(1) Diltiazem

(a) Absorption. Oral bioavailability appears to be good.

(b) Metabolism. Diltiazem is metabolized extensively. Some metabolites are pharmacologically active.

(i) Peak plasma levels occur 30–60 minutes after oral dosing.

(ii) Peak effects are seen within 2 hours of oral dosing. Effects last at least 6 hours.

(iii) In cats, Cardizem-CD reaches a peak serum level 6 hours after oral dosing, and effects last approximately 24 hours.

(c) Elimination. In dogs, the half-life of diltiazem is just over 2 hours. Because of enterohepatic circulation, long-term oral dosing can prolong diltiazem's half-life. Metabolites and the parent drug are excreted in the urine.

(2) Verapamil

(a) Absorption. Verapamil is poorly absorbed and undergoes first-pass hepatic metabolism, resulting in low oral bioavailability.

(b) Fate. In dogs, the volume of distribution is 2.4–4.5 L/kg, the total body clearance is 36–65 ml/min/kg, and the half-life is approximately 1.0–2.5 hours.

d. Pharmacologic effects. Calcium channel blockers cause dose-related slowing of sinus rate and A-V conduction. As a group, they cause coronary and systemic vasodilation, enhanced myocardial relaxation, and reduced cardiac contractility. Some calcium channel blockers have antiarrhythmic effects.

(1) Diltiazem causes potent coronary and mild peripheral vasodilation. It has less negative inotropic effect than verapamil.

(2) Verapamil has significant negative inotropic and some vasodilating effects that can cause serious decompensation, hypotension, and even death if underlying myocardial disease is present.

e. Therapeutic uses

(1) Diltiazem and verapamil are effective against re-entrant supraventricular and atrial tachycardias.

(2) Diltiazem is also used to slow the ventricular response rate in atrial fibrillation, usually in combination with digoxin.

f. Adverse effects

(1) Diltiazem. At therapeutic dosages, adverse effects are uncommon, although anorexia, nausea, and bradycardia may occur.

(2) Verapamil. Toxic effects of verapamil include sinus bradycardia, A-V block, hypotension, reduced myocardial contractility, and cardiogenic shock. Overdosage or exaggerated response to calcium channel blockers is treated with supportive care.

(a) Atropine is used for bradycardia or A-V blocks.

(b) Dopamine or dobutamine and furosemide are used for heart failure.

(c) Dopamine or intravenous calcium salts are used for hypotension.

g. Contraindications include congestive heart failure (verapamil), sick sinus syndrome, A-V conduction disturbances, and digitalis glycoside toxicity.

h. Drug interactions

(1) Concurrent use of verapamil or diltiazem and a β-blocker can cause either a sudden fall in the sinus rate or a complete heart block.

(2) Verapamil reduces the renal clearance of digoxin, thereby raising its serum concentration.

(3) Concurrent administration of diltiazem and propranolol increases the effects of diltiazem by increasing its oral bioavailability.

(4) Cimetidine may reduce the negative dromotropic effect of diltiazem.

(5) Amiodarone reduces the clearance of diltiazem.

5. Digoxin (see I D 1) is commonly used to treat frequent supraventricular or atrial premature beats and tachycardias. It is also used to slow A-V conduction in atrial fibrillation.

C. **Drugs used for bradyarrhythmias**

1. Anticholinergic (vagolytic) drugs

a. Preparations

(1) Atropine

(2) Glycopyrrolate

(3) Propantheline bromide

    b. **Mechanism of action.** Anticholinergic drugs competitively antagonize the action of acetylcholine (ACh) at muscarinic receptors.

    c. **Pharmacokinetics**

        (1) Absorption. Atropine is well absorbed after oral or intramuscular administration and is widely distributed.

        (2) Elimination is mainly renal.

    d. **Pharmacologic effects**

        (1) An increase in heart rate is the main cardiac effect of anticholinergic drugs. Heart rate effects in dogs last 60–90 minutes with atropine.

        (2) Atropine injection may cause a transient centrally mediated worsening of a bradyarrhythmia.

    e. **Therapeutic uses**

        (1) Indications for parenteral atropine or glycopyrrolate include bradycardia and A-V block induced by anesthesia, CNS lesions, and other diseases or toxicities.

        (2) An atropine response test is often used in dogs and cats presenting with a bradyarrhythmia to determine the extent of vagal influence.

        (3) Propantheline bromide or other oral anticholinergic therapy may be useful in treating sinus bradycardia, sick sinus syndrome, and partial A-V blocks that are responsive to parenteral atropine.

    f. **Adverse effects**

        (1) Vagolytic drugs may aggravate paroxysmal supraventricular tachyarrhythmias (as in sick sinus syndrome) and should not be used as long-term therapy in patients with evidence of such tachyarrhythmias.

        (2) Other side effects of anticholinergic therapy include vomiting, diarrhea, dry mouth, keratoconjunctivitis sicca, and drying of respiratory secretions.

2. Sympathomimetic drugs (see also Chapter 2)

    a. **Pharmacokinetics.** Oral administration is not usually effective because of marked first-pass hepatic metabolism.

    b. **Therapeutic uses.** Isoproterenol is occasionally used for symptomatic A-V block or bradycardia refractory to atropine.

    c. **Adverse effects.** Isoproterenol can cause serious tachyarrhythmias.

    d. **Contraindications.** Because of its affinity for β_2 receptors, isoproterenol can cause hypotension and is not used in heart failure or cardiac arrest.

III. ANTIHYPERTENSIVE DRUGS

A. Introduction

1. Systemic arterial hypertension has been associated with renal disease, hyperadrenocorticism, and pheochromocytoma in dogs and with renal disease and hyperthyroidism in cats. In some cases, no underlying cause is identified.

2. Therapy usually includes dietary salt restriction and management of underlying diseases. Drug therapy is individualized for each patient, usually using one or more of the following agents.

B. Diuretics (see Chapter 7)

1. Mechanism of action. Diuretics may reduce blood pressure by promoting sodium and water excretion.

2. Furosemide is most commonly used, although hydrochlorothiazide may be helpful in nonazotemic dogs.

C. β-Blockers (see also II B 2; Chapter 2)

1. Mechanism of action. β-Blockers may reduce blood pressure by slowing heart rate, decreasing cardiac contractility, or by other peripheral and central mechanisms.

2. Propranolol and atenolol are used most commonly in animals.

D. **Vasodilators**

1. **ACE inhibitors** (see I C 2)
   a. **Mechanism of action.** ACE inhibitors may help control blood pressure by reducing angiotensin II formation, vasodilator kinin degradation, and aldosterone release.
   b. In dogs and cats, ACE inhibitors may be used alone, with a diuretic, or with a diuretic and a β-blocker.

2. **Hydralazine** and **α-blockers** (e.g., **prazosin, phentolamine, phenoxybenzamine**) have been tried in some dogs with uncertain success.

E. **Calcium channel blockers** decrease intracellular calcium in vascular smooth muscle, reducing vascular resistance. Some agents also reduce cardiac output by slowing heart rate, decreasing contractility, or both. **Nifedipine** and **diltiazem** may be useful. Recently, **amlodipine besylate** has produced positive results in hypertensive cats.

IV. DRUGS USED FOR HEARTWORM DISEASE PREVENTION AND TREATMENT (see also Chapter 13)

A. **Drugs used for heartworm disease prevention**

1. **Preparations**
   a. **Diethylcarbamazine** (Filaribits, Caricide, Difil, Nemacide)
   b. **Ivermectin** (Heartgard-30)
   c. **Milbemycin oxime** (Interceptor)

2. **Therapeutic uses**
   a. Prevention of heartworm disease in uninfected dogs living in endemic areas
   b. Prevention of heartworm disease after successful microfilaricide treatment

3. **Contraindications.** Diethylcarbamazine is contraindicated in dogs with microfilaremia.

B. **Adulticide drugs**

1. **Thiacetarsamide 1%** (Caparsolate) has been the only drug approved for treating adult heartworm infections. It must be very carefully administered and has many serious potential adverse effects in dogs and cats.

2. **Melarsomine dihydrochloride** (Immiticide), another arsenical drug, is being evaluated for use as an adulticide. It appears to be effective, safer than thiacetarsamide, and easier to administer. It is expected to become commercially available soon.

C. **Microfilaricide drugs**

1. **Preparations**
   a. **Dithiazanine iodide** (Dizan) is the only microfilaricide approved by the Food and Drug Administration (FDA). Its effectiveness may vary.
   b. **Other commonly used drugs** have various adverse effects. These drugs include **ivermectin** (Ivomec), **levamisole** (Levasol), and **fenthion** (Spotton) used topically.

2. **Therapeutic uses.** These drugs are used to kill microfilaria following adulticide therapy. Ivermectin has become popular as an effective microfilaricide. A single oral dose 4 weeks after adulticide therapy may be all that is needed. An additional benefit is the prevention of reinfection during the treatment period.

3. **Contraindications.** Ivermectin is not used as a microfilaricide in **collie** and **collie-mix** dogs.

V. DRUGS USED IN THE TREATMENT OF FELINE THROMBOEMBOLISM

A. **Drugs used to treat acute thromboembolism**

1. **Heparin**
   a. **Mechanism of action.** Heparin, a cofactor for antithrombin III, inhibits coagulation. The antithrombin III–heparin complex neutralizes factors IX, X, XI, XII, and thrombin (factor II), preventing further coagulation. Existing thromboemboli are not affected.
   b. **Administration.** Heparin is given initially intravenously, followed by subsequent subcutaneous doses, which are adjusted to prolong the activated coagulation time to 1.5–2.5 times the pretreatment level.

2. **Streptokinase** and other nonspecific thrombolytic agents
   a. **Mechanism of action.** These drugs enhance the production of plasmin and cause generalized clot lysis. A potential for excess bleeding exists.
   b. **Administration.** Intra-arterial administration close to the clot would probably have greater positive effects than intravenous administration, but is usually impractical.

3. **Tissue plasminogen activator (TPA)**
   a. **Mechanism of action.** TPA, in the presence of fibrin within a clot, activates the conversion of plasminogen to plasmin at the site of the clot. Plasmin then breaks down fibrin, leading to clot lysis. TPA has a higher specificity of action against fibrin within thrombi, with low affinity for circulating plasminogen.
   b. **Adverse effects.** Variable results have occurred. High subsequent mortality rate is thought to be related to reperfusion injury in some cats.

4. **Vasodilators** (e.g., hydralazine, acetylpromazine maleate)
   a. **Pharmacologic effects**
      (1) These drugs may improve collateral circulation after acute thromboembolism; however, it is not known whether these agents truly reduce vasoconstriction caused by vasoactive substances released by platelet activation.
      (2) Hydralazine does not increase skeletal muscle blood flow as much as it does splanchnic, coronary, cerebral, and renal blood flow.
   b. **Adverse effects.** Potential adverse effects include exacerbation of preexisting hypothermia and hypotension.

B. **Drugs used to inhibit further thromboembolism**

1. **Aspirin**
   a. **Mechanism of action.** Aspirin acts by irreversibly inhibiting cyclooxygenase, thereby reducing thromboxane A_2 synthesis and subsequent platelet aggregation, serotonin release, and vasoconstriction.
   b. **Therapeutic uses**
      (1) Aspirin has been used to reduce further platelet aggregation after a thromboembolic event.
      (2) Aspirin therapy has improved collateral circulation in experimentally induced feline aortic thrombosis.

2. **Warfarin** (Coumarin)
   a. **Mechanism of action.** Warfarin inhibits the synthesis of vitamin K–dependent clotting factors (i.e, factors II, VII, IX, and X).
   b. **Therapeutic uses.** Warfarin is sometimes used orally in cats that survive an acute thromboembolic event.
   c. **Administration.** The dose is adjusted to maintain the prothrombin time at twice the baseline value at 8–10 hours after dosing. Up to 72 hours may be needed before clinical response is noted.
   d. **Adverse effects.** The potential for spontaneous bleeding is high.

STUDY QUESTIONS

DIRECTIONS: Each of the numbered items or incomplete statements in this section is followed by answers or by completions of the statement. Select the **one** numbered answer or completion that is **best** in each case.

1. A purely venous vasodilator would be most useful in treating which of the following conditions?

(1) Chronic, stable dilated cardiomyopathy
(2) Aortic regurgitation from endocarditis
(3) Cardiac tamponade with ascites
(4) Mitral regurgitation with acute pulmonary edema
(5) Pulmonic stenosis with syncope

2. A 7-year-old cat has been diagnosed with hypertrophic cardiomyopathy. Which of the following drugs would be most effective for treating the diastolic dysfunction caused by this disease?

(1) Furosemide
(2) Captopril
(3) Digoxin
(4) Hydralazine
(5) Diltiazem

3. Which of the following statements regarding hydralazine is true?

(1) Hydralazine dilates both arterioles and veins.
(2) Hydralazine directly dilates arteriolar smooth muscle.
(3) Vasodilation with hydralazine is most pronounced in skeletal muscle and skin.
(4) Hypotension and reflex tachycardia are uncommon side effects.
(5) Hydralazine dampens the neurohumoral compensatory response in heart failure.

4. In general, digoxin would be indicated only for a dog with which one of the following conditions?

(1) Dilated cardiomyopathy
(2) Moderate mitral regurgitation
(3) Pericardial effusion
(4) Hypertrophic cardiomyopathy
(5) Constrictive pericarditis

5. Drugs that act by blocking β-adrenergic receptors comprise which class of antiarrhythmic agents?

(1) Class I
(2) Class II
(3) Class III
(4) Class IV

6. A 10-year-old cat has frequent ventricular premature contractions and paroxysmal ventricular tachycardia associated with cardiomyopathy. Initial treatment with propranolol and low-dose lidocaine has been ineffective. Which would be the best drug to try next?

(1) Quinidine
(2) Phenytoin
(3) Digitoxin
(4) Digoxin
(5) Verapamil

DIRECTIONS: Each of the numbered items or incomplete statements in this section is negatively phrased, as indicated by an italicized word such as *not*, *least*, or *except*. Select the **one** numbered answer or completion that is **best** in each case.

7. All of the following angiotensin converting enzyme (ACE) inhibitors are excreted mainly by the kidneys *except:*

(1) captopril.
(2) enalapril.
(3) lisinopril.
(4) benazepril.

8. Regarding digoxin, all of the following are true *except:*

(1) in dogs, elimination is primarily renal.
(2) in cats, elimination is by renal and hepatic routes equally.
(3) dosage should be based on lean body weight because of poor lipid solubility.
(4) in dogs, serum concentration is closely correlated with the dose administered.
(5) cachectic animals may easily become toxic.

9. Regarding dopamine and dobutamine, all of the following statements are true *except:*

(1) both agents have a half-life of 10–20 minutes.
(2) both agents have extensive hepatic metabolism.
(3) long-term use is limited by β receptor down-regulation.
(4) dopamine, but not dobutamine, stimulates vasodilatory dopaminergic receptors.
(5) dopamine is more arrhythmogenic than dobutamine.

10. All of the following are true regarding amrinone *except:*

(1) it acts by inhibiting phosphodiesterase III.
(2) peak effects occur after 45 minutes of infusion in dogs.
(3) it can be used orally twice a day.
(4) vasodilation is an effect.
(5) it may worsen ventricular arrhythmias.

11. Which antiarrhythmic drug is *incorrectly* matched with its classification?

(1) Lidocaine - class IA
(2) Procainamide - class IA
(3) Tocainide - class IB
(4) Quinidine - class IA
(5) Flecainide - class IC

12. All of the statements regarding the adverse effects of class I antiarrhythmic drugs are true *except*:

(1) central nervous system (CNS) excitement is the most common toxic effect of lidocaine.
(2) cats and horses are very sensitive to the toxic effects of lidocaine.
(3) exacerbation of arrhythmias is not a problem with class IA drugs.
(4) gastrointestinal upset can occur with quinidine and procainamide.
(5) marked QT interval prolongation can occur with quinidine.

13. Heparin is used in cats after acute thromboembolism because of its inhibitory effects on coagulation. In combination with antithrombin III, it neutralizes all the following factors *except:*

(1) XII.
(2) XI.
(3) X.
(4) IX.
(5) VIII.

ANSWERS AND EXPLANATIONS

1. The answer is 4 [I C 1 a (2), 4 e (2)].
Cases of acute, fulminant cardiogenic pulmonary edema are most likely to benefit from preload reduction with a venodilator. In general, a mixed or arteriolar vasodilator is of more benefit in most other cases and would be of benefit here, as well. Preload reduction could be harmful in cardiac tamponade.

2. The answer is 5 [I E 2].
Treatment of diastolic dysfunction centers on slowing heart rate, decreasing myocardial oxygen consumption, and enhancing relaxation. Diltiazem, a calcium channel blocker, causes coronary and systemic vasodilation and enhances myocardial relaxation; therefore, it can be used to treat hypertrophic cardiomyopathy in cats. Hydralazine may increase the heart rate and possibly worsen any outflow obstruction. Digoxin may also worsen outflow obstruction and increase oxygen consumption by increasing contractility. Furosemide and captopril may be useful for treating congestive signs, but they would not address the diastolic abnormality.

3. The answer is 2 [I C 3].
Hydralazine is a direct arteriolar dilator. Vasodilation is more pronounced in cerebral, coronary, and splanchnic circulations. Hypotension and reflex tachycardia are common side effects. Enhancement of the neurohumoral response is thought to occur.

4. The answer is 1 [I D 1 d; Table 6-1].
Digoxin is most often used in the treatment of myocardial failure. Mitral regurgitation is usually associated with good myocardial function until very advanced disease. Pericardial effusion, hypertrophic cardiomyopathy, and constrictive pericarditis are not characterized by systolic dysfunction.

5. The answer is 2 [II B 2].
β-Blockers are considered Class II agents (Vaughn-Williams classification system). Class I drugs are the local anesthetics. Class III drugs prolong action potential duration. Class IV drugs are the calcium channel blockers.

6. The answer is 1 [II B 1 e (1)]
Quinidine may be effective, but intravenous use should be avoided. Phenytoin and digitoxin should not be used in cats. Digitalis glycosides in general may exacerbate ventricular arrhythmias. Class IV agents such as verapamil are usually not effective for ventricular arrhythmias.

7. The answer is 4 [I C 2 c].
Benazepril has approximately equal biliary and renal excretion. Captopril, enalapril, and lisinopril are excreted mainly by the kidneys.

8. The answer is 4 [I D 1].
With digoxin therapy, there is only weak correlation between dose and serum concentration. Because of extensive binding to skeletal muscle, animals with reduced muscle mass as well as those with renal dysfunction easily become toxic.

9. The answer is 1 [I D 2].
Catecholamines such as dopamine and dobutamine have a half-life of less than 2 minutes. Their short half-life, as well as their rapid hepatic metabolism, means they are effectively given only by intravenous infusion.

10. The answer is 3 [I D 3].
Amrinone's short half-life necessitates intravenous administration, usually by constant infusion. Peak effects occur after 45 minutes of constant rate infusion. Amrinone inhibits phosphodiesterase III [an intracellular enzyme that degrades cyclic adenosine monophosphate (cAMP)]. Amrinone improves contractility and stimulates vasodilation. It may exacerbate ventricular arrhythmias.

11. The answer is 1 [II B 1; Table 6-3].
Lidocaine is a class IB drug, as is tocainide. Procainamide and quinidine are class IA agents. Flecainide is a class IC agent.

12. The answer is 3 [II B 1 g].
All antiarrhythmic drugs can have proarrhythmic effects. Central nervous system (CNS) excitement is the most common toxic effect of lidocaine. Cats and horses are particularly sensitive to the toxic effects of lidocaine. Quinidine and procainamide can cause gastrointestinal upset, and marked QT interval prolongation can occur with quinidine.

13. The answer is 5 [V A 1 a].
The antithrombin III–heparin complex neutralizes factors XII, XI, X, IX and II (thrombin).

Chapter 7

Diuretics

Franklin A. Ahrens

I. INTRODUCTION

A. **Mechanism of action.** Diuretics increase urinary excretion of sodium ions (Na^+) and water. The resultant extracellular fluid (ECF) volume depletion removes fluid that has accumulated in the interstitial space (edema) and restores normal tissue perfusion and organ function.

B. **Sites of action.** All diuretic agents (except osmotics) act directly on renal tubular epithelia at specific sites in the nephron (Table 7-1).

1. **Proximal convoluted tubule.** Sixty-five percent of the filtered Na^+ and water is reabsorbed from this segment. Activation of the renin-angiotensin system in response to volume depletion or a fall in blood pressure increases Na^+ and water reabsorption from this segment.
   a. Na^+ is reabsorbed by active transport, coupled transport with glucose and amino acids, and passive diffusion. High concentrations of carbonic anhydrase (CA) in tubule cells generate hydrogen ions (H^+):

   $$CO_2 + H_2O \Leftrightarrow H_2CO_3 \Leftrightarrow H^+ + HCO_3^-$$

   The hydrogen ions are exchanged with luminal Na^+ in a process known as **$Na^+ - H^+$ antiport.**
   b. Filtered bicarbonate (HCO_3^-) is reabsorbed from the lumen by a reversal of the reaction shown in I B 1 a. Brush border CA and the diffusion of carbon dioxide (CO_2) into the proximal tubule cell catalyze this reaction.
   c. Chloride (Cl^-) and potassium (K^+) ions are passively reabsorbed. Absorption is isosmotic because water is reabsorbed with ions.

2. **Descending loop of Henle.** Na^+ and Cl^- ions are not reabsorbed; rather, they are concentrated in luminal fluid when water osmotically moves into the hypertonic medullary interstitium.

3. **Thick portion of the ascending loop of Henle.** Twenty-five percent of the filtered Na^+ is reabsorbed in this segment.
   a. The tubule epithelium is impermeable to water. The movement of ions but not water out of the lumen in this segment is essential to the countercurrent multiplier system of the kidney, which generates the hypertonic medullary interstitium.
   b. Na^+, K^+, and Cl^- are coupled and actively transported out of the lumen as Na^+-K^+-$2Cl^-$. Calcium (Ca^{2+}) and magnesium (Mg^{2+}) are passively reabsorbed.
   c. Luminal fluid is hypotonic as it leaves this segment.

4. **Distal convoluted tubule, diluting segment.** Ten percent of the filtered Na^+ is reabsorbed in this segment.
   a. Cl^- is transported with Na^+ (symport).
   b. Ca^{2+} reabsorption is controlled by parathyroid hormone (PTH) acting at this segment of the nephron.
   c. The tubule epithelium is impermeable to water, resulting in further dilution of tubular urine.

5. **Late distal tubule and collecting duct.** Four percent of the filtered Na^+ is actively reabsorbed in this segment, and K^+ and H^+ are actively secreted.

TABLE 7-1. Sites of Action of Diuretics

Nephron Segment	Diuretics
Proximal convoluted tubule	CA inhibitors (e.g., acetazolamide) Osmotic agents (e.g., mannitol) Xanthines (e.g., aminophylline)
Ascending loop of Henle	Loop diuretics (e.g., furosemide)
Early distal convoluted tubule	Thiazides (e.g., hydrochlorothiazide)
Late distal convoluted tubule and collecting duct	K^+-sparing diuretics (e.g., triamterine, spironolactone)

CA = carbonic anhydrase; K^+ = potassium.

a. An increase in the Na^+ load reaching this segment tends to increase K^+ and H^+ secretions as Na^+ is reabsorbed. Therefore, loop and thiazide diuretics indirectly increase urinary loss of K^+ and H^+ and tend to produce hypokalemia and metabolic alkalosis.

b. Aldosterone acts at this segment to increase Na^+ absorption and K^+ excretion.

c. Water is reabsorbed only if antidiuretic hormone (ADH) is present.

C. **Therapeutic uses.** Diuretics are primarily used in the prevention and treatment of generalized edema or severe local edema.

1. **Generalized edema** may result from congestive heart failure, liver disease, renal disease, or protein-losing enteropathies. The latter three conditions are characterized by low levels of plasma albumin, which result from impaired synthesis (liver disease) or excessive loss (renal or intestinal disease). The resulting fall in plasma oncotic pressure results in transudation of fluid from plasma to the interstitial space.

2. **Localized edema** may be cerebral, pulmonary, ocular, or mammary (udder) and may result from infection, inflammation, trauma, or poisons.

II. LOOP (HIGH-CEILING) DIURETICS

A. **Preparations** include **furosemide,** the most commonly used loop diuretic in veterinary medicine, **bumetanide,** and **ethacrynic acid.**

B. **Chemistry.** All loop diuretics are carboxylic acids.

1. Furosemide and bumetanide are structurally related to sulfonamides.

2. Ethacrynic acid is a derivation of phenoxyacetic acid.

C. **Mechanism of action**

1. Loop diuretics inhibit electrolyte, Ca^{2+}, and Mg^{2+} reabsorption in the thick ascending limb of the loop of Henle. They act at the luminal surface of the epithelial cell to inhibit Na^+-K^+-2Cl^- cotransport into the cell.

2. Their diuretic action is independent of urinary pH.

3. Loop diuretics increase systemic venous capacitance, possibly by stimulating the juxtaglomerular apparatus to release prostaglandins (PGs).

D. **Pharmacokinetics**

1. **Absorption.** Furosemide, bumetanide, and ethacrynic acid are well absorbed orally.

2. **Fate**
   a. Loop diuretics are actively secreted into urine by the organic acid transport system of the proximal convoluted tubule. Thus, they rapidly reach the loop of Henle, leading to a rapid onset of action.
   b. Peak diuresis is greater than with the other classes of diuretics because compensatory mechanisms for increased Na^+ reabsorption are limited beyond the loop of Henle.
   c. In most species, a single oral dose produces a plasma half-life of 1–2 hours and a diuresis of 3–6 hours. Intravenous administration produces diuresis within 2–20 minutes, lasting 2 hours.

3. **Excretion**
   a. Furosemide is excreted in the urine as unchanged drug (80%) or as glucuronide (20%).
   b. Ethacrynic acid is excreted in both urine (65%) and bile (35%).

E. **Therapeutic uses**

1. Loop diuretics are the drugs of choice for the rapid mobilization of **edema.**

2. Furosemide may be combined with osmotic diuretics (e.g., mannitol) to maintain urine flow in cases of severe **oliguria** and **acute renal failure.**

3. Furosemide increases urinary Ca^{2+} excretion and is used in the treatment of **hypercalcemia** and **hypercalciuric nephropathy** in dogs and cats.

4. In race horses, furosemide is used to prevent **exercise-induced pulmonary hemorrhage** and **epistaxis.** This effect may be related to increased blood vessel capacitance and decreased left atrial pressure.

F. **Administration.** Furosemide is administered **orally** or **intravenously.**

1. **Treatment of edema**
   a. In dogs and cats, furosemide is administered 3 times a day.
   b. In cattle and horses, it is administered twice daily. Treatment for udder edema in cattle should not continue for longer than 48 hours postpartum because extended treatment can impair lactation.

2. **Treatment of oliguric renal failure.** To treat oliguric renal failure, furosemide is administered intravenously at hourly intervals until diuresis occurs.

3. **Prevention of exercise-induced pulmonary hemorrhage.** Furosemide is administered intravenously to horses 1–2 hours prior to a race, subject to state racing authority regulations.

4. **Treatment of hypercalcemia.** To treat hypercalcemia in dogs and cats, furosemide is administered intravenously in saline supplemented with potassium chloride, 1–2 times a day.

G. **Adverse effects.** Cats are more sensitive than dogs to the effects of loop diuretics, and lower doses should be given.

1. **Fluid** and **electrolyte imbalances** (especially hypokalemia) are the most common adverse effects. High or prolonged doses may produce:
   a. Dehydration
   b. Muscle weakness
   c. Central nervous system (CNS) depression
   d. Volume depletion
   e. Cardiovascular collapse

2. **Deafness** may occur if loop diuretics are administered concomitantly with ototoxic drugs (e.g., aminoglycoside antibiotics). Loop diuretics may cause electrolyte alterations in the endolymph of the inner ear that exacerbate ototoxicity.

3. **Transient granulocytopenia** and **thrombocytopenia** may occur.

III. THIAZIDE DIURETICS (BENZOTHIADIAZIDES)

A. **Preparations** include **chlorothiazide, hydrochlorothiazide,** and **trichlormethiazide.**

B. **Chemistry.** The thiazides are heterocyclic compounds with a benzene ring and an unsubstituted sulfonamide group ($-SO_2NH_2$).

C. **Mechanism of action**

1. The thiazide diuretics block Na^+-Cl^- symport and increase Ca^{2+} absorption in the early part of the distal tubule, increasing excretion of Na^+, Cl^-, Mg^{2+}, and K^+ and decreasing excretion of Ca^{2+}.
   a. Thiazide diuresis tends to be moderate because 90% of the filtered Na^+ has been reabsorbed from the nephron by the time it reaches the distal segment.
   b. Urinary excretion of ions tends to be in physiologic ratios; therefore, thiazides have a minimal effect on ECF ion balance.

2. Paradoxically, thiazides reduce urine output in animals with diabetes insipidus. The mechanism of action is unknown, but it is related to their natriuretic (Na^+-excreting) effect.

3. Thiazides weakly inhibit CA, but this does not contribute to their diuretic action at normal doses.

D. **Pharmacokinetics** of thiazides in animals are not reported.

1. In humans, oral absorption occurs at rates of 10%–20% for hydrochlorothiazide and 65%–75% for chlorothiazide. These drugs, which are not metabolized, are excreted in the urine by active tubular secretion.

2. In dogs and cats, a diuretic response occurs in 2–3 hours and lasts 6–12 hours.

E. **Therapeutic uses**

1. **Long-term diuretic therapy**
   a. Chlorothiazide and hydrochlorothiazide are useful adjuncts in the treatment of **congestive heart failure** in dogs and cats.
   b. Hydrochlorothiazide and trichlormethiazide are used in the treatment of **udder edema** in cattle.

2. **Nephrogenic diabetes insipidus.** Thiazide diuretics are effective in reducing urine output in dogs with this condition.

3. **Calcium oxalate uroliths.** In dogs, hydrochlorothiazide reduces urinary Ca^{2+} excretion.

F. **Administration**

1. Chlorothiazide and hydrochlorothiazide are administered orally twice daily to dogs and cats.

2. To treat udder edema in cattle, hydrochlorothiazide is administered intravenously or intramuscularly twice daily. Trichlormethiazide combined with dexamethasone in a proprietary preparation (Naquasone) is administered orally once daily.

G. Adverse effects

1. **Minimal ECF electrolyte balance disturbance.** This effect is less with thiazides than with other classes of diuretics because thiazides produce only a moderate diuresis.

2. **Hypokalemia** and **hypochloremia** may result from prolonged thiazide therapy.

3. **Hyperglycemia** and **glycosuria.** Thiazides may induce hyperglycemia and glycosuria in diabetic or prediabetic animals by inhibiting the conversion of proinsulin to insulin.

IV. OSMOTIC DIURETICS

A. **Preparations. Mannitol** is the most commonly used osmotic diuretic. **Glycerol** and **urea** are used less often.

B. **Chemistry.** Mannitol is a six-carbon sugar alcohol.

C. Mechanism of action

1. Osmotic diuretics are filtered at the glomerulus but are poorly reabsorbed from the lumen of the nephron. These unabsorbed solutes in the proximal tubule cause decreased reabsorption of water, resulting in a large volume of urine. There is a small increase in Na^+ and Cl^- excretion.

2. Mannitol causes an increase in renal medullary blood flow via a PG-mediated mechanism.

D. Pharmacokinetics

1. **Absorption.** Mannitol is poorly absorbed orally, necessitating intravenous administration.

2. **Fate.** Mannitol is distributed to the ECF. The plasma half-life is 1–2 hours.

3. **Excretion.** The unmetabolized drug is excreted by renal glomerular filtration.

E. Therapeutic uses

1. **Poisonings.** In dogs and cats, forced diuresis using mannitol hastens the elimination of poisons excreted by the kidney.

2. **Oliguric renal failure.** In dogs and cats, mannitol may be used as an adjunct to furosemide therapy. The osmotic expansion of the plasma increases glomerular filtration volume and maintains urine flow.

3. **Acute glaucoma.** In dogs and cats, increased intraocular pressure is reduced by osmotic diuretics such as mannitol or glycerol.

4. **Cerebral edema.** When used as an adjunct to furosemide, mannitol may prevent the hypovolemic shock commonly observed in large and small animals with cerebral edema.

F. **Administration.** Mannitol solutions (5%–20%) are administered by slow intravenous infusions over a period of 15–30 minutes in all species. Infusions may be repeated every 6–8 hours.

G. Adverse effects and contraindications

1. Osmotic diuretics rarely produce toxicity; but fluid and electrolyte balance and urine output should be monitored, especially in the treatment of oliguric renal failure.

    2. Mannitol is **contraindicated in animals with generalized or acute pulmonary edema.** Its saluretic effect (i.e., ability to promote Na^+ and Cl^- excretion) is small, and it produces an initial expansion of the ECF that may exacerbate the edema and cause decompensation in animals with congestive heart failure.

V. CARBONIC ANHYDRASE (CA) INHIBITORS

A. **Preparations** include **acetazolamide, methazolamide, dichlorphenamide,** and **ethazolamide.**

B. **Chemistry.** CA inhibitors are sulfonamide derivatives.

C. **Mechanisms of action**

    1. In the kidney. These agents reversibly inhibit CA enzymes, predominantly in the proximal convoluted tubules, reducing the number of hydrogen ions available for $Na^+ - H^+$ exchange. CO_2 reabsorption from the glomerular filtrate is decreased and $Na^+ - HCO_3^-$ excretion is increased, resulting in an alkaline urine. To maintain ionic balance, Cl^- is retained by the kidney, resulting in a hyperchloremic acidosis. This metabolic acidosis (low plasma HCO_3^-) eventually induces a refractory state and decreased diuresis.

    2. In the eye. CA is found in high concentrations in the ciliary process of the eye, and it is involved in aqueous humor formation. CA inhibitors reduce intraocular pressure in animals with glaucoma by decreasing the production of aqueous humor.

D. **Pharmacokinetics**

    1. Absorption. CA inhibitors are absorbed orally.

    2. Distribution. They are distributed to tissues with high CA concentrations (renal cortex, eye, erythrocytes). In small animals, the onset of diuresis occurs in 30 minutes and effects last 6–12 hours.

    3. Excretion. They are excreted by the kidney by active secretion and passive reabsorption.

E. **Therapeutic uses.** CA inhibitors are used in the treatment of **glaucoma** and as an adjunct therapy for **metabolic alkalosis.**

F. **Administration.** To treat glaucoma, oral doses of acetazolamide, methazolamide, ethazolamide, or dichlorphenamide are given 2–3 times daily. In acute cases, a single intravenous dose of acetazolamide is administered, followed by an oral dosage regimen.

G. **Adverse effects and contraindications**

    1. Rarely, oral administration causes **vomiting.**

    2. CA inhibitors are **contraindicated in the presence of liver disease** because they divert ammonia from the urine to the systemic circulation, leading to **hepatic coma.**

VI. K$^+$-SPARING DIURETICS

A. **Preparations** include **triamterene, amiloride,** and **spironolactone.**

B. **Mechanism of action**

    1. Triamterene and **amiloride** inhibit active Na^+ reabsorption in the late distal convoluted tubule and collecting duct, reducing the driving force for K^+ secretion. They cause a small increase in Na$^+$ and Cl$^-$ excretion without increasing K$^+$ excretion. Their action is independent of aldosterone.

2. **Spironolactone** is a competitive antagonist of the mineralocorticoid aldosterone. It interferes with the aldosterone-mediated Na$^+$ − K$^+$ exchange at the late distal convoluted tubule, increasing Na$^+$ loss while decreasing K$^+$ loss. Spironolactone is most effective when circulating aldosterone levels are high.

C. Pharmacokinetics

1. Triamterene, amiloride, and spironolactone are **absorbed orally.**

2. **Spironolactone** has a **slow onset of action.** The maximal effect occurs within 48–72 hours.

D. Therapeutic uses

1. **Chronic edema.** Triamterene or amiloride in combination with thiazide or loop diuretics increase the natriuretic effect while decreasing K$^+$ loss.

2. **Refractory edema.** Spironolactone is occasionally used as an adjunct to other diuretics when excessive K$^+$ loss is a concern.

3. **Adrenal gland tumors.** Spironolactone is used to counter the aldosterone-induced Na$^+$ and K$^+$ changes produced by adrenal gland tumors.

E. Administration

1. **Triamterene** and **spironolactone** are administered orally twice daily in dogs and cats.

2. **Amiloride** is administered orally once daily.

F. Adverse effects and contraindications

1. **Hyperkalemia.** K$^+$-sparing diuretics should not be given in combination with one another. They are contraindicated in hyperkalemic patients, especially in those with diabetes mellitus, renal disease, or thromboembolic disease.

2. **Gastrointestinal disturbances** may occur.

VII. METHYLXANTHINES

A. Preparations include **aminophylline, theophylline, caffeine,** and **theobromine.**

B. Mechanisms of action

1. Methylxanthines increase renal blood flow and glomerular filtration rate and inhibit Na$^+$ reabsorption in the proximal convoluted tubule. Diuresis is enhanced by an alkaline urine and thus is greater in herbivores than in carnivores.

2. Methylxanthines dilate bronchi by inhibiting adenosine receptors.

3. They stimulate the CNS.

C. Therapeutic uses

1. **Respiratory disease.** Aminophylline and theophylline are bronchodilators.

2. **Diuresis.** Methylxanthines are rarely used solely for diuresis, but increased urine output is observed when they are employed as bronchodilators.

D. Adverse effects. High or prolonged dosage of methylxanthines may produce excitement, skeletal muscle fasciculation, vomiting, and cardiovascular toxicity (e.g., palpitations, hypotension).

VIII. ACIDIFYING SALTS (AMMONIUM CHLORIDE)

A. **Mechanism of action.** Ammonium chloride (NH_4Cl^-) lowers the pH of extracellular fluid and urine. The liver converts NH_4Cl^- to urea, H^+, and Cl^-. H^- is buffered by HCO_3^- in plasma, which leads to acidosis. The increased Cl^- load to the kidney produces urinary loss of Na^+ and Cl^- and a mild diuresis.

B. **Therapeutic uses**
 1. **Urinary acidification** to promote excretion of ionizable drugs or poisons
 2. **Urolith dissolution** and **prevention**

C. **Administration.** NH_4Cl^- is administered orally 2–3 times per day. It may be added to the diets of dogs and cats.

D. **Adverse effects**
 1. **Severe, uncompensated acidosis** may result if renal function is impaired.
 2. **Nausea** and **gastric irritation** may result from oral administration.

STUDY QUESTIONS

DIRECTIONS: Each of the numbered items or incomplete statements in this section is followed by answers or by completions of the statement. Select the **one** numbered answer or completion that is **best** in each case.

1. In cases of severe generalized edema, which of the following fluid compartments is increased in volume?

(1) Intracellular
(2) Interstitial
(3) Transcellular
(4) Plasma

2. Urinary excretion of ions in physiologic ratios with little distortion of extracellular fluid ion balance characterizes the moderate diuretic action of:

(1) triamterene.
(2) ethacrynic acid.
(3) acetazolamide.
(4) hydrochlorothiazide.
(5) spironolactone.

3. Which one of the following diuretics produces an alkaline urine and decreases the rate of aqueous humor formation?

(1) Ethacrynic acid
(2) Dichlorphenamide
(3) Mannitol
(4) Triamterene

4. Which one of the following diuretics decreases calcium (Ca^{2+}) excretion via increased absorption in the distal tubule and is thus used to prevent calcium oxalate bladder stones?

(1) Hydrochlorothiazide
(2) Ethacrynic acid
(3) Urea
(4) Spironolactone
(5) Triamterene

5. Hyperglycemia via inhibition of the conversion of proinsulin to insulin may occur with:

(1) thiazide diuretics.
(2) loop (high-ceiling) diuretics.
(3) carbonic anhydrase (CA) inhibitors.
(4) methylxanthines.

6. Which of the following diuretic agents is contraindicated in animals with liver disease because it may precipitate hepatic coma?

(1) Hydrochlorothiazide
(2) Acetazolamide
(3) Furosemide
(4) Spironolactone

7. Fluid and electrolyte imbalance leading to dehydration, muscle weakness, hypokalemia, and central nervous system (CNS) depression may result from high or prolonged dosage with:

(1) chlorothiazide.
(2) amiloride.
(3) furosemide.
(4) theophylline.

DIRECTIONS: Each of the numbered items or incomplete statements in this section is negatively phrased, as indicated by an italicized word such as *not, least,* or *except.* Select the **one** numbered answer or completion that is **best** in each case.

8. Hypoalbuminemia underlies the edema arising from all of the following causes *except:*

(1) hepatic disease.
(2) congestive heart failure.
(3) renal disease.
(4) protein-losing enteropathy.

9. All of the following statements concerning furosemide are true *except:*

(1) it tends to produce a metabolic alkalosis via urinary loss of hydrogen (H^+), potassium (K^+), and chloride (Cl^-).
(2) it decreases calcium (Ca^{2+}) reabsorption in the loop of Henle and increases urinary Ca^{2+} loss.
(3) it may increase capacitance of pulmonary blood vessels and reduce epistaxis in racehorses.
(4) it blocks Na^+-K^+-$2Cl^-$ coupled transport in the ascending loop of Henle.
(5) it is less potent than agents that act at the proximal convoluted tubule.

10. All of the following statements about methylxanthine diuretics are true *except:*

(1) they increase the glomerular filtration rate.
(2) they are less effective than loop (high-ceiling) diuretics.
(3) they can produce central nervous system (CNS) stimulation.
(4) they are most effective in an acid urine.

ANSWERS AND EXPLANATIONS

1. The answer is 2 [I A].
Generalized edema results from accumulation of fluid in the interstitial space. In severe edema, this compartment may nearly double in volume. Intracellular, transcellular, and plasma volumes are minimally affected.

2. The answer is 4 [III C 1].
The thiazides tend to produce less distortion of the ionic composition of the extracellular fluid because of their moderate potency and mechanism of action, which results in the urinary excretion of sodium (Na^+), potassium (K^+), and chloride (Cl^-) in physiologic ratios. Ethacrynic acid tends to produce hypokalemia. Triamterene and spironolactone are K^+-sparing diuretics and may produce hyperkalemia. Acetazolamide tends to produce hyperchloremia.

3. The answer is 2 [V C 1–2].
Dichlorphenamide is a carbonic anhydrase (CA) inhibitor that reduces sodium–hydrogen ($Na^+ - H^+$) exchange in the proximal convoluted tubule; thus, bicarbonate (HCO_3^-) is excreted and the urine becomes alkaline. CA activity is required for aqueous humor formation; therefore, inhibition of this enzyme by dichlorphenamide reduces intraocular pressure in animals with glaucoma. Ethacrynic acid, mannitol, and triamterene do not inhibit CA.

4. The answer is 1 [III E 3].
The thiazide diuretics stimulate calcium (Ca^{2+}) reabsorption in the early distal tubule and reduce urinary Ca^{2+} concentrations. This action may aid in preventing the formation of calcium oxalate uroliths. Loop diuretics increase Ca^{2+} excretion. Excretion of Ca^{2+} is not affected by spironolactone, triamterene, or urea.

5. The answer is 1 [III G 3].
Thiazides may produce hyperglycemia by slowing the conversion of proinsulin to insulin, particularly in diabetic or prediabetic animals. This effect does not occur with loop diuretics, carbonic anhydrase (CA) inhibitors, or the methylxanthines.

6. The answer is 2 [V G 2].
Carbonic anhydrase (CA) inhibitors (e.g., acetazolamide) are contraindicated in patients with liver disease. CA inhibitors increase urinary bicarbonate excretion and produce alkaline urine, eliminating the driving force for ammonia excretion into the urine. The ammonia produced by the distal tubules is reabsorbed by the blood stream instead of excreted in urine. Ammonia is converted to urea by the liver. If liver function is impaired, blood levels of ammonia rise and may precipitate hepatic coma.

7. The answer is 3 [II G 1].
The toxic effects of loop (high-ceiling) diuretics such as furosemide are an extension of their therapeutic effects. High or prolonged dosages produce a potent diuretic action that may deplete the body of water and electrolytes and lead to dehydration, hypokalemia, muscle weakness, and central nervous system (CNS) depression. These adverse effects are less likely to occur with less potent diuretics such as chlorothiazide, amiloride, or theophylline.

8. The answer is 2 [I C 1].
Plasma albumin concentrations are not changed in congestive heart failure. Renal disease and protein-losing enteropathy result in loss of plasma proteins, and plasma protein synthesis by the liver is decreased in hepatic disease. These conditions result in hypoalbuminemia, decreased plasma oncotic pressure, and transudation of fluid from blood vessels to the interstitial space.

9. The answer is 5 [II C, E 4].
Furosemide increases hydrogen (H^+), potassium (K^+), and chloride (Cl^-) excretion rates, which produces a metabolic alkalosis. Calcium (Ca^{2+}) reabsorption in the loop of Henle is decreased because of the loss of transcellular potential produced by blockade of Na^+-K^+-$2Cl^-$ cotransport. Blood vessel capacitance is increased, and this may prevent exercise-induced pulmonary hemorrhage in horses. Loop diuretics are more potent than agents that act at the proximal tubules because compensatory mechanisms for Na^+ reabsorption are limited beyond the loop of Henle.

10. The answer is 4 [VII B 1].
The action of methylxanthine diuretics is enhanced by an alkaline urine; thus, they are not very potent in carnivores. The methylxanthine diuretics increase glomerular filtration rate and renal blood flow by increasing cardiac output. They are less effective than other diuretics in promoting sodium (Na^+) and chloride (Cl^-) excretion. They are central nervous system (CNS) stimulants.

Chapter 8

Endocrine Pharmacology

Walter H. Hsu

I. **ENDOCRINE FUNCTION.** Hormones are natural secretions of endocrine glands that can exert powerful effects on other tissues. Synthetic compounds that produce hormone-like effects have important therapeutic uses.

A. **Hypothalamic–pituitary relationship**

1. **Releasing hormones.** The hypothalamus produces neurohumoral substances, or releasing hormones, which affect both the synthesis and the release of pituitary hormones.
   a. **Four releasing hormones** have been well characterized:
      (1) **Gonadotropin-releasing hormone (GnRH)**
      (2) **Growth hormone-releasing hormone (GHRH)**
      (3) **Thyrotropin-releasing hormone (TRH)**
      (4) **Corticotropin-releasing hormone (CRH)**
   b. Most hormones regulate their releasing hormones through **feedback inhibition.** This mechanism can be manipulated for therapeutic or diagnostic purposes.

2. **Inhibitory hormones** are also produced by the hypothalamus.
   a. **Somatostatin** suppresses **growth hormone (GH)** release.
   b. **Dopamine** suppresses **prolactin** release.

3. **Vasopressin** and **oxytocin** are also produced by the hypothalamus. The active hormones are released from the posterior pituitary.

B. **Classification of pituitary hormones**

1. **Somatomammotropins** include **GH, prolactin,** and **placental lactogen.**

2. **Glycoproteins** include:
   a. **Luteinizing hormone (LH)**
   b. **Follicle-stimulating hormone (FSH)**
   c. **Human chorionic gonadotropin (HCG)**
   d. **Pregnant mare serum gonadotropin (PMSG)**
   e. **Thyroid-stimulating hormone (TSH)**

3. **Corticotropin and related peptides**
   a. **ACT (corticotropin)**
   b. **α-Melanocyte-stimulating hormone (α-MSH)**
   c. **β-Melanocyte-stimulating hormone (β-MSH)**
   d. **β-Lipotropin (β-LPH)**
   e. **γ-Lipotropin (γ-LPH)**

C. **Mechanism of action.** Many hormones effect signal transduction through one of three major mechanisms:

1. **Guanosine triphosphate (GTP)-binding proteins (G proteins)**
   a. **G_s** couples to adenylyl cyclase, which increases the formation of cyclic adenosine monophosphate (cAMP). cAMP activates protein kinase A, which phosphorylates cellular constituents. Glucagon, glucagon-like peptides, and β-adrenergic agonists use this mechanism.
   b. **G_i** and **G_o** couple negatively to adenylyl cyclase and voltage-dependent calcium channels (VDCCs) to decrease cAMP formation and calcium influx, respectively. They may couple to potassium channels to increase efflux, causing membrane hyperpolarization and closure of VDCCs. Somatostatin, galanin, and α_2-adrenergic agonists use this mechanism.

c. G_q proteins couple to phospholipase C, which increases the formation of inositol triphosphate (IP_3) and diacylglycerol (DAG). IP_3 elevates intracellular calcium concentrations by increasing calcium release from the endoplasmic reticulum and calcium influx through receptor-operated cation channels or VDCCs (or both). DAG activates protein kinase C, which phosphorylates cellular constituents. Vasopressin and oxytocin use this mechanism.

2. Tyrosine kinase receptors. Some hormones (e.g., insulin, certain growth factors) act at tyrosine kinase receptors in the plasma membrane. The insulin receptor is used as an example to explain how tyrosine kinase works.

    a. The activated insulin receptor (tyrosine kinase) phosphorylates its substrates [e.g., insulin receptor substrate-1 (IRS-1)].

    b. Activated IRS-1 is thought to be involved in the movement of glucose transporters to the plasma membrane for actions.

3. Cytosolic or **nuclear receptors.** Steroid hormones and thyroid hormones bind to these proteins to act on deoxyribonucleic acid (DNA), increasing transcription processes (and thereby increasing protein synthesis). In addition, recent evidence indicates that steroid hormones may bind to receptors in the plasma membrane that can cause rapid changes by means other than increasing transcription (e.g., via coupling to VDCCs to rapidly increase calcium influx).

D. **Pharmacokinetics**

1. Polypeptides

    a. Absorption. Polypeptides are destroyed in the gastrointestinal tract following oral administration. They are well absorbed from injection sites.

    b. Fate

        (1) Distribution. Polypeptides are evenly distributed in the body. Most of them do not penetrate the central nervous system (CNS).

        (2) Metabolism. Polypeptides are usually rapidly metabolized in the liver and kidney and are also destroyed by peptidases in the plasma. Despite their short half-lives (5–10 minutes), their biological actions usually last several hours.

    c. Excretion. Few polypeptides are excreted in the urine or feces.

2. Glycoproteins

    a. Absorption. Glycoproteins are destroyed in the gastrointestinal tract following oral administration. They are well absorbed from injection sites.

    b. Fate

        (1) Distribution. Glycoproteins are evenly distributed in the body; however, they cannot penetrate the CNS when given parenterally.

        (2) Metabolism. Glycoproteins are slowly metabolized by the liver and kidney. Generally, the more carbohydrates in the chemical structure, the more resistant the compound is to metabolism. Their plasma half-lives range from 1–12 hours.

    c. Excretion. Glycoproteins are usually not detectable in the urine or feces following parenteral administration.

3. Steroids and thyroid hormones

    a. Absorption. Both the steroids and thyroid hormones are well absorbed from the gastrointestinal tract following oral administration, but because the natural steroids are rapidly metabolized in the liver following oral administration, only thyroid hormones and synthetic steroids that are resistant to liver enzymes can be effectively administered orally.

    b. Fate. The circulating steroids and thyroid hormones are bound to plasma binding proteins (albumin and specific globulins) and are evenly distributed throughout the body, including the CNS. At least 90% of steroids and thyroid hormones are bound to binding proteins. Consequently, these substances have much longer half-lives (hours to days) than polypeptide hormones.

    c. Excretion. When steroids and thyroid hormones are metabolized, they are hydroxylated and then undergo conjugation to form glucuronides and sulfates, which are water soluble and therefore readily excreted in the urine and feces.

II. ENDOCRINE DYSFUNCTION

A. Anterior pituitary disorders

1. **Hypopituitarism** (pituitary dwarfism)

2. **Acquired growth hormone deficiency**

3. **Neoplasia** (functional and nonfunctional)

4. **Hypersecretion of pituitary hormones**
   a. **Acromegaly** results from **excess GH.**
   b. **Cushing's syndrome** results from **excess ACTH.**
   c. **Galactorrhea** results from **excess prolactin.**

B. Posterior pituitary disorders. Diabetes insipidus results from a vasopressin deficiency.

C. Thyroid disorders

1. **Hypothyroidism** is usually seen in dogs and horses and can be treated with thyroid hormones.

2. **Hyperthyroidism** is usually seen in cats. Hyperthyroidism in species other than cats is frequently caused by adenocarcinoma, and the prognosis in these animals is usually poor. Thus, antithyroid agents are only recommended for cats.

D. Parathyroid disorders

1. **Hypoparathyroidism** leads to **hypocalcemia,** which is characterized by neuromuscular dysfunction, bradycardia, and convulsions.

2. **Hyperparathyroidism** causes **hypercalcemia,** which has renal, skeletal, gastrointestinal, and neurologic ramifications.

E. Adrenal dysfunction

1. **Hypoadrenocorticism.** Addison's disease is the result of primary insufficiency; secondary insufficiency can occur as well.

2. **Hyperadrenocorticism** manifests itself as Cushing's syndrome.

3. **Pheochromocytoma** causes excessive production of catecholamines, resulting in hypertension.

F. Pancreatic dysfunction results in carbohydrate metabolism disorders.

1. **Hyperglycemia. Diabetes mellitus** is the most common cause; other causes are also possible.

2. **Hypoglycemia (hyperinsulinemia)** may be caused by an **insulinoma.**

G. Gonadal dysfunction results in hypogonadism and ovarian cystic disorders (e.g., follicular cysts, luteal cysts).

III. HORMONES AND AGENTS AFFECTING ENDOCRINE FUNCTION

A. Growth hormone (GH) is a large polypeptide molecule containing 191 amino acids. Because it resembles prolactin and placental lactogen in structure, it is thought that these three polypeptides evolved from a common ancestral cell.

1. **Preparations. Bovine growth hormone (BGH) [bovine somatotropin (BST)]** is a prolonged-release injectable formulation of a recombinant DNA-derived BGH analog.

2. The **mechanism of action** of BGH is not completely understood. It does not use any

of the currently recognized second messengers (e.g., cAMP, calcium). GH may act by stimulating secretion of **somatomedins** (also known as **insulin-like growth factors**).

3. **Pharmacologic effects.** BGH promotes growth of all tissues of the body that are capable of growing, especially bone and muscle.
   a. It increases uptake of glucose and amino acids into cells and promotes lipolysis.
   b. It increases synthesis of DNA and ribonucleic acid (RNA).

4. **Therapeutic uses.** BGH has recently been approved for use in cattle to promote milk production.

5. **Administration.** It is injected subcutaneously (500 mg) once every 14 days.

6. **Adverse effects**
   a. Mild hyperthermia
   b. Clinical and subclinical mastitis
   c. Reduced feed intake
   d. Mild, transient swelling at the injection site
   e. Mild anemia
   f. Reduced pregnancy rates, as a result of cystic ovaries and disorders of the uterus caused by BGH
   g. Shorter gestation periods, decreased birth weights, and increased rates of twinning and placental retention

B. Gonadotropins

1. **Synthesis, secretion, and actions**
   a. **FSH** and **LH** are produced and secreted by the gonadotropic cells of the pituitary. Production of FSH and LH is under hypothalamic control; it is stimulated by GnRH.
      (1) In **male animals**, FSH increases the diameter of the seminiferous tubules and promotes spermatogenesis. LH increases testosterone synthesis from Leydig cells. Secretion of FSH and LH is rather consistent.
      (2) In **female animals**, FSH stimulates graafian follicle development and estrogen synthesis. LH evokes ovulation and increases luteinization, leading to increased progesterone synthesis. Secretion varies with the stage of the estrous cycle.
         (a) **Proestrus** (the **follicular phase**). Rising FSH levels are followed by rising LH levels, which mediate follicular growth and ovulation, respectively. Production of ovarian estrogens increases. The reproductive tract is hypertrophied and hyperemic.
         (b) **Estrus (ovulation)** is associated with an LH spike.
         (c) **Metestrus–diestrus** (the **luteal phase**) is characterized by proliferation of the reproductive tract mucosa as a result of increased progesterone production from the corpus luteum. As the corpus luteum involutes, ovarian steroid levels decline, causing endometrial degeneration.
   b. **HCG** has LH-like activity. It is secreted from the placenta and extracted from the urine of pregnant women.
   c. **PMSG** has FSH-like activity. It is secreted from the placenta and extracted from the serum of pregnant mares.

2. **Preparations and therapeutic uses**
   a. **Gonadorelin** is the drug name for GnRH. It is administered intramuscularly (100 μg) to induce LH release for **treatment of follicular cysts in cows.**
   b. **LH and HCG**
      (1) In female animals, LH and HCG are used to control ovulation and to treat **persistent infertility.**
      (2) In male animals, they are used to treat **cryptorchidism.** LH increases testosterone production, which causes descent of the testicles into the scrotum.
   c. **FSH** and **PMSG**
      (1) In females, FSH and PMSG are used to **stimulate graafian follicle development,** which leads to **estrus** and may increase the incidence of multiple births.

(2) In males, FSH and PMSG are used to treat **infertility.** These hormones may improve libido and spermatozoa counts.

3. Adverse effects. Anaphylactic shock may develop after repeated interspecies administration of a gonadotropin.

C. **Sex steroids**

1. Estrogens
  a. Synthesis, secretion, and actions. Endogenous estrogens are secreted from the ovaries, testicles (especially in stallions), adrenal cortex, and placenta. Approximately 90% are bound by plasma proteins (i.e., sex steroid-binding globulin and albumin).
    (1) Estrogens stimulate and maintain the reproductive tract and cause hyperemia, hypertrophy, and edema during estrus.
    (2) They cause cervical dilation.
    (3) They stimulate growth of the mammary glands.
    (4) They increase ossification of epiphysial lines to limit growth.
    (5) They increase sexual receptivity.
    (6) They have protein anabolic effects (i.e., they stimulate protein synthesis).
    (7) They antagonize androgen receptors.
  b. Classification
    (1) Steroidal estrogens include **estradiol, estrone,** and **estriol.** Estradiol is the most potent endogenous estrogen that is also used therapeutically.
    (2) Nonsteroidal estrogens include **zeranol,** a mycotoxin, and **diethylstilbestrol (DES).**
  c. Preparations include **estradiol, zeranol,** and **DES.**
    (1) Pharmacokinetics
      (a) Estradiol cypionate. Following intramuscular administration, estradiol cypionate is absorbed slowly over several days. It is distributed throughout the body and accumulates in adipose tissue. Estradiol cypionate undergoes hepatic metabolism. The metabolite is excreted into the urine and the bile, where most of it is reabsorbed from the gastrointestinal tract.
      (b) Zeranol. No information about the pharmacokinetics of zeranol is available.
      (c) DES is well absorbed from the gastrointestinal tract of monogastric animals. It is slowly metabolized (primarily to a glucuronide) by the liver, and then it is excreted in the urine and feces.
    (2) Therapeutic uses
      (a) Mismating therapy in dogs. Estrogen preparations decrease implantation and interfere with ovum transport by increasing contraction of the utero-tubal sphincter.
      (b) Correction of anestrus in cows. Estrogen therapy is sometimes effective.
      (c) Treatment of persistent corpus luteum in cows. Estrogen therapy is occasionally successful, depending on the cause.
      (d) Treatment of pyometra and **mummified fetus**
      (e) Treatment of problems associated with spaying (e.g., urinary incontinence, vaginitis, dermatitis)
      (f) Treatment of prostatic hyperplasia or tumors associated with increased androgenic activity. Estrogens are used as androgen receptor antagonists.
      (g) Growth promotion (mainly in ruminants)
        (i) Estradiol is usually combined with progesterone or testosterone for parenteral administration to promote growth in calves, heifers, or steers. There is no preslaughter withdrawal time indicated for this use.
        (ii) Zeranol is also used to promote growth in cattle and sheep. The preslaughter withdrawal time of zeranol is 65 days in cattle and 40 days in sheep.
    (3) Adverse effects include vaginal and rectal prolapse, abortion, follicular cysts, bone fractures (as a result of excessive ossification), aplastic anemia and leuko-

penia (a unique toxic effect of estrogens in dogs and cats caused by bone marrow suppression), and pyometritis.

(4) Contraindications include **pregnancy.** High estrogen levels may cause fetal genitourinary malformations and may induce abortion.

2. Progestins

a. **Synthesis, secretion, and action. Progesterone** is secreted from the corpus luteum and placenta of mares and ewes and from the adrenal cortex. Approximately 90% of progesterone is bound by plasma proteins (corticosteroid-binding globulin and albumin).

(1) Progesterone **increases glandular growth** after priming with estrogens.

(2) It **desensitizes the myometrium to oxytocin** (i.e., it prevents uterine contractions during pregnancy).

(3) It has **anabolic effects** (e.g. increased appetite, decreased physical activity).

b. **Preparations** include **progesterone** and the synthetic progestins, **medroxyprogesterone, megestrol, melengestrol,** and **altrenogest.**

(1) Pharmacokinetics

(a) Progesterone is rapidly inactivated by liver enzymes following gastrointestinal absorption. The synthetic analogs of progesterone are more resistant to metabolism than progesterone.

(b) Medroxyprogesterone acetate. No information about the pharmacokinetics of this preparation is available. However, the duration of action is at least 30 days when used to treat behavior problems in cats.

(c) Megestrol acetate is well absorbed from the gastrointestinal tract of monogastric animals and is metabolized in the liver to conjugates. The half-life is 8 days in dogs.

(d) Melengestrol and **altrenogest.** No information about the pharmacokinetics of these agents is available.

(2) Therapeutic uses

(a) Altrenogest is administered orally to mares (0.044 mg/kg, one dose daily for 15 consecutive days) to synchronize or suppress estrus and extend the luteal phase.

(b) Progestins are used (with limited success) to treat implantation failure and habitual abortion.

(c) Megestrol acetate (2.2 mg/kg/day orally for 32 days starting in anestrus) is used as a contraceptive in bitches.

(d) Medroxyprogesterone acetate (intramuscularly or subcutaneously) is used to control aggressiveness and inappropriate urination or spraying.

(e) Progesterone combined with an estrogen increases receptivity in bitches and ewes.

(f) Melengestrol and progesterone are used as growth promoters in cattle.

(i) Melengestrol is used as a feed additive. A withdrawal period of at least 48 hours should be implemented when using melengestrol in cattle.

(ii) Progesterone is used parenterally and no preslaughter withdrawal time is required.

(3) Adverse effects

(a) Endometrial hyperplasia, endometritis, and pyometra may occur.

(b) The glucocorticoid-like activity of the progestins may induce diabetes mellitus in animals that already have marginal disease.

(c) Inhibition of adrenal cortical function is also an adverse effect associated with the glucocorticoid-like activity of the progestins.

3. Androgens

a. **Synthesis, secretion, and action. Testosterone** is secreted by the testis and adrenal cortex. Ninety-eight percent is bound by the sex steroid binding globulin and albumin. In target tissues (e.g., Sertoli cells, prostate gland), testosterone is reduced to dihydrotestosterone, which has twice the biologic activity of testosterone. Testosterone is metabolized in the liver to form conjugates and is excreted predominantly in the urine.

(1) Testosterone is responsible for **masculinization.**

    (a) Testosterone is responsible for the development of the accessory sex organs, epididymis, vas deferens, prostate, and seminal vesicles, and the secondary sex characteristics.

    (b) Acting in conjunction with FSH and LH, it promotes spermatogenesis.

    (c) It increases libido.

(2) It has **anabolic effects,** leading to increased protein synthesis (particularly in skeletal muscle), retention of potassium and phosphorus, and increased growth of bone, cartilage, and other tissues.

(3) It increases **erythropoiesis** by promoting the secretion of erythropoietin.

b. Preparations include **testosterone esters, mibolerone, boldenone,** and **stanozolol.** The latter two are weak androgens and are called anabolic steroids.

    (1) Pharmacokinetics

        (a) Testosterone esters are administered intramuscularly. The duration of action may persist for 2–4 weeks. The plasma half-life of testosterone cypionate is 8 days.

        (b) Mibolerone is well absorbed from the gastrointestinal tract after oral administration and is rapidly metabolized in the liver to over ten metabolites. Excretion is equally divided between urine and feces.

        (c) Boldenone and **stanozolol** are well absorbed after intramuscular administration; stanozolol may also be administered orally. The effects of boldenone persist up to 8 weeks, while those of stanozolol persist for at least 1 week.

    (2) Therapeutic uses

        (a) Testosterone has been used:

            (i) To treat impotency and infertility, with variable success

            (ii) To treat urinary incontinence and dermatitis in castrated males

            (iii) To produce a teaser animal in cull cows, heifers, and steers

        (b) Mibolerone, which inhibits gonadotropin secretion, is used as a contraceptive in bitches (2.6 μg/kg/day orally).

        (c) Stanozolol and **boldenone** are used for growth promotion, muscle buildup, and reversal of tissue depletion (e.g., cachexia) and to treat anemia.

    (3) Adverse effects include:

        (a) Infertility or oligospermia

        (b) Perianal adenomas, perineal hernias, prostatic disorders, and behavioral changes (following long-term androgen administration)

        (c) Masculinization of females and female fetuses

        (d) Hepatotoxicity

D. **Uterine contractants.** When used to induce labor, these agents are called **oxytocic** or **ecbolic agents.** When they are used to induce abortion, they are called **abortifacients.**

1. General uterine physiology

    a. Hormonal influence. Estrogen and progesterone influence uterine activity.

        (1) During proestrus and estrus, under the influence of estrogens, the uterus shows large and slow contractions.

        (2) During metestrus–diestrus, under the influence of progesterone, the uterus shows weak and rapid contractions.

        (3) At parturition, a surge of fetal cortisol secretion stimulates estrogen synthesis from progesterone.

            (a) As a result, prostaglandin (PG) synthesis increases, promoting luteolysis.

                (i) The presence of corpus luteum in prepartum animals may inhibit the action of an oxytocic agent; therefore, luteolysis may need to be induced.

                (ii) Because prepartum mares do not have a functional corpus luteum, oxytocic agents alone can effectively induce foaling.

            (b) Oxytocin secretion and the density of oxytocin receptors increase, leading to large and effective uterine contractions that expel the fetuses from the genital tract.

b. Autonomic influence. Adrenergic and cholinergic activities also influence smooth muscle contraction.
   (1) α_1- **and** α_2-**Adrenergic receptors** mediate excitatory responses, whereas β_2-adrenergic receptors mediate inhibitory responses.
   (2) **M_3 muscarinic receptors** mediate excitatory responses.

2. Preparations
   a. Oxytocin is a nonapeptide hypothalamic hormone stored in and released from the posterior pituitary. It is released in response to signals from the genital tract and mammary gland.
   (1) **Actions.** Oxytocin increases uterine contractions and milk ejection and facilitates the transport of sperm in the female genital tract.
   (2) **Therapeutic uses**
      (a) Oxytocin is used to **induce labor** and **reverse uterine inertia.** The cervix must be dilated and the fetus must be in normal presentation position.
      (b) It is used to treat **agalactia** through stimulation of milk ejection. Oxytocin is not a galactopoietic agent.
   (3) **Adverse effects.** Oxytocin may cause **uterine dystocia.**
   b. Ergonovine is an ergot alkaloid that causes prolonged contraction of smooth muscle, including the myometrium and blood vessels.
   (1) **Mechanism of action.** Its effect on smooth muscle is mainly through activation of α-adrenergic receptors and possibly also through serotonergic and dopaminergic receptors.
   (2) **Therapeutic uses**
      (a) Induction of uterine involution
      (b) Postpartum hemorrhage control
      (c) Expulsion of placenta (particularly in cows and bitches) when oxytocin is ineffective
   (3) **Administration.** Ergonovine is administered intramuscularly.
   (4) **Adverse effects.** Ergonovine is safe when given as directed; however, overdosage may cause CNS excitation, muscle weakness, hypertension, and vomiting. It may cause agalactia through inhibition of prolactin release.
   c. Bromocriptine is an ergot alkaloid.
   (1) **Mechanism of action.** Bromocriptine has dopaminergic agonistic activity that inhibits prolactin secretion, resulting in luteolysis. (Prolactin is a luteotropic hormone.)
   (2) **Therapeutic uses**
      (a) It is used to treat **galactorrhea.**
      (b) Bromocriptine has been used **experimentally as a canine abortifacient** because of its luteolytic effect. It is given orally (10–15 μg/kg) twice daily for 3–5 days for this purpose.
   (3) **Adverse effects.** Bromocriptine is safe when used as directed. It has minimal vascular and uterotonic effects. It may cause agalactia in milking animals.
   d. Prostaglandin $F_{2\alpha}$ ($PGF_{2\alpha}$, dinoprost tromethamine) and analogs (e.g., **cloprostenol, fluprostenol, fenprostalene**)
   (1) **Pharmacologic effects**
      (a) PGs cause strong vasoconstriction. The resultant decreased blood supply causes luteolysis and reduction of progesterone synthesis.
      (b) PGs have a strong oxytocic effect, especially in mares.
   (2) **Pharmacokinetics**
      (a) **$PGF_{2\alpha}$ (dinoprost)** is distributed rapidly to tissues after intramuscular administration. In cattle, the serum half-life may be only minutes.
      (b) **Cloprostenol, fenprostalene,** and **fluprostenol.** No information is available. Fenprostalene is apparently more slowly absorbed and eliminated than other PGs.
   (3) **Therapeutic uses**
      (a) **Estrous cycle control in cows.** PGs induce luteolysis of mature corpora lutea, leading to estrus within 2–3 days.

   (b) Early abortion usually occurs within 7 days of injection as a result of luteo-
       lysis.
   (c) Labor induction. In waxing (lactating) mares, PGs induce labor in 30 min-
       utes.
   (d) Pyometra. $PGF_{2\alpha}$ can be used to treat pyometra and effect the **expulsion
       of mummified fetuses.**
   (e) Ovarian cysts. Following treatment with gonadorelin to cause ovulation,
       $PGF_{2\alpha}$ is administered to induce luteolysis.
   (4) Administration. PGs are administered intramuscularly or subcutaneously. The
       dosages of $PGF_{2\alpha}$ analogs are only 5%–20% those of dinoprost because they
       are more resistant to metabolism.
   (5) Adverse effects include placental retention, dystocia, and acute systemic toxic-
       ity (i.e., colic, tachycardia, tachypnea, sweating, decreased rectal tempera-
       ture).
   e. Long-acting glucocorticoids [e.g., **dexamethasone;** see III E 3 e (1) (c)].
      (1) Mechanism of action. These agents can mimic the action of fetal cortisol
          surge, thereby inducing parturition.
      (2) Therapeutic uses and administration. Dexamethasone has been used to in-
          duce parturition in cows, ewes, and sows. In prepartum cows, dexamethasone
          (20 mg intramuscularly) may induce parturition within 48 hours. If dexametha-
          sone administration is followed in 40 hours by dinoprost (30 mg intramuscu-
          larly), calving occurs within 2–5 hours.
      (3) Adverse effects. Placental retention may occur. The adverse effects are usually
          not a problem when glucocorticoids are used as oxytocic agents.

E. | **Corticotropin and adrenal corticosteroids**

   1. General considerations
      a. The **adrenal cortex** serves as a **homeostatic organ,** regulating reactions to stress.
      b. Corticosteroid pathway. The release of adrenal corticosteroids is controlled by a
         pathway that includes the CNS.
         (1) A number of stimuli, including trauma, chemicals, diurnal rhythms, and stress,
             can cause the hypothalamus to release CRH.
         (2) CRH moves down the hypophyseal portal system and stimulates the anterior
             pituitary gland to release **ACTH.**
         (3) ACTH stimulates the adrenal cortex to produce **corticosteroids.**
             (a) Endogenous glucocorticoids include **cortisol** and **corticosterone.**
             (b) Endogenous mineralocorticoids
                 (i) Deoxycorticosterone is produced by the adrenal cortex in response
                     to ACTH stimulation.
                 (ii) Aldosterone secretion is stimulated by serum angiotensin and high po-
                     tassium levels.
         (4) A **negative feedback pathway** maintains homeostasis. When the levels of en-
             dogenous corticosteroids increase, the pituitary–adrenal axis is suppressed and
             the production of CRH and ACTH is decreased.

   2. ACTH is a polypeptide hormone consisting of 39 amino acids.
      a. Preparations. Synthetic ACTH [ACTH (1-24)] possesses the biological activity of
         ACTH and is identical for all species.
      b. Mechanism of action. ACTH receptors are coupled to the G_s–adenylyl cyclase
         system.
      c. Therapeutic uses. ACTH is used mainly as a diagnostic tool for distinguishing the
         two types of adrenal insufficiency.
         (1) Primary adrenal insufficiency. Intramuscular administration of ACTH produces
             little or no increase in cortisol secretion because of the underlying adrenal cor-
             tical dysfunction.
         (2) Secondary adrenal insufficiency (i.e., anterior pituitary dysfunction). ACTH ad-
             ministration produces a large increase in cortisol secretion.
      d. Adverse effects. ACTH (1-24) is safe when used as directed.

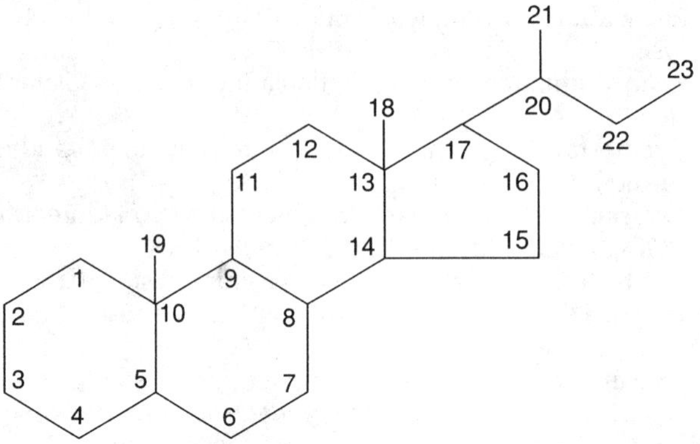

FIGURE 8-1. General structure of the adrenal corticosteroids. Certain structural features relevant to activity. *Positions 1 and 2:* The presence of a double bond (delta group) prolongs the activity, especially glucocorticoid activity. (Most synthetic glucocorticoids have this change.) *Position 3:* The presence of a keto group is essential for corticoid function. *Positions 4 and 5:* The presence of a double bond (delta group) is essential for corticoid function. *Position 6 or 9:* Halogenation or methylation potentiates activity, especially glucocorticoid activity. *Position 11:* The presence of OH increases glucocorticoid activity and the absence of OH increases mineralocorticoid activity. The presence of a keto group abolishes corticoid activity. The 11-keto group has to be converted to 11-OH for action. *Position 16:* The presence of OH or CH_3 increases glucocorticoid activity. (Many synthetic glucocorticoids have this change.) *Position 17:* The presence of OH increases glucocorticoid activity. The presence of acetonide on positions 16 or 17 further enhances and prolongs glucocorticoid activity (many synthetic glucocorticoids for topical use have this change).

3. **Corticosteroids**
    a. **Chemistry.** The general structure of corticosteroids is shown in Figure 8-1.
    b. **Mechanism of action.** Like other steroid hormones, corticosteroids act by controlling the rate of protein synthesis (e.g., aldosterone increases the synthesis of Na^+-K^+-ATPase in the distal renal tubule).
    c. **Pharmacokinetics** (Table 8-1)
        (1) **Absorption.** Corticosteroids are readily absorbed from the gastrointestinal tract, mucous membranes, and skin.

TABLE 8-1. Corticosteroids: Anti-inflammatory and Sodium-retaining Potencies (Oral Administration)

Corticosteroid	Anti-inflammatory Potency	Sodium-retaining Potency
Short-acting (≤12 hr)*		
Hydrocortisone	1	1
Cortisone	0.8	0.8
Fludrocortisone	10	125
Intermediate-acting (12–36 hr)*		
Prednisone	4	0.8
Prednisolone	5	0.8
Methylprednisolone	5	0.5
Triamcinolone	5	0
Long-acting (36–72 hr)*		
Paramethasone	10	0
Betamethasone	25	0
Dexamethasone	25	0
Flumethasone	30	0

* Biologic half-life.

(2) Fate. The majority of corticosteroids are bound by plasma proteins (corticosteroid-binding globulin and albumin).

(3) Metabolism

   (a) The C3 keto group is reduced to an -OH group, which then undergoes conjugation.

   (b) Reduction of the C11 keto group to an -OH group is necessary to convert cortisone to cortisol (hydrocortisone) and prednisone to prednisolone, their biologically active forms.

(4) Excretion. The conjugates are excreted by the kidneys.

d. Activity

(1) Glucocorticoids

   (a) Metabolic effects. Glucocorticoids increase liver glycogen synthesis and storage, gluconeogenesis, and lipolysis and redistribution of lipids.

   (b) CNS effects. They stimulate the CNS, leading to euphoria.

   (c) Cardiovascular effects. They maintain cardiovascular function by potentiating catecholamines.

   (d) Muscular effects. At physiologic doses, glucocorticoids maintain skeletal muscle function; however, at pharmacologic doses, wasting of muscle mass occurs.

   (e) Effects on blood

   (i) Polycythemia results from decreased erythrophagocytosis.

   (ii) Neutrophilia results from increased entry of neutrophils into the circulation, combined with decreased removal of cells from the circulation. The function of neutrophils, however, is suppressed.

   (iii) Eosinopenia, monocytopenia, and **lymphocytopenia** result from redistribution of these cells to systems other than blood. Proliferation of B lymphocytes and activation of T lymphocytes are suppressed.

   (f) Anti-inflammatory and antiallergic effects occur with **pharmacologic doses.**

   (i) Involution of the lymph nodes, thymus, and spleen occurs.

   (ii) Leukocyte migration and function are suppressed.

   (iii) Plasma and lysosomal membranes are stabilized, resulting in decreased autacoid release. This membrane-stabilizing effect is attributed to a decrease in phospholipase A_2 activity.

   (iv) PG and leukotriene (LT) syntheses are suppressed as a result of inhibition of phospholipase A_2.

   (v) Fibroblast activity, collagen synthesis, and tissue repair are reduced in inflamed areas.

   (vi) Glucocorticoids decrease capillary permeability, which is associated with the release of autacoids (especially histamine).

   (vii) At massive doses, the production of antibodies and lymphokines may be inhibited.

(2) Mineralocorticoids. Mineralocorticoids increase sodium and bicarbonate retention and decrease retention of potassium and chloride by changing reabsorption activity in the renal tubules and, to a lesser extent, in the gastrointestinal tract.

e. Preparations and therapeutic uses

(1) Glucocorticoids

   (a) Short-acting drugs (see Table 8-1) are available without prescription for topical use.

   (b) Intermediate-acting drugs (see Table 8-1) are used for long-term control of allergy, chronic inflammation (e.g., arthritis), and immunosuppression.

   (c) Long-acting drugs (see Table 8-1)

   (i) Long-acting drugs are used for the immediate relief of hypersensitivity and shock and the long-term control of allergy in cats. They are used topically to treat pruritus and inflammation associated with allergy.

   (ii) They may be used to induce parturition [see III D 2 e (2)].

(2) Mineralocorticoids

        (a) **Aldosterone** is not available as a pharmacologic agent because of its short duration of action.

        (b) **Deoxycorticosterone** and **fludrocortisone** are used as mineralocorticoid replacements in hypoadrenocorticism. Fludrocortisone has high mineralocorticoid and glucocorticoid potency; thus, it is the preferred drug for the treatment of hypoadrenocorticism.

  f. Administration

    (1) Oral. All synthetic corticosteroids can be administered orally. Alternate-day oral administration of an intermediate-acting drug helps reduce the inhibition of ACTH secretion.

    (2) Intravenous. Water-soluble drugs (e.g., the succinate, phosphate, and polyethylene glycol forms) may be given intravenously.

    (3) Intramuscular administration of steroids may be performed at weekly intervals for chronic use.

    (4) Topical. Water-insoluble drugs are available in cream and ointment forms.

  g. Adverse effects

    (1) Iatrogenic hypoadrenocorticism may follow withdrawal from long-term use of high doses.

    (2) Toxic effects following continued use of high doses are extensions of the pharmacologic effects and include:

      (a) Decreased wound healing

      (b) Increased susceptibility to infection

      (c) Fluid and electrolyte imbalance

      (d) Myopathy

      (e) Osteoporosis, as a result of calcium absorption from the gastrointestinal tract and reabsorption from the kidney

      (f) Edema (from increased sodium retention)

      (g) Liver degeneration in dogs

      (h) Gastrointestinal ulceration

      (i) Diabetes mellitus, particularly when used chronically in animals that already have mild diabetes

      (j) Abortion in late pregnancy

  h. Contraindications include uncontrolled infections, diabetes mellitus, corneal ulcers, cardiac disorders, burns, and pregnancy.

4. Adrenal steroid inhibitors

  a. Mitotane (o,p'-DDD)

    (1) Chemistry. Mitotane is related to DDT, an insecticide. It is a lipophilic drug.

    (2) Mechanism of action. Its mechanism of action is not understood. Mitotane is cytotoxic to the zonae fasciculata and reticularis of the adrenal cortex, which secrete all endogenous steroids except aldosterone. The zona glomerulosa, which secretes aldosterone, is not affected by mitotane.

    (3) Pharmacokinetics. No information related to use in domestic animals is available.

    (4) Therapeutic uses include hyperadrenocorticism (Cushing's syndrome) and adrenal adenoma and carcinoma.

    (5) Administration. Mitotane is administered orally (25 mg/kg twice daily for 10–14 days, followed by 25–50 mg/kg once per week).

    (6) Adverse effects

      (a) Animals may show lethargy, ataxia, weakness, anorexia, vomiting, or diarrhea, attributable to lowered corticosteroid secretion.

      (b) Hepatotoxicity (i.e., congestion, centrolobular atrophy, and fatty degeneration) may be seen.

      (c) Mitotane-induced hypoadrenocorticism may occur.

        (i) In approximately 5% of dogs treated with mitotane, fludrocortisone may be needed as replacement therapy.

        (ii) All animals treated with mitotane should receive glucocorticoid supplementation when undergoing stress.

  b. Ketoconazole (see Chapter 11 XII B) inhibits adrenal steroidogenesis and is being studied for use in the treatment of hyperadrenocorticism that is resistant to mitotane. The recommended dose is 15 mg/kg twice daily for as long as necessary.

F. Antidiabetic agents

1. **Introduction. Diabetes mellitus** is usually seen in adult animals, particularly dogs and cats older than 7 years of age.
   a. **Insulin-dependent diabetes (IDD)** is the most frequently seen type of diabetes. Animals with this disease do not have any significant secretion of insulin from β cells.
   b. **Non–insulin-dependent diabetes (NIDD).** Animals with this disease do have significant insulin-secreting ability. They may or may not be obese. Their basal insulin levels may be lower or higher than those of unaffected animals; however, their responses to glucose are usually poor. As β cells are destroyed by high plasma glucose concentrations, NIDD may progress to IDD.

2. **Insulin** remains the most frequently used antidiabetic agent in veterinary medicine.
   a. **Synthesis, secretion, and action**
      (1) **Synthesis.** Insulin consists of two peptide chains joined by disulfide linkages.
         (a) Pancreatic β cells synthesize insulin from a single-chain precursor, proinsulin, which possesses little biologic activity.
         (b) The amino acid sequence of insulin varies among species.
            (i) Porcine and canine insulin are identical, and are similar to human insulin.
            (ii) Feline and bovine insulin are similar in structure.
      (2) **Secretion.** Insulin secretion is controlled by blood glucose levels, gastrointestinal hormones, and the autonomic nervous system.
         (a) **Stimulation.** Insulin secretion is increased by glucose, amino acids, fatty acids (especially butyric acid in ruminants), calcium, and gastrointestinal hormones (e.g., secretin, gastrin, cholecystokinin, glucagon, glucagon-like polypeptides, gastric inhibitory polypeptides, vasoactive intestinal polypeptides). Amino acids may stimulate the secretion of gastrointestinal hormones.
         (b) **Inhibition.** Insulin secretion is inhibited by somatostatin, galanin, and epinephrine.
         (c) **Autonomic influences**
            (i) Epinephrine and norepinephrine inhibit insulin secretion by activating α_2-adrenergic receptors.
            (ii) In the presence of α_2-receptor blockade, epinephrine and norepinephrine stimulate insulin secretion by activating β_2-adrenergic receptors.
            (iii) Acetylcholine (ACh) stimulates insulin secretion by activating M_3 receptors.
      (3) **Actions**
         (a) **Carbohydrate metabolism.** Insulin decreases blood glucose concentrations by increasing glycogen synthesis, decreasing hepatic glycogenolysis, decreasing gluconeogenesis, and increasing glucose transport into cells. Hepatocytes, erythrocytes, leukocytes, adrenal medullary chromaffin cells, and brain cells do not require insulin for glucose transport.
         (b) **Fat metabolism.** Insulin increases lipid synthesis and decreases lipolysis.
         (c) **Protein metabolism.** Insulin increases the uptake of amino acids and protein synthesis.
         (d) **Potassium metabolism.** Insulin increases uptake of potassium ions into cells through activation of the Na^+-K^+-ATPase pump.
   b. **Mechanism of action.** Insulin binds to its receptors and stimulates tyrosine kinase, which is a part of the receptor. The activation of tyrosine kinase causes phosphorylation of the insulin receptor and other proteins, generating mediators of insulin action (see also I C 2).
   c. **Pharmacokinetics.** Insulin is metabolized by enzymes in the liver and kidney. Peptidases in the blood also inactivate insulin. The plasma half-life of insulin is approximately 5 minutes, but the biologic half-life is longer (several hours).

d. Preparations. Commercial insulin preparations are mostly of human origin and are produced using a recombinant DNA technique.

(1) **Crystalline zinc insulin (regular insulin)** is a short-acting, soluble insulin that is prepared in a phosphate buffer with zinc at a pH of 3.5.

    (a) **Pharmacokinetics.** Onset of effect occurs within 15 minutes of subcutaneous injection, peaks within 2–4 hours, and lasts 5–7 hours.

    (b) **Administration.** It can be administered subcutaneously or intravenously. Injections must be given 4–5 times daily.

    (c) **Therapeutic uses.** Crystalline zinc insulin is useful for rapidly resolving diabetic ketoacidosis. The frequency with which regular insulin must be administered makes it inconvenient for maintenance of normal plasma glucose levels.

(2) **Isophane insulin (NPH)** is an intermediate-acting insulin that contains a small amount of protamine (0.3–0.4 mg/100 U insulin), a basic protein that slows down the absorption of insulin. The onset of action for NPH insulin occurs within 2 hours. Peak effect occurs in 8–12 hours and lasts 24–48 hours.

(3) **Lente insulins** do not contain protamine. Their insolubility results from the addition of zinc in an acetate, rather than a phosphate, buffer. The onset of action for the lente insulin depends on the physical state, the zinc concentration, and the pH.

    (a) **Semilente insulin** is a microamorphous form of insulin. Peak effect occurs in 4–8 hours and has a duration of action of 12–16 hours.

    (b) **Ultralente insulin** is a large crystalline form of insulin with a high zinc content. Its onset and duration of action are similar to those of protamine zinc insulin [see III F 2 d (4)].

    (c) **Lente insulin** is seven parts ultralente and three parts semilente. It is quite similar to isophane insulin in its onset and duration of action.

(4) **Protamine zinc insulin.** The addition of protamine to crystalline zinc insulin causes the formation of large crystals.

    (a) **Pharmacokinetics.** When injected, this formulation serves as a tissue depot, producing slow absorption into the blood stream. The action of protamine zinc insulin begins in 4 hours, peaks in 16–18 hours, and lasts up to 36 hours.

    (b) **Therapeutic uses.** Fine control of hyperglycemia is difficult with such a long-acting preparation. However, because of its prolonged action, protamine zinc insulin is convenient for use in veterinary medicine.

e. Adverse effects

(1) **Hypoglycemia.** Early signs of hypoglycemia (e.g., tachycardia, hunger) result from epinephrine release. "**Insulin shock,**" the worst sequela of hypoglycemia, is characterized by CNS disturbances, including convulsions and coma. Hypoglycemia is best treated with intravenous glucose administration.

(2) **Insulin resistance.** Some diabetic animals may experience insulin resistance at the receptor level.

    (a) Insulin antibodies may attenuate responses to exogenous insulin. They are more likely to develop in cats than in dogs given human or porcine insulin preparations.

    (b) Stress may induce acute insulin resistance by increasing secretion of epinephrine and corticosteroids.

3. Sulfonylureas (e.g., **glipizide**) are rarely used in veterinary medicine.

a. Mechanism of action. Sulfonylureas stimulate insulin secretion of pancreatic β cells.

(1) They block ATP-sensitive potassium channels, which decreases potassium exit from β cells.

(2) Retention of intracellular potassium leads to depolarization of the plasma membrane, which activates VDCCs.

(3) Opening of the VDCCs promotes calcium entry and elevates intracellular calcium concentrations. Calcium evokes exocytosis, resulting in insulin release.

b. **Therapeutic uses.** Glipizide has been used with some success to treat NIDD in cats.

c. **Adverse effects.** Glipizide is safe when used as directed. Overdose-induced hypoglycemia is milder than that induced by insulin and is usually not life-threatening.

G. Thyroid hormones and antithyroid agents

1. **Thyroid hormones**
   a. **Synthesis** (Figure 8-2)
      (1) **Thyroglobulin (TG),** a large glycoprotein, is synthesized in the thyroid gland and transported into the follicular lumen (colloid).
      (2) The tyrosines on TG are iodinated to form **monoiodotyrosine (MIT)** and **diiodotyrosine (DIT).**
         (a) **Thyroxine (T$_4$)** is formed by the coupling of DITs.
         (b) **Triiodothyronine (T$_3$)** is formed from MIT and DIT.
      (3) Endocytosis and proteolysis of TG from colloid release T$_3$ and T$_4$ into follicular cells. The hormones are then transported out of the cells into the circulation.
   b. **Secretion. Thyrotropin (TSH)** stimulates thyroid hormone secretion by increasing sodium iodide uptake, oxidation and coupling processes, and endocytosis and proteolysis of TG.
      (1) Other anions, such as nitrate, thiocyanate, and perchlorate, inhibit sodium iodide uptake by competing with iodide for active transport.
      (2) Thioureylene drugs (e.g., methimazole) inhibit oxidation and coupling processes.
   c. **Pharmacokinetics**
      (1) **Absorption.** T$_3$ and T$_4$ are readily absorbed from the gastrointestinal tract when given orally.

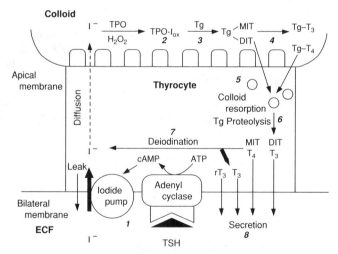

FIGURE 8-2. Iodide uptake, organification, and secretion by the thyroid cell. (*1*) Inorganic iodide (*I⁻*) is transported into the follicular cell from the extracellular fluid (*ECF*) via active transport. The maintenance of the sodium gradient via the Na⁺-K⁺-ATPase pump appears to be important for this process. This step is stimulated by the interaction of thyroid-stimulating hormone (*TSH*) with its receptor, which leads to the activation of adenylyl cyclase. (*2*) After diffusing to the apical plasma membrane, the iodide is oxidized by thyroid peroxidase enzyme (*TPO*). (*3*) The oxidized iodide is then organified onto tyrosine residues of preformed thyroglobulin (*TG*) to form monoiodotyrosine (*MIT*) and diiodotyrosine (*DIT*). (*4*) The MIT and DIT residues on TG couple to form triiodothyronine (*T$_3$*). Two DIT residues couple to form thyroxine (*T$_4$*). (*5*) Under the stimulus of TSH, follicular colloid containing TG is resorbed into the thyroid cell. (*6*) Thyroid hormones, MIT, and DIT are released from TG under the stimulus of TSH. (*7*) At the time of secretion, TSH also stimulates deiodinase enzymes, which convert T$_4$ to T$_3$ and rT$_3$ and deiodinate the iodotyrosines, allowing the recycling of iodide. (*8*) T$_4$, T$_3$, and rT$_3$ are released into the circulation. (Redrawn with permission from Peterson ME: *Hyperthyroid diseases*. In *Textbook of Veterinary Internal Medicine*, 4th ed. Edited by Ettinger SJ and Feldman EC. Philadelphia, WB Saunders, 1995, p 1479.) *ATP* = adenosine triphosphate; *cAMP* = cyclic adenosine monophosphate.

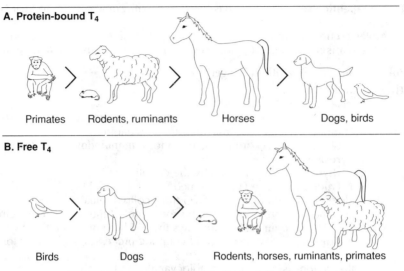

A. Protein-bound T$_4$

Primates   Rodents, ruminants   Horses   Dogs, birds

B. Free T$_4$

Birds   Dogs   Rodents, horses, ruminants, primates

FIGURE 8-3. Thyroxine (T$_4$) binding activity by species.

(2) Fate
  (a) Both T$_3$ and T$_4$ are bound by plasma proteins [e.g., thyroxine-binding globulin (TBG) and albumin]. High estrogen levels promote synthesis of TBG, leading to increased total T$_3$ and T$_4$ concentrations in the plasma.
  (b) Plasma protein-binding activities of thyroid hormones differ among animal species (Figure 8-3).
(3) Metabolism
  (a) Thirty to forty percent of T$_4$ is converted to T$_3$, thereby increasing biologic activity in the liver, kidney, and other peripheral tissues.
  (b) Fifteen to twenty percent of T$_4$ and nearly 100% of T$_3$ form conjugates with glucuronic acid and sulfuric acid in the liver. These conjugates are then excreted in the bile. Through enterohepatic circulation, some T$_3$ and T$_4$ are liberated and reabsorbed from the GI tract.
  (c) Fifty percent of T$_4$ is converted in peripheral tissues to reverse T$_3$, which is an inactive metabolite.
(4) Plasma half-lives
  (a) In humans, the plasma half-lives of T$_4$ and T$_3$ are 6–7 days and 1 day, respectively.
  (b) In dogs, the plasma half-lives of T$_4$ and T$_3$ are 12–24 hours and 6 hours, respectively.
  (c) Factors affecting plasma half-lives
     (i) Hyperthyroidism and hypothyroidism shorten and lengthen the plasma half-life of T$_4$, respectively.
     (ii) Increased TBG levels increase plasma half-lives.
     (iii) Decreased plasma protein levels decrease plasma half-lives.
     (iv) Other drugs that compete for albumin binding sites increase T$_3$ and T$_4$ levels, leading to decreased plasma half-lives.
  (5) Excretion. Twenty to forty percent of administered T$_4$ is excreted in the feces.
 d. Activity. T$_3$ is three to five times as active as T$_4$.
  (1) Thyroid hormones **promote growth and development.**
  (2) Thyroid hormones **increase the basal metabolic rate;** therefore, they are **calorigenic.**
  (3) They are **cardiac stimulants.** In addition to being directly inotropic, they increase cardiac output and enhance the susceptibility of the heart to catecholamines.
  (4) They **enhance carbohydrate utilization** and **lipolysis** (the latter effect leads to a decrease in plasma cholesterol).

e. Preparations
   (1) Levothyroxine is **T$_4$**.
   (2) Liothyronine is the drug name for **T$_3$**.
f. Administration. Because of different plasma protein-binding activities of thyroid hormones in humans and dogs, human dosages should not be used in dogs.
   (1) Levothyroxine. The initial dose in dogs is 20 μg/kg/day, orally.
   (2) Liothyronine. The initial dose in dogs is 5 μg/kg orally, two to three times daily.
   (3) Doses may need to be adjusted following the initial dose.

2. Antithyroid agents
   a. Thioureylenes (methimazole)
      (1) Mechanism of action. Methimazole inhibits the synthesis of T$_3$ and T$_4$ [III G b (2)].
      (2) Pharmacokinetics
         (a) After oral administration, the elimination half-life is 2.3–10.2 hours. Because of the high plasma-binding activity of thyroid hormones, plasma levels of T$_3$ and T$_4$ decline slowly. Significant reductions are usually reported within 1–3 weeks.
         (b) Bioavailability and volume of distribution are variable.
      (3) Adverse effects. Anorexia, vomiting, lethargy, pruritus, hepatopathy, bleeding, thrombocytopenia, agranulocytosis, leukopenia, eosinophilia, and lymphocytosis may occur.
   b. Radioactive iodide (Na^{131}I)
      (1) Mechanism of action. Na^{131}I destroys thyroid follicular cells. Therefore, it is an alternative to surgical thyroidectomy, which can be risky.
      (2) Pharmacokinetics. Na^{131}I is rapidly incorporated into the thyroid follicles. It has a half-life of 8 days and emits β particles and γ ray. Control of hyperthyroidism may be delayed.
      (3) Administration. Na^{131}I is administered intravenously or orally.
      (4) Adverse effects. Hypothyroidism may result.
      (5) Contraindications. Na^{131}I is contraindicated in pregnant and nursing queens.

H. Agents for the treatment of hypocalcemia

1. Regulation of serum calcium
   a. Secretion and actions of parathyroid hormone (PTH). PTH is secreted from the parathyroid gland. Its secretion is increased in response to hypocalcemia and decreased in response to hypercalcemia. PTH increases calcium and decreases phosphate levels in the extracellular fluid (ECF).
      (1) It acts on the bone, small intestine, and kidneys to transfer calcium to the ECF.
      (2) It increases the absorption of calcium from the small intestine. (This is a vitamin D-dependent process.)
      (3) It increases the rate of resorption of calcium and phosphate from bone.
      (4) It increases renal tubular reabsorption of calcium and the excretion of phosphate.
   b. Secretion and actions of calcitonin. Calcitonin is secreted from the parafollicular cells of the thyroid gland. Its secretion is increased in response to hypercalcemia and decreased in response to hypocalcemia. Calcitonin decreases calcium and phosphate levels in the ECF.
      (1) Calcitonin acts on the bone and kidneys to decrease the transfer of calcium and phosphate to the ECF.
      (2) It decreases the rate of resorption of calcium and phosphate from the bone.
      (3) It decreases renal tubular reabsorption of calcium and phosphate.

2. Preparations used to treat hypocalcemia
   a. Calcium gluconate
      (1) Pharmacokinetics
         (a) Absorption. Calcium is absorbed from the small intestine.
            (i) Vitamin D$_3$, PTH, and an acidic pH facilitate absorption.
            (ii) Dietary fiber, phytates, fatty acids, steatorrhea, and uremia interfere with absorption.

        (b) Fate. After absorption, calcium enters the ECF and then is readily incorporated into bone. Nearly 99% of total body calcium is found in bone. Of circulating calcium, approximately 50% is bound to serum proteins or complexes with anions and the other 50% is in free calcium ion, which is distributed to all tissues, including the CNS and placenta.

        (c) Excretion. Both unabsorbed calcium and calcium excreted into the bile and pancreatic juice are eliminated primarily in the feces. Only a small amount of calcium is excreted in the urine because most of it is reabsorbed from the renal tubules.

    (2) Therapeutic uses include **hypocalcemia** and **cardiac arrhythmias** induced by hyperkalemia.

    (3) Administration

        (a) Calcium gluconate is usually administered to effect by **slow intravenous injection.**

        (b) Intraperitoneal injection may also be used.

        (c) Long-term therapy can be accomplished by increasing dietary calcium and administering vitamin D (dihydrotachysterol; see III H 2 b).

    (4) Adverse effects

        (a) Hypercalcemia may occur, particularly in animals with cardiac or renal disease.

        (b) Rapid intravenous injections of calcium gluconate can cause **hypotension, arrhythmias,** and **cardiac arrest.** Treatment should be discontinued in the presence of elevated ST segments, shortened QT intervals, or arrhythmias.

    (5) Contraindications include ventricular fibrillation, hypercalcemia, renal or cardiac disease, and concurrent treatment with digitalis.

  b. Dihydrotachysterol (DHT)

    (1) Chemistry. DHT is a vitamin D_2 analog.

    (2) Mechanism of action

        (a) Vitamin D and its analogs increase the synthesis of calcium-binding proteins through promotion of mRNA synthesis.

        (b) Vitamin D metabolites rapidly increase calcium influx by activating the receptors in the plasma membrane.

    (3) Pharmacologic effects. DHT increases serum concentrations of calcium and phosphate by:

        (a) Increasing calcium and phosphorus absorption

        (b) Decreasing calcium and phosphorus excretion from the kidney

        (c) Increasing bone resorption

    (4) Pharmacokinetics

        (a) Absorption. Vitamin D analogs are absorbed from the small intestine when lipid absorption is normal. The presence of steatorrhea or hepatic or renal disease will decrease absorption.

        (b) Fate

            (i) Vitamin D and its analogs circulate in plasma tightly bound to a carrier protein, the vitamin D-binding globulin.

            (ii) DHT is hydroxylated in the liver to 25(OH)DHT, which is the active form of the drug. DHT does not need to undergo 1-hydroxylation in the kidney for further activation.

            (iii) Excess DHT is stored in adipose tissue.

        (c) Excretion. The metabolic clearance rate of DHT is not known.

    (5) Therapeutic uses. DHT is used to treat **hypocalcemia** associated with hypoparathyroidism or severe renal failure.

    (6) Adverse effects include **hypercalcemia, hyperphosphatemia,** and **nephrocalcinosis.**

STUDY QUESTIONS

DIRECTIONS: Each of the numbered items or incomplete statements in this section is followed by answers or by completions of the statement. Select the **one** numbered answer or completion that is **best** in each case.

1. Oxytocin without a preceding prostaglandin $F_{2\alpha}$ treatment can consistently induce parturition in:

(1) mares.
(2) sows.
(3) cows.
(4) bitches.

2. Which of the following is a preferred drug for the treatment of postpartum hemorrhage and uterine involution?

(1) Oxytocin
(2) Bromocriptine
(3) Cloprostenol
(4) Dexamethasone
(5) Ergonovine

3. Chronic administration of a glucocorticoid may:

(1) induce anemia.
(2) increase the amount of adipose tissue in the body by decreasing lipolysis.
(3) induce osteoporosis.
(4) induce lymphocytosis.

4. Frequent administration of which one of the following sex steroids in animals would most likely inhibit growth of the adrenal cortex and adrenocorticotropic hormone (ACTH) secretion?

(1) Boldenone
(2) Estradiol
(3) Megestrol
(4) Stanozolol

5. Which of the following steroids is used to treat anemia?

(1) Deoxycorticosterone
(2) Estradiol
(3) Medroxyprogesterone
(4) Boldenone

6. Administration of mibolerone in bitches as an oral contraceptive may cause:

(1) masculinization.
(2) pyometra.
(3) aplastic anemia.
(4) bone fracture.
(5) diabetes mellitus.

7. All of the following statements concerning agents for treatment of hypocalcemia are true *except*:

(1) only a small amount of calcium administered is excreted in the urine.
(2) calcium gluconate is also used for the treatment of cardiac arrhythmias induced by hyperkalemia.
(3) dihydrotachysterol (DHT), like parathyroid hormone (PTH), elevates serum calcium concentrations and lowers serum phosphate concentrations.
(4) DHT is metabolized in the liver to a 25(OH)-metabolite, which is the active form of the drug.

8. Use of a glucocorticoid is contraindicated in all of the following conditions *except*:

(1) diabetes mellitus.
(2) corneal ulceration.
(3) anaphylactic shock.
(4) infection uncontrolled by antibiotics.
(5) burns.

9. All of the following statements concerning antidiabetic agents are true *except*:

(1) commercial insulin preparations are mostly of human origin.
(2) hepatocytes, erythrocytes, leukocytes, adrenal medullary chromaffin cells, and brain cells do not require insulin to transport glucose.
(3) dogs are more likely than cats to develop insulin antibodies to porcine or human insulin preparations.
(4) glipizide, a sulfonylurea, has been used with some success to treat non–insulin-dependent diabetes (NIDD) in cats.

10. All of the following progestins are effective when administered orally to an animal *except*:

(1) progesterone.
(2) megestrol.
(3) melengestrol.
(4) altrenogest.

ANSWERS AND EXPLANATIONS

1. The answer is 1 [*III D 1 a (3) (a)*].
The presence of a corpus luteum may inhibit the action of an oxytocic agent. Because prepartum mares do not have a functional corpus luteum, oxytocin can effectively induce foaling. All prepartum sows, cows, and bitches have corpora lutea; therefore, luteolysis must occur [or be induced, for example, with prostaglandin $F_{2\alpha}$ ($PGF_{2\alpha}$)] before an oxytocic agent can work effectively.

2. The answer is 5 [*III D 2 b (2)*].
Ergonovine causes prolonged contraction of myometrium and uterine blood vessels; therefore, it is a preferred drug for the treatment of postpartum hemorrhage and uterine involution. Oxytocin is a peptide hormone that evokes short-term uterine contractions. Bromocriptine at therapeutic doses has an insignificant effect on smooth muscle contraction. Cloprostenol is a prostaglandin $F_{2\alpha}$ ($PGF_{2\alpha}$) analog that is used to induce parturition and abortion, to treat pyometra, and to expel mummified fetuses. Dexamethasone is used to induce parturition.

3. The answer is 3 [*III E 3 g*].
Glucocorticoids may create a negative calcium balance by inhibiting calcium absorption from the gastrointestinal tract and reabsorption from the kidney. Glucocorticoids induce polycythemia, lipolysis, and lymphocytopenia.

4. The answer is 3 [*III C 2 b (3) (c)*].
Progestins, such as megestrol, have glucocorticoid-like activities that can inhibit adrenocorticotropic hormone (ACTH) secretion, inducing iatrogenic hypoadrenocorticism. Estrogens (e.g., estradiol) and androgens (e.g., stanozolol, boldenone) do not have significant glucocorticoid activities.

5. The answer is 4 [*III C 3 a (3), b (2) (c)*].
Androgens increase erythropoiesis by promoting erythropoietin synthesis. Therefore, androgens such as boldenone can be used to treat anemia.

6. The answer is 1 [*III C 3 b (3) (c)*].
Mibolerone, an androgen, may cause masculinization of females and female fetuses.

7. The answer is 3 [*III H 1 a (4), 2 b (3)*].
Dihydrotachysterol (DHT) elevates both serum calcium and phosphate concentrations. Like parathyroid hormone (PTH), DHT increases serum calcium concentrations by promoting calcium and phosphorus resorption from the gastrointestinal tract and bone and by deceasing calcium excretion from the kidney. However, unlike PTH, DHT decreases phosphorus excretion from the kidney.

8. The answer is 3 [*III E 3 h*].
Glucocorticoids are not contraindicated in anaphylactic shock. They should not be used in animals with corneal ulceration, diabetes mellitus, infections uncontrolled by antibiotics, or burns.

9. The answer is 3 [*III F 2 d, e (2), 3 b*].
Following administration of a human or porcine insulin preparation, cats are more likely than dogs to develop insulin antibodies. Most commercial products are developed using recombinant DNA techniques and are of human origin. Hepatocytes, erythrocytes, leukocytes, adrenal medullary chromaffin cells, and brain cells do not require insulin for glucose transport. Glipizide, a sulfonylurea, has been used with some success to treat non–insulin-dependent diabetes (NIDD).

10. The answer is 1 [*III C 2 b (1)*].
Progesterone is a natural steroid that is rapidly inactivated by liver enzymes following absorption from the gastrointestinal tract. Synthetic progestins (e.g., megestrol, melengestrol, altrenogest) are more resistant to liver enzymes.

Chapter 9

Nonnarcotic Analgesics and Nonsteroidal Anti-inflammatory Drugs

Walter H. Hsu

I. PROSTAGLANDIN (PG) SYNTHESIS INHIBITORS

A. Overview

1. **Pharmacologic effects** (Table 9-1)
   a. **Analgesia.** By blocking cyclooxygenase (PG synthase), PG inhibitors prevent the formation of PGE_2, PGI_2, and $PGF_{2\alpha}$. These substances are thought to play a role in the vasodilation, pain, and edema associated with inflammation.
   b. **Antipyretic action.** PG inhibitors impair the ability of pyrogens to raise the set point of the temperature-regulating mechanism in the hypothalamus. As a result, cutaneous vasodilation, sweating, and panting are stimulated.
   c. **Anti-inflammatory action.** The anti-inflammatory effect of PG inhibitors is attributed to stabilization of lysosomal membranes, inhibition of the complement system, phagocytosis, leukocyte accumulation, synthesis of mucopolysaccharides and histamine, antagonism of bradykinin's actions, induction of oxygen radical scavenger action, and uncoupling of oxidative phosphorylation to deprive inflammatory tissues of energy.
   d. **Anticoagulant effect.** PG inhibitors inhibit synthesis of thromboxanes, which encourage platelet aggregation.

2. **Adverse effects.** PG inhibitors frequently cause gastrointestinal erosions and ulcers.

B. Aspirin (acetylsalicylate) and other salicylates

1. **Mechanism of action.** Aspirin irreversibly blocks cyclooxygenase.

2. **Pharmacokinetics**
   a. **Absorption.** Salicylates are readily absorbed from the stomach and upper intestine. Gastric acidity enhances absorption by favoring deionization.
   b. **Fate**
      (1) Salicylates are inactive but quickly convert to **salicylic acid,** which is active.
      (2) In animals, salicylate metabolism is primarily through conjugation with glucuronic acid **(glucuronidation).**
         (a) Because of varying glucuronidation capabilities plasma half-lives ($t_{1/2}$) vary extensively among species (e.g., from 30 hours in cats to 5 hours in horses).
         (b) Cats are highly sensitive to aspirin toxicity because they have limited glucuronidation capabilities. When glucuronidation is exhausted, salicylates form conjugates with glutathione.

3. **Therapeutic uses.** Aspirin is more readily available than other salicylates.
   a. Aspirin is used primarily for relief of minor pain, particularly that of musculoskeletal origin (e.g., arthritis).
   b. Because of its activity in inhibiting platelet aggregation, aspirin is used for treatment of **disseminated intravascular coagulation secondary to malignancy, pancreatitis, chronic hepatitis, heat stroke,** and **sepsis.**
   c. Aspirin is useful as **adjunct therapy for septic and endotoxic shock.**
      (1) It is especially helpful in animals with severe infections.
      (2) Aspirin increases the survival rate by decreasing the formation of mediators (e.g., PGs) and inhibiting platelet aggregation.

TABLE 9-1. Nonnarcotic Analgesics

Class	Therapeutic Uses	Advantages
PG inhibitors	Relief of mild to moderate pain (e.g., cephalgia, myalgia, arthralgia); fever reduction; inflammation reduction*; anticoagulation	Do not produce tolerance or physical dependence
α_2-Adrenergic agonists	Relief of moderate to severe superficial and deep visceral pain as well as sharp, intense pain; sedation	Sedative effect particularly useful in veterinary medicine

PG = prostaglandin.
* Except acetaminophen.

      d. Aspirin is used as an **adjunct to thiacetarsamide therapy** in the treatment of heartworm in dogs. Aspirin may reduce the incidence of pulmonary thromboembolism associated with thiacetarsamide.

  4. Administration
    a. For **cats,** 10 mg/kg of aspirin are administered every 48 hours.
    b. For **dogs,** 10 mg/kg of aspirin are administered every 12 hours.

  5. Adverse effects
    a. Gastrointestinal signs (e.g., vomiting, anorexia, gastric ulceration)
    b. Depression
    c. Bone marrow hypoplasia
    d. Pulmonary edema may occur in sheep.
    e. Toxicity. Higher salicylate dosages cause toxic effects; therefore, dosages should not be increased in an attempt to relieve intense pain.
      (1) Effects
        (a) Hyperpyrexia may occur because of uncoupling of oxidative phosphorylation.
        (b) Acid–base disturbances
          (i) Respiratory alkalosis, the result of hyperventilation caused by direct stimulation of the medullary receptor center, may occur first.
          (ii) Respiratory acidosis may follow, as a result of central nervous system (CNS) depression.
          (iii) Metabolic acidosis may result from: the release of H^+ from salicylic acid; uncoupling of oxidative phosphorylation, which increases the buildup of pyruvic and lactic acids; increased fat metabolism, which leads to ketoacidosis; or depression of renal function, which results in accumulation of sulfuric and phosphoric acids.
        (c) Dehydration may result from vomiting, sweating, or hyperpyrexia.
      (2) Treatment for toxicity includes:
        (a) Gastric lavage followed by administration of activated charcoal or **peritoneal dialysis** may be used to remove the drug.
        (b) Administration of sodium bicarbonate raises the urinary pH, thereby increasing urinary excretion of aspirin.
        (c) Fluid therapy corrects metabolic acidosis and dehydration.

  6. Drug interactions
    a. Salicylates often displace other drugs from plasma protein binding sites.
    b. Coumarin and aspirin have additive anticoagulant effects.

C. **Acetaminophen**

  1. Mechanism of action. Acetaminophen reversibly blocks cyclooxygenase.

  2. Pharmacokinetics
    a. Absorption. Acetaminophen is rapidly absorbed from the gastrointestinal tract.

    b. Fate. Acetaminophen is 80%–90% conjugated in the liver, mostly with glucuronic acid and to a much lesser extent with sulfuric acid and cysteine. It is then excreted within 24 hours in the urine.

      (1) Small amounts of hydroxylated metabolites are ordinarily excreted. At high doses of acetaminophen, one of these metabolites forms **N-acetyl-p-benzoquinone,** the metabolite thought to be responsible for toxicity.

      (2) Because cats have very limited ability for glucuronidation, glutathione conjugation takes over. Upon depletion of glutathione, *N*-acetyl-*p*-benzoquinone accumulates, producing adverse effects.

3. Pharmacologic effects. Acetaminophen has analgesic and antipyretic actions, but it does not have apparent anti-inflammatory action.

4. Therapeutic uses. Acetaminophen has little value in veterinary medicine and is not recommended for use in cats.

5. Adverse effects

    a. Hemolytic anemia and **hepatic necrosis** result from acetaminophen-induced methemoglobin formation and denaturation of red blood cell membranes.

    b. Toxicity. Cats are particularly sensitive to acetaminophen toxicity.

      (1) Effects include Heinz body formation, hemolytic anemia, and methemoglobin formation.

      (2) Signs include hypoxia, cyanosis, and icterus.

      (3) Treatment involves:

        (a) Emptying of the stomach and administration of activated charcoal

        (b) Administration of acetylcysteine to replenish hepatic stores of glutathione

        (c) Supportive and symptomatic therapy

        (d) Oxygen therapy to counteract methemoglobinemia and anemia

        (e) Administration of ascorbic acid to combat methemoglobinemia

D. **Naproxen** is approved for use in horses only.

1. Mechanism of action. Naproxen irreversibly binds cyclooxygenase.

2. Pharmacokinetics. Naproxen is metabolized into a glucuronide conjugate. In horses, the plasma half-life is 4 hours.

3. Therapeutic uses. Naproxen is recommended for **soft tissue problems** (e.g., myositis).

4. Administration. Naproxen is administered orally.

5. Adverse effects. Naproxen may cause gastric erosions when administered on an empty stomach.

E. **Flunixin meglumine (Banamine)** is approved for use in horses only.

1. Mechanism of action. Flunixin meglumine irreversibly binds cyclooxygenase.

2. Pharmacokinetics

    a. Fate. Onset of action occurs within 2 hours; the peak effect occurs at 12–16 hours; and the duration of action is 24–36 hours.

      (1) When administered intravenously, flunixin meglumine has a plasma half-life of 1.6 hours in horses and can be detected in plasma for 8 hours and in urine for more than 48 hours.

      (2) PGE_2 is absent from exudate for 12–24 hours after a single intravenous dose, making flunixin meglumine an effective anti-inflammatory agent.

    b. Elimination is primarily through the kidneys. Urine concentration of both conjugate and free forms is approximately 40 times higher than the plasma concentration.

3. Therapeutic uses. Flunixin meglumine, which is considered to be a more potent analgesic than other currently available inhibitors of PG synthesis, pentazocine, meperidine, or codeine, is used to alleviate pain associated with **musculoskeletal disorders, gastrointestinal spasm** (e.g., colic), and **endotoxic shock.** It is a preferred drug for the treatment of colic.

4. Administration. Flunixin meglumine is administered intravenously or intramuscularly.

5. Adverse effects. Flunixin meglumine overdose may cause:
   a. Ulceration of the tongue, gingiva, palate, lips, or stomach
   b. CNS depression
   c. Listlessness
   d. Anorexia

F. **Meclofenamic acid**

1. **Chemistry.** Meclofenamic acid is a derivative of anthranilic acid, which is an analog of salicylic acid.

2. **Mechanism of action.** Meclofenamic acid irreversibly binds cyclooxygenase.

3. **Pharmacokinetics**
   a. After oral dosing, plasma levels peak within 1–4 hours.
   b. In two independent studies, the plasma half-life was reported to be 2.6 and 6–8 hours in horses.
   c. The onset of action is slow (36–96 hours).
   d. Meclofenamic acid can be detected in urine 96 hours after the final dose.

4 **Therapeutic uses**
   a. In horses, meclofenamic acid is used in the treatment of **osteoarthritic disease** and **soft tissue inflammation** affecting the locomotor system.
   b. It is used in **dogs with hip dysplasia** to improve mobility.
   c. It is effective in the **control of anaphylaxis,** especially that attributed to kinins, PGs, and leukotrienes.

5. **Administration**
   a. Meclofenamic acid is approved for oral use in dogs and horses.
   b. With long-term use, the lowest dosage that maintains a satisfactory anti-inflammatory effect (as evidenced by normal locomotor activity) should be used.

6. **Adverse effects**
   a. In horses, **overdoses** may induce buccal erosions, anorexia, gastrointestinal disturbances, and a low packed cell volume (PCV).
   b. In horses heavily infested with bots, **therapeutic dosages** may induce colic and diarrhea.
   c. In dogs, **chronic use** may induce vomiting, tarry stools, leukocytosis, low hemoglobin levels, and erosion of the small intestine mucosa.

G. **Phenylbutazone**

1. **Mechanism of action.** Phenylbutazone irreversibly binds to cyclooxygenase.

2. **Pharmacokinetics**
   a. Fate
      (1) In dogs and horses, the plasma half-life is 3.5–6 hours following intravenous administration of therapeutic doses.
      (2) In animals, **binding** of phenylbutazone to plasma proteins **exceeds 99%.**
      (3) The **major metabolites** are **oxyphenbutazone** and *r*-**hydroxyphenylbutazone.**
         (a) In horses, phenylbutazone is almost completely metabolized.
         (b) In dogs, oxyphenbutazone persists in the urine for 48 hours or more following oral dosing with phenylbutazone; however, the unchanged drug cannot be detected in urine after 36 hours.
         (c) Administration of oxyphenbutazone inhibits metabolism of phenylbutazone, thereby extending the plasma half-life of phenylbutazone.
      (4) The **long duration of action** (24–72 hours) may be attributed to the following factors.
         (a) Because phenylbutazone irreversibly binds to cyclooxygenase, new enzyme production at the inflammation site needs to occur before PGs can be synthesized.

        (b) The plasma protein that binds phenylbutazone may penetrate inflamed tissues; consequently, plasma levels of phenylbutazone may be underestimated in inflamed tissues.

        (c) The active metabolite oxyphenbutazone persists in the body.

   (5) Phenylbutazone induces the production of hepatic microsomal enzymes, which promote the breakdown of phenylbutazone, resulting in progressively lower plasma levels during long-term administration.

  b. Elimination

   (1) In horses, 25% of phenylbutazone is excreted by the kidneys within 24 hours.

   (2) Because of its weak acid property, phenylbutazone is excreted at a more rapid rate in alkaline urine and at a slower rate in acidic urine.

3. Therapeutic uses

  a. Phenylbutazone is the most widely used **analgesic in race horses** in the United States.

   (1) It is used to treat various forms of **lameness** as well as **osteoarthritis** or other painful conditions of the limbs, including **soft tissue conditions** or **nonarticular rheumatism.**

   (2) Phenylbutazone should not be used to conceal equine lameness.

  b. Phenylbutazone is used for **nonspecific inflammation** (e.g., **thrombophlebitis, pericarditis, pleurisy**).

4. Administration

  a. Phenylbutazone is approved for oral and intravenous administration in dogs and horses.

  b. Other parenteral routes are not recommended because phenylbutazone can cause local irritation. For example, perivascular injection may result in phlebitis.

5. Adverse effects include anorexia, depression, colic, hypoproteinemia, diarrhea, petechial hemorrhages of the mucous membranes, oral and gastrointestinal tract erosions and ulcers, and renal papillary necrosis and anuria. Death may occur as the result of a protein-losing enteropathy that leads to decreased blood volume, hemoconcentration, hypovolemic shock, and circulatory collapse. If gastrointestinal tract ulceration is prominent, the shock syndrome may be complicated by sepsis.

6. Contraindications to phenylbutazone use include cardiac dysfunction, renal dysfunction, hepatic dysfunction, and certain hematocytologic disorders (e.g., aplastic anemia, leukopenia, agranulocytosis, thrombocytopenia).

H. Dipyrone

1. Chemistry. Dipyrone is chemically related to phenylbutazone and isopyrin.

2. Mechanism of action. Dipyrone irreversibly blocks cyclooxygenase.

3. Pharmacokinetics. The pharmacokinetics of dipyrone are not well understood.

4. Therapeutic uses. Dipyrone is approved for use in dogs, cats, and horses.

  a. It is used as an analgesic and an antipyretic.

  b. In both **small and large animals,** it is used to treat conditions of **gastrointestinal spasm** or **hypermotility;** however, the value of dipyrone in the treatment of hypermotility has been challenged. Dipyrone antagonizes intestinal spasms induced by bradykinin but not spasms induced by other substances.

5. Administration. Dipyrone may be administered intravenously, intramuscularly, or orally.

6. Adverse effects

  a. Dipyrone may induce **agranulocytosis** and **leukopenia.**

  b. It has a tendency to **increase bleeding.**

  c. Overdose may result in **convulsions.**

7. Drug interactions
  a. Dipyrone is contraindicated for use in conjunction with barbiturates or phenylbutazone. These drugs induce hepatic microsomal enzymes that degrade dipyrone.
  b. Use of dipyrone with chlorpromazine can cause severe hypothermia.

I. **Ibuprofen** and **indomethacin** are not approved for use in animals.

II. α_2-ADRENERGIC AGONISTS

A. Overview

  1. Pharmacologic effects (see Table 9-1)
    a. Analgesia
      (1) Mechanism of action
        (a) α_2-Adrenergic agonists activate α_2-adrenergic receptors in the CNS. These receptors are located on the dorsal horn neurons of the spinal cord, where they inhibit the release of nociceptive neurotransmitters (e.g., substance P, calcitonin gene-related peptide).
        (b) These agents may play a role in modulating spinal pain processing.
        (c) α_2-Adrenergic mechanisms do not work through opioidergic mechanisms, because cross-tolerance is not universally present. α_2-Adrenergic agonist–mediated analgesia may not be reversed by opioid antagonists.
      (2) α_2-Adrenergic agonists are **potent analgesic agents.** They are very effective against head, neck, and body pain, but they are only minimally effective for pain in the extremities.
    b. Sedation
      (1) Mechanism of action. Postsynaptic α_2 receptors in the locus ceruleus of the brain mediate α_2-adrenergic agonist–induced sedation.
      (2) Sedative properties vary among species and agents.
        (a) Ruminants are most sensitive to α_2-adrenergic agonist–induced sedation; cats, dogs, and horses are somewhat sensitive, and pigs are least sensitive.
        (b) Medetomidine, which is not yet available in the United States, has the most powerful sedative effects of the α_2-adrenergic agonists.
      (3) High doses of α_2-adrenergic agonists may induce CNS excitation, which is attributable to activation of α_1-adrenergic receptors.
    c. Skeletal muscle relaxation. α_2-Adrenergic agonists produce skeletal muscle relaxation by inhibiting intraneuronal transmission of impulses at the central level of the CNS. These drugs do not work at the neuromuscular junction.
    d. Emesis. α_2-Adrenergic agonists activate the α_2 receptors in the chemoreceptor trigger zone of the area postrema to induce emesis (see Chapter 10 V B 2).
    e. Reduction of gastrointestinal motility and secretions
      (1) Mechanism of action. α_2-Adrenergic agonists may inhibit acetylcholine (ACh) release to produce these gastrointestinal effects.
      (2) Because of these gastrointestinal effects, α_2-adrenergic agonists are useful in the **treatment of diarrhea.**
    f. Hypertension, hypotension, bradycardia
      (1) Intravenous injection of an α_2-adrenergic agonist causes mild hypertension for up to 10 minutes, followed by hypotension for several hours. **Intramuscular injection** of an α_2-adrenergic agonist usually causes only hypotension.
        (a) **Hypertension** is caused by activation of postsynaptic α_2 receptors in vascular smooth muscle.
        (b) **Hypotension** is caused by decreased norepinephrine release to vascular smooth muscle, attributable to the decreased sympathetic outflow from the CNS as well as activation of presynaptic α_2 receptors in the sympathetic nerve terminal.

(2) Bradycardia accompanied by sinus arrhythmia, atrioventricular (A-V) block, or both usually occurs with hypotension and hypertension.

(a) Bradycardia results from decreased norepinephrine release to the myocardium, particularly the sinus node [see II A 1 i (1)]. There are no postsynaptic α_2 receptors in the myocardium.

(b) The barcreceptor reflex, which may be stimulated by hypertension, causes slowing of the heart and vasodilation. Therefore, atropine administration may change the α_2-adrenergic agonist–induced bradycardia into a tachycardia while potentiating the α_2-adrenergic agonist–induced hypertension.

g. **Diuresis.**

(1) α_2-Adrenergic agonists may inhibit the release of antidiuretic hormone (ADH).

(2) They may inhibit the action of ADH on free water reabsorption from the collecting ducts of the kidneys.

h. **Hypoxemia.** In ruminants, α_2-adrenergic agonists cause hypoxemia by activating peripheral α_2 receptors, thereby increasing airway resistance. This respiratory effect has not been noted in other species.

i. **Neuroendocrine effects**

(1) α_2-Adrenergic agonists inhibit sympathoadrenal outflow to decrease the release of norepinephrine and epinephrine.

(2) α_2-Adrenergic agonists inhibit insulin release, which is associated with a moderate to severe hyperglycemia lasting up to 24 hours, depending on the dosage. This effect is prominent in ruminants.

(3) α_2-Adrenergic agonists increase growth hormone release by inhibiting the release of somatostatin from the hypothalamus.

2. **Therapeutic uses.** In addition to their applications as analgesics and sedatives, α_2-adrenergic agonists are commonly used for immobilization, preanesthetic treatment, anesthesia in combination with other agents, and induction of epidural analgesia (xylazine). When using α_2-adrenergic agonists as preanesthetics, anesthetic dosages usually can be reduced by 70% or more.

3. **α_2-Adrenergic antagonists (α_2-receptor blockers).** α_2-Adrenergic receptor activation has adverse effects, such as bradycardia and decreased gastrointestinal motility.

a. α_2-Adrenergic antagonists greatly increase the safety of α_2-adrenergic agonists.

b. α_2-Receptor blockers have been used to reverse the pharmacologic and toxicologic effects of α_2-adrenergic agonists.

(1) For nonruminants, 0.1 mg/kg of yohimbine is administered.

(2) For ruminants, 1–2 mg/kg of tolazoline is used.

B. **Xylazine** is approved for use in cats, dogs, horses, and wildlife (e.g., deer and elk); however, it is also frequently used in other species (particularly cattle).

1. **Pharmacokinetics**

a. **Fate.** After a rapid distribution, with a half-life of 1.2–6 minutes, the apparent volume of distribution for xylazine is 1.9–2.7 L/kg in dogs, horses, sheep, and cattle. The pharmacologic effects of xylazine may last much longer than its plasma half-life.

b. **Elimination.** The half-life of elimination after intravenous administration of xylazine is 49.5 minutes in horses, 36.5 minutes in cattle, 30 minutes in dogs, and 23 minutes in sheep.

2. **Therapeutic uses**

a. Xylazine is used to **induce epidural analgesia.**

b. Xylazine and ketamine are commonly used together as a **parenteral anesthetic.**

3. **Administration.** Xylazine may be injected intramuscularly, intravenously, or subcutaneously.

4. **Adverse effects**

a. **Gastrointestinal stasis** and **bloat** can be associated with xylazine administration.

   b. Xylazine affects the thermoregulation center in the hypothalamus.
      (1) It produces **hypothermia** when the ambient temperature is low.
      (2) It produces **hyperthermia** when the ambient temperature is high.
   c. Xylazine may precipitate **seizures** in susceptible animals.
   d. Sudden death has occurred in horses when xylazine has been inadvertently injected into the carotid artery.

5. Contraindications
   a. Xylazine should be used cautiously in the presence of:
      (1) Cardiac aberrations
      (2) Hypotension, shock, or dehydration
      (3) Renal impairment or urinary obstruction
      (4) Hepatic impairment
      (5) Epilepsy
      (6) Advanced pregnancy (because it may induce abortion)
   b. Use of xylazine in combination with ketamine must be used with caution in animals with cardiopulmonary complications, because these agents synergistically suppress cardiopulmonary function.
   c. Xylazine should be used with caution in the treatment of colic.
      (1) Xylazine's powerful analgesic effect can mask the underlying problem.
      (2) Xylazine can paralyze the gastrointestinal tract.

C. Detomidine (Dormosedan)

1. Pharmacokinetics
   a. Fate. In horses, intravenous injection of detomidine produces a first distribution phase with a half-life of 3 minutes, a redistribution phase with a half-life of 47 minutes, and an elimination half-life of 9.7 hours.
   b. Elimination. Metabolism to hydroxylated products and their conjugates and excretion in the urine seems to be the major elimination route, although a small amount of the drug is excreted in the feces.

2. Administration. Detomidine is approved for intramuscular or intravenous use in horses.

3. Adverse effects
   a. The **recommended dose** of 40 μg/kg may produce piloerection, sweating, partial penis prolapse, salivation, and, occasionally, slight muscle tremors.
   b. Overdose
      (1) Detomidine at 10 times the recommended dose (400 μg/kg) daily for 3 consecutive days produces microscopic foci of myocardial necrosis in 1 of 8 horses tested.
      (2) Excessive doses of detomidine can induce CNS excitation.

4. Drug interactions. Intravenous sulfonamides used in horses being treated with detomidine may produce potentially fatal cardiac dysrhythmias.

III. NONSTEROIDAL ANTI-INFLAMMATORY DRUGS

A. Orgotein

1. Chemistry. Orgotein is a copper- and zinc-containing protein that is isolated from the bovine liver.

2. Mechanism of action
   a. Orgotein exerts anti-inflammatory effects through its superoxide dismutase activity. The increased cellular respiration associated with inflammation leads to excessive production of superoxide. Superoxide depolymerizes hyaluronic acid, reducing the viscosity and lubricating qualities of synovial fluid. Superoxide dismutase

breaks down superoxide free radicals into peroxide, which is then broken down to water and oxygen.

   b. Orgotein stimulates the chemotactic activity of polymorphonuclear leukocytes and prevents the disruption of lysosomal membranes.

3. Pharmacokinetics. No information regarding the pharmacokinetics of orgotein is available.

4. Therapeutic uses. Orgotein is approved for use in dogs and horses.

   a. In **dogs,** orgotein is used in the treatment of spondylosis, ankylosing spondylitis, and vertebral disk diseases.

   b. In **horses,** orgotein is used to treat soft-tissue inflammation and arthritis; however, there is a fair amount of controversy regarding orgotein's efficacy in equine medicine.

5. Administration. Orgotein is supplied as a lyophilized powder (5 mg); 2 ml of sterile saline are used to dissolve the powder for intramuscular, subcutaneous, or intra-articular injection.

6. Adverse effects

   a. Occasionally, a **transient paradoxical exacerbation of signs** occurs, especially with intra-articular administration.

   b. Because orgotein is a foreign protein to dogs and horses, **hypersensitivity reactions** may occur.

7. Contraindications include previous hypersensitivity to orgotein or to other bovine proteins.

B. | **Dimethyl sulfoxide (DMSO)**

1. Chemistry. DMSO is a solvent for many aromatic and unsaturated hydrocarbons as well as organic nitrogen compounds and inorganic salts.

   a. DMSO is a clear, colorless to straw-yellow liquid.

   b. Because of its hygroscopic characteristics, DMSO can absorb greater than 70% of its weight in water from the air at a temperature of 70°F and 65% relative humidity. Therefore, the container should be tightly sealed.

2. Pharmacologic effects. DMSO possesses anti-inflammatory, analgesic, antimicrobial, antifungal, antidiuretic, and anticholinesterase activity. In addition, DMSO is able to rapidly penetrate the skin (but not nail or tooth enamel) following topical application.

3. Mechanisms of action

   a. Anti-inflammatory effect. DMSO, like orgotein, traps free radicals such as superoxide.

   b. Analgesic effect. DMSO produces a thermal effect that may account for its alleviation of muscle and joint pain.

   c. Skin penetrating effect. DMSO increases the permeability of the skin by altering the plasma membrane of the epithelial cells. As it rapidly penetrates the membrane barriers, DMSO carries dissolved compounds (e.g., another drug) with it, regardless of the size and characteristics of the molecule.

   d. Other effects. DMSO has antidiuretic, anticholinesterase, and weak antibacterial and antifungal effects (when used topically). The mechanisms by which DMSO exerts these effects are not understood.

4. Pharmacokinetics

   a. Absorption. DMSO is well-absorbed after topical application.

   b. Fate

      (1) DMSO is extensively and rapidly distributed to every part of the body.

      (2) The half-life in horses is approximately 9 hours following intravenous administration.

      (3) DMSO is rapidly metabolized to dimethyl sulfide (DMS), methyl sulfinic acid, and dimethyl sulfone.

    c. Excretion. DMSO and its metabolites are excreted primarily by the kidneys; some biliary and respiratory excretion also occurs. DMS and methyl sulfinic acid are believed to be responsible for the obnoxious oyster-like odor detectable on the breath seconds after the application of DMSO to the skin.

  5. Therapeutic uses
    a. DMSO is used to reduce acute swelling resulting from musculoskeletal trauma.
    b. Other possible indications include:
      (1) Acute traumatic conditions of the CNS and posterior paralysis resulting from spinal cord trauma
      (2) Cystitis associated with urethral obstruction in the cat
      (3) Superficial burns
      (4) Skin grafts
      (5) Edema of the limbs resulting from fractures
      (6) Swelling and engorgement of the mammary glands in the nursing bitch
      (7) Severe inflammation resulting from the extravascular injection of irritating drugs
    c. A mixture of diethylcarbamazine and DMSO is effective in killing fly larvae that cause skin sores in the horse.

  6. Administration. DMSO is administered topically only. Rubber gloves should be worn during application, and DMSO should be applied only to clean and dry areas to avoid carrying other chemicals into the systemic circulation.

  7. Adverse effects. When used as labeled, DMSO appears to be an extremely safe drug.
    a. Local effects (e.g., a burning sensation, erythema, vesiculation, dry skin, and allergic reactions) and a garlicky or oyster-like breath odor are the most likely adverse effects. These effects are transient and quickly resolve when therapy is discontinued.
    b. Lenticular changes, which may result in myopia, have been noted when high doses of DMSO are used chronically (i.e., longer than 14 days in dogs or 30 days in horses).

  8. Contraindications. DMSO must not be used in animals that are being treated concurrently with anticholinesterases.

C. Polysulfated glycosaminoglycan (Adequan)

  1. Chemistry. This anti-arthritic compound is chemically similar to the mucopolysaccharides of cartilage.

  2. Mechanisms of action
    a. Through proteolytic enzyme inhibition, polysulfated glycosaminoglycan decreases or reverses the mechanisms that result in loss of cartilaginous mucopolysaccharides.
    b. Polysulfated glycosaminoglycan apparently improves joint articular function by enhancing synovial membrane activity and by increasing the viscosity of synovial fluid.

  3. Pharmacokinetics. No information regarding the pharmacokinetics of polysulfated glycosaminoglycan is available.

  4. Therapeutic uses. Polysulfated glycosaminoglycan is used in horses to treat traumatic joint dysfunction and noninfectious degeneration of the carpal joint.

  5. Administration. Polysulfated glycosaminoglycan is administered intra-articularly or intramuscularly. When administered intra-articularly, the joint area must be shaved, cleansed, and sterilized prior to injection.

  6. Adverse effects. When used as labeled, polysulfated glycosaminoglycan is safe.
    a. Rarely, animals show inflammatory joint reactions consisting of joint pain, effusion, swelling, and lameness (aseptic arthritis). This reaction may result from hy-

persensitivity, trauma sustained during injection, overdose or excessively frequent administration, or drug interactions.

b. Septic arthritis may be induced if the sterile injection procedure is not followed. Excessive inflammation accompanied by lameness, swelling, and edema extending beyond the joint limits should alert the practitioner to the possibility of sepsis.

7. Contraindications. Intra-articular injections must not be administered when the overlying skin shows lesions of infection, or in cases of septic arthritis.

STUDY QUESTIONS

DIRECTIONS: Each of the numbered items or incomplete statements in this section is followed by answers or by completions of the statement. Select the **one** numbered answer or completion that is **best** in each case.

1. Which one of the following enzymes influences the half-life of aspirin in domestic animals?

(1) Glutathione reductase
(2) Cyclooxygenase
(3) N-acetyl transferase
(4) Glucuronide transferase
(5) Cytochrome oxidase

2. Bioavailability of aspirin can be increased by:

(1) increasing urine pH.
(2) using enteric-coated tablets.
(3) administering sodium bicarbonate orally.
(4) maintaining a low pH in the stomach.
(5) increasing the particle size of aspirin in oral formulation.

3. The most widely used analgesic in racehorses in the United States is:

(1) aspirin.
(2) phenylbutazone.
(3) naproxen.
(4) xylazine.
(5) mecloflenamic acid.

4. Which one of the following analgesics can be used to induce epidural analgesia?

(1) Aspirin
(2) Phenylbutazone
(3) Naproxen
(4) Xylazine
(5) Meclofenamic acid

5. Which one of the following nonsteroidal anti-inflammatory drugs acts through proteolytic enzyme inhibition to reverse the loss of cartilaginous mucopolysaccharides that occurs in arthritis?

(1) Orgotein
(2) Dimethyl sulfoxide (DMSO)
(3) Polysulfated glycosaminoglycan
(4) Phenylbutazone
(5) Flunixin meglumine

6. Naproxen is approved by the Food and Drug Administration (FDA) for use in:

(1) horses.
(2) dogs.
(3) cats.
(4) cattle.
(5) pigs.

7. Which one of the following analgesics has an extremely slow onset of action?

(1) Acetaminophen
(2) Aspirin
(3) Dipyrone
(4) Meclofenamic acid
(5) Naproxen

8. Which of the following is the most frequently seen adverse effect of the prostaglandin (PG) inhibitors?

(1) Agranulocytosis
(2) Gastric erosions
(3) Renal papillary necrosis
(4) Anemia
(5) Diarrhea

9. Which one of the following nonsteroidal anti-inflammatory drugs has superoxide dismutase activity?

(1) Orgotein
(2) Dimethyl sulfoxide (DMSO)
(3) Polysulfated glycosaminoglycan
(4) Phenylbutazone
(5) Naproxen

DIRECTIONS: Each of the numbered items or incomplete statements in this section is negatively phrased, as indicated by an italicized word such as *not*, *least*, or *except*. Select the **one** numbered answer or completion that is **best** in each case.

10. Salicylates alleviate all of the following types of pain *except:*

(1) headache.
(2) muscle pain.
(3) joint pain.
(4) colic.

11. Which one of the following drugs has the *least* anti-inflammatory effect?

(1) Hydrocortisone
(2) Meclofenamic acid
(3) Acetaminophen
(4) Aspirin
(5) Phenylbutazone

12. The treatment for acetaminophen intoxication in cats includes all of the following *except:*

(1) atropine.
(2) oxygen therapy.
(3) ascorbic acid.
(4) acetylcysteine.

13. Musculoskeletal pain in animals can be treated with all of the following drugs *except:*

(1) aspirin.
(2) phenylbutazone.
(3) naproxen.
(4) xylazine.
(5) flunixin meglumine.

14. The antipyretic effect of nonnarcotic analgesics can result from all of the following *except:*

(1) prevention of prostaglandin (PG) synthesis in the central nervous system (CNS).
(2) dilation of the peripheral vasculature.
(3) sweating.
(4) raising the set point of the temperature-regulating mechanism in the hypothalamus.

15. All of the following statements regarding the administration of a nonnarcotic analgesic to a 6-year-old cat are true *except:*

(1) the nonnarcotic analgesic may cause complications if the animal is dehydrated.
(2) acetaminophen is contraindicated.
(3) aspirin should be administered following a meal.
(4) aspirin should be administered every 8 hours.

16. Which of the following statements concerning α_2-adrenergic agonists is *incorrect*?

(1) Ruminants are more sensitive to the sedative properties of these drugs than nonruminants.
(2) Intramuscular administration of these drugs induces vomiting more frequently than does intravenous administration.
(3) They increase insulin secretion.
(4) Concurrent administration of ketamine may synergistically suppress cardiopulmonary function.

ANSWERS AND EXPLANATIONS

1. The answer is 4 [I B 2 b (2)].
Glucuronidation is the main biotransformation process for aspirin and dictates the plasma half-life of the compound. Aspirin is primarily metabolized by glucuronidation. Because the ability to conjugate glucuronic acid varies among species, the plasma half-life of aspirin also varies. Aspirin irreversibly binds cyclooxygenase to inhibit the formation of prostaglandins. When glucuronidation capabilities are exhausted, salicylates form conjugates with glutathione. N-Acetyl transferase and cytochrome oxidase are not involved in the biotransformation of aspirin.

2. The answer is 4 [I B 2 a].
Aspirin is a weak acid that crosses biologic membranes most readily in an acidic environment and least readily in an alkaline environment. Increasing the pH of the urine or administering sodium bicarbonate decreases the bioavailability of aspirin because these measures induce an alkaline environment. Enteric coatings or large particles decrease the gastrointestinal absorption of aspirin.

3. The answer is 2 [I G 3 a].
Phenylbutazone is widely used as an equine analgesic because it is effective against many types of lameness.

4. The answer is 4 [II B 2 a].
The α_2-adrenergic agonists, such as xylazine, activate the receptors on the dorsal horn neurons of the spinal cord. A high degree of analgesia can be achieved by injecting these drugs into the epidural space of the spinal cord.

5. The answer is 3 [III C 2].
Polysulfated glycosaminoglycan is chemically similar to the mucopolysaccharides of cartilage; therefore, it can reverse the mechanisms that cause the loss of these mucopolysaccharides. Orgotein and dimethyl sulfoxide (DMSO) exert anti-inflammatory effects by scavenging free radicals. Phenylbutazone and flunixin meglumine are nonnarcotic analgesics.

6. The answer is 1 [I D].
Naproxen is approved for use in horses only and is recommended for soft tissue problems (e.g., myositis).

7. The answer is 4 [I F 3 c].
Meclofenamic acid is an unusual drug among the nonnarcotic analgesic agents in that its onset of action is slow, taking 36–96 hours to develop.

8. The answer is 2 [I A 2].
Gastrointestinal erosions and ulcers are the most frequently seen adverse effects of the prostaglandin (PG) inhibitors.

9. The answer is 1 [III A 1, 2 a].
Orgotein is a copper- and zinc-containing protein derived from the bovine liver that has superoxide dismutase activity. Superoxide dismutase degrades free radicals that are involved in the inflammatory process. Dimethyl sulfoxide (DMSO), polysulfated glycosaminoglycan, phenylbutazone, and naproxen do not have superoxide dismutase activity.

10. The answer is 4 [Table 9-1].
The inhibitors of prostaglandin (PG) synthesis do not relieve deep visceral pain, such as colic. They usually alleviate pain from the integument, including skeletal muscles and joints.

11. The answer is 3 [I C 3].
Acetaminophen does not have apparent anti-inflammatory action. Hydrocortisone, mecloflenamic acid, aspirin, and phenylbutazone all have anti-inflammatory properties.

12. The answer is 1 [I C 5 b (3)].
Cholinergic stimulation is not involved in acetaminophen toxicosis; thus, the use of atropine is not justified. Acetaminophen induces methemoglobin formation and hemolytic anemia; ascorbic acid and oxygen therapy counteract these conditions. Because glutathione is depleted during acetaminophen intoxication, acetylcysteine replenishes hepatic stores of glutathione.

13. The answer is 4 [II B].
Xylazine is one of the α_2-adrenergic agonists, which are not suitable for treatment of musculoskeletal pain because of their short duration of action, marked central nervous system (CNS) depressant effect, and lack of anti-inflammatory effects. Aspirin, phenylbutazone, naproxen, and flunixin meglumine are inhibitors of prostaglandin (PG) synthesis and are preferred for musculoskeletal pain, particularly when inflammation is involved.

14. The answer is 4 [I A 1 b].
Prostaglandin (PG) synthesis inhibitors lower the set point of the thermoregulatory center of the hypothalamus, causing vasodilation sweating, and panting.

15. The answer is 4 [I B 4, 5 a, C 4].
Because of its long half-life in cats, aspirin should be administered every 48 hours, not every 8 hours. The standard dosage for cats is 10 mg/kg. Inhibitors of prostaglandin (PG) synthesis can cause profuse sweating and gastrointestinal hemorrhage, and α_2-adrenergic agonists can cause diuresis, all of which are detrimental to dehydrated animals. Acetaminophen is contraindicated in cats. Aspirin is irritating to the gastrointestinal mucosa and thus should be given after a meal.

16. The answer is 3 [II A 1 b, d, i, B 5 b].
α_2-Adrenergic agonists can inhibit insulin release and hence induce hyperglycemia. Ruminants are most sensitive to α_2-adrenergic agonist–induced sedation. Intramuscular injection of these drugs induces vomiting more frequently than intravenous injection. Concurrent administration of ketamine and an α_2-adrenergic agonist may synergistically suppress cardiopulmonary function.

Chapter 10

Drugs Acting on the Gastrointestinal Tract

Franklin A. Ahrens

I. **INTRODUCTION.** Gastrointestinal disease or dysfunction is a common clinical problem in veterinary practice, and accurate diagnosis is essential for effective therapy. Nonspecific therapy includes correction of fluid and electrolyte imbalance, ensuring rest of the gastrointestinal tract to allow healing, diet modification, and nutritional support.

A. **Correction of fluid and electrolyte balance.** Prolonged vomiting or diarrhea produces dehydration, electrolyte loss, and disturbances in acid–base balance that must be corrected by **parenteral fluid therapy.**

1. With severe vomiting, loss of sodium, chloride, potassium, hydrogen, and bicarbonate leads to a metabolic acidosis.

2. If the pylorus is obstructed, duodenal bicarbonate is retained and the loss of gastric chloride, potassium, and hydrogen leads to a metabolic alkalosis.

B. **Ensuring rest of the gastrointestinal tract. Fasting** for 24–48 hours is often effective in small animals suffering acute gastrointestinal disturbances of vomiting and diarrhea. Fasting permits decreased gastric secretion and increased time for mucosal healing (enterocyte regeneration) and results in fewer osmotically active particles in the gut lumen.

C. **Diet modification**

1. **Bland diet.** A bland, easily digested, low-fat diet such as 1 part boiled hamburger or chicken with 4 parts of cooked rice should be offered after the 24–48-hour fast. Limiting dietary fat is important because unabsorbed fatty acids are hydroxylated by colonic bacteria, resulting in decreased absorption and osmotic retention of water, which increases fecal water loss.

2. **Lactose-free diet.** Milk products should be eliminated from the diet if the animal suffers from lactose intolerance or loss of mucosal brush border lactase as a result of invasive enteritis.

3. **Insoluble fiber.** Fiber absorbs water and normalizes intestinal transit. Increasing the insoluble fiber content of the diet is useful when treating constipation, chronic diarrhea, or idiopathic colitis.

4. **Gluten-free diet.** Gluten-sensitive enteropathy has been observed in Irish setters. Clinical improvement occurs with a cereal-free diet.

D. **Provision of nutritional support.** Calories, protein, and vitamins should be supplied to maintain a positive energy and protein balance. For example, the addition of medium-chain triglycerides to the diet of dogs with intestinal lymphangiectasis provides calories because medium-chain triglycerides are absorbed in the portal vasculature, not the lymphatics.

E. **Alleviation of visceral pain**

1. **Mild visceral pain** may be alleviated by alimentary protectives or absorbants (e.g., **aluminum or magnesium silicates, kaolin-pectin, bismuth salts**). These agents may reduce pain by reducing gastric acidity, coating inflamed mucosae, or absorbing noxious agents in the lumen.

2. **Severe visceral pain** is alleviated by morphine or other μ-receptor opioid agonists that inhibit nociceptive reflexes at spinal and supraspinal sites within the central nervous system (CNS).
   a. **Opiates**
      (1) **Morphine** is administered intramuscularly in dogs and cats.
         (a) Morphine's duration of action is 6 hours in dogs and cats.
         (b) High doses of morphine produce excitement in cats and horses.
      (2) **Butorphanol**, an opioid agonist/antagonist similar to pentazocine, is administered intravenously to horses for the control of **colic pain.** Its duration of action is 1–2 hours.
   b. **Nonsteroidal anti-inflammatory drugs. Flunixin meglumine, dipyrone,** or **phenylbutazone** are given intravenously or intramuscularly to horses for the control of **colic pain.** Their duration of action is 1–8 hours, depending on the cause and severity of the pain.
   c. **Sedatives. Xylazine** and **detomidine** produce sedation and analgesia in horses suffering from **colic.** Their duration of action is 1–4 hours following intravenous or intramuscular administration.

II. **APPETITE STIMULANTS.** Inappetence or anorexia is common in disease states, and the resultant malnutrition can delay recovery and may exacerbate the underlying disease.

A. **Enteral alimentation with liquid supplements** is useful in small animals.

B. **Small amounts of palatable food** should be offered at frequent intervals. Warming the food may enhance appetite in carnivores.

C. **Various drugs** are used for the short-term stimulation of appetite.

1. **Benzodiazepines** (e.g., diazepam, oxazepam)
   a. **Mechanism of action.** Benzodiazepines increase γ-aminobutyric acid (GABA) activity. The resultant antiserotonergic effect depresses the satiety center in the hypothalamus.
   b. **Therapeutic uses.** Benzodiazepines are used for short-term stimulation of appetite most frequently in cats, and less frequently in horses, dogs, and goats. After two to three treatments, the effect of benzodiazepines on appetite is diminished.
   c. **Administration**
      (1) **Diazepam** is administered orally, intravenously, or intramuscularly once or twice daily.
      (2) **Oxazepam** is administered orally once daily.
   d. **Adverse effects** include **sedation** and **ataxia.**

2. **Cyproheptadine**
   a. **Mechanism of action.** Cyproheptadine acts as a serotonin and a histamine$_1$ (H$_1$) antagonist. It suppresses the satiety center in the hypothalamus.
   b. **Therapeutic use.** Cyproheptadine stimulates appetite in cats and in humans, but not in dogs.
   c. **Adverse effects.** CNS excitement and marked aggressive behavior occur in 20% of the cats administered cyproheptadine.

3. **Glucocorticoids** (e.g., **prednisolone, dexamethasone**)
   a. **Mechanism of action.** The mechanism by which glucocorticoids stimulate appetite is unknown. Stimulation of appetite may result from glucocorticoid-induced euphoria, which in part results from the anti-inflammatory action of glucocorticoids.
   b. **Administration**

    (1) Small animals. Prednisolone or dexamethasone is administered intramuscularly once daily or every other day.

    (2) Large animals. Prednisolone or dexamethasone is administered intramuscularly once daily.

  c. Adverse effects

    (1) Immunosuppression may delay recovery from the underlying disease.

    (2) Gastric ulcers may result from decreased gastric mucus production.

4. Bitters are plant-derived compounds containing alkaloids, such as nux vomica.

  a. Mechanism of action. Bitters stimulate salivation.

  b. Therapeutic uses. The effect of bitters on appetite is questionable and they are seldom used in this capacity; however, bitters are a component of tonics for appetite stimulation in large animals.

5. Zinc is essential for the sensation of taste; therefore, zinc supplements may increase appetite in zinc-deficient animals.

III. | **ANTACIDS** reduce the hydrochloric acid content of the stomach by inhibiting acid secretion, neutralizing acid, or coating and protecting the gastric mucosa.

A. | **Acid secretion inhibitors**

1. Histamine$_2$ (H$_2$)-blockers (e.g., **cimetidine, ranitidine**)

  a. Chemistry. H$_2$-blockers are structurally similar to histamine.

  b. Mechanism of action. H$_2$ stimulates the proton (acid) pump in parietal cells. H$_2$-blockers competitively block the H$_2$ receptors on parietal cells, thereby decreasing hydrochloric acid secretion.

  c. Pharmacokinetics

    (1) Absorption. H$_2$-blockers are well absorbed by the gastrointestinal tract.

    (2) Fate. They are widely distributed in body tissues with only 10%–20% bound to plasma proteins. Up to 50% of the drug is metabolized by the liver.

    (3) Excretion. Metabolites and the parent drug are excreted by the kidneys.

  d. Therapeutic uses

    (1) H$_2$-blockers are used in **dogs and cats** with **gastritis, gastric ulcers, esophagitis,** and **gastrinomas.**

    (2) They are used to prevent destruction of replacement pancreatic enzymes by gastric acid in **dogs and cats** with **exocrine pancreatic disease.**

    (3) H$_2$-blockers are used in **horses** with **gastritis** and **gastric erosions.**

  e. Administration. Low doses are effective in dogs and cats because gastric hydrochloric acid secretion is intermittent in carnivores.

    (1) Cimetidine is administered orally, intramuscularly, or intravenously every 6–8 hours.

    (2) Ranitidine is administered orally, intramuscularly, or intravenously every 12 hours.

  f. Drug interactions. Cimetidine inhibits hepatic microsomal enzymes and may slow the metabolism of drugs requiring hepatic metabolism (e.g., phenytoin, phenobarbital).

2. Proton pump inhibitors (e.g., **omeprazole**)

  a. Mechanism of action. Proton pump inhibitors reduce hydrogen secretion by inhibiting the H$^+$-K$^+$-ATPase pump on the luminal membrane of parietal cells. Binding to adenosine triphosphatase (ATPase) is irreversible; therefore, cells must synthesize new ATPase to restore hydrochloric acid secretion.

  b. Pharmacokinetics

    (1) Absorption. Omeprazole is absorbed by the gastrointestinal tract.

    (2) Fate

    (a) Omeprazole enters gastric parietal cells, where it is protonated and trapped in the acidic intracellular fluid. **The protonated drug is the active form;** thus, ATPase in non–acid-producing cells is not affected.

    (b) Because the drug slowly accumulates in parietal cells with repeated doses, **pharmacologic action is not correlated with plasma half-life.**

    (c) Omeprazole is **metabolized by hepatic microsomal enzymes.**

  (3) Excretion. Omeprazole is excreted by the kidneys.

 c. Therapeutic uses

  (1) Omeprazole is used in **dogs, cats, and horses** to limit acid secretion in **gastritis, gastric ulcers,** and **esophagitis.**

  (2) It is used in the **prevention and treatment of gastric erosions by nonsteroidal anti-inflammatory drugs.**

 d. Administration. Omeprazole is administered orally once daily.

 e. Drug interactions. Omeprazole inhibits hepatic microsomal metabolism and may prolong the actions of drugs requiring hepatic metabolism.

B. **Locally acting antacids**

1. Preparations

 a. Aluminum salts (e.g., aluminum hydroxide, aluminum carbonate, aluminum silicate) are the most common preparations.

 b. Magnesium salts [e.g., magnesium oxide (milk of magnesia), magnesium trisilicate] have a laxative effect in addition to their potent antacid activity.

2. Mechanism of action. Locally acting antacids **neutralize gastric hydrochloric acid** and **inhibit pepsin section.**

 a. Most are colloidal compounds that have a protective or adsorbent action on the mucosa of the gastrointestinal tract following oral administration.

 b. A mucosal cytoprotective action results from their ability to stimulate mucosal prostaglandins (PGs).

3. Therapeutic uses

 a. Locally acting antacids are administered as **adjuncts to H_2-blockers or proton pump inhibitors** in the **treatment of gastric and duodenal ulcers.**

 b. They are used in **nonspecific therapy of acute gastritis** and **gastroenteritis** in **small animals.**

 c. Because aluminum salts increase fecal excretion of phosphate, they are used in the treatment of **hyperphosphatemia.**

4. Adverse effects

 a. Rebound hydrochloric acid secretion. Aluminum salts do not raise the gastric pH above 4, so there is no rebound hydrochloric acid secretion. Rebound hydrochloric acid secretion may be a problem with **magnesium salts,** which can raise the gastric pH to 7.

 b. Constipation. Aluminum salts increase fecal phosphate excretion, which tends to produce constipation. Combination with laxative magnesium salts offsets this effect.

 c. Impaired absorption of other drugs. Locally acting antacids may impair absorption of other oral drugs for at least 2 hours.

5. Contraindications. Approximately 20% of the magnesium ions in **magnesium salts** are absorbed and excreted by the kidneys. Impaired excretion may result in CNS depression; therefore, magnesium salts should be avoided in the presence of **renal disease.**

C. **Gastric protectives**

1. Preparations. Sucralfate is a sucrose sulfate–aluminum hydroxide complex.

2. Mechanism of action. Sucralfate polymerizes to a viscous gel at a pH less than 4. The sulfate groups bind to proteins in ulcerated tissue and protect ulcers from acid and pepsin.

3. **Therapeutic use.** Sucralfate is used in the treatment of gastric and duodenal ulcers in dogs, cats, and foals.

4. **Adverse effects.** Constipation may occur with long-term therapy.

IV. DIGESTANTS

A. Pancrelipase

1. **Chemistry.** Pancrelipase consists of pancreatic enzymes (e.g., lipase, amylase, trypsin) derived from porcine pancreatic tissue.

2. **Therapeutic uses.** Pancrelipase treats **exocrine pancreatic insufficiency** in **dogs, cats, and birds.**

3. **Administration**
   a. Pancrelipase powder preparations are administered orally, mixed with food.
   b. Use of enteric-coated preparations or pretreatment with H_2-blockers prevents pancrelipase destruction by gastric hydrochloric acid.

B. Bile acids and salts

1. **Preparations**
   a. **Bile acids** (e.g., cholic acid, chenodeoxycholic acid)
   b. **Semisynthetic bile acid derivatives** (e.g., dehydrocholic acid)
   c. **Sodium salts of bile acids**

2. **Mechanism of action**
   a. **Bile acids** stimulate choleresis (bile flow).
   b. **Bile salts** emulsify dietary lipids, enhancing the digestion of fats and the absorption of long-chain fatty acids.

3. **Therapeutic uses.** Bile salts and acids treat various **maldigestion syndromes characterized by steatorrhea** (e.g., pancreatitis, bile salt deficiency).

V. EMETICS

A. General considerations

1. **Vomiting reflex**
   a. Vomiting is **triggered by the vomiting center,** which receives central or peripheral stimulation from the:
      (1) **Chemoreceptor trigger zone** (via dopaminergic input)
      (2) **Gastrointestinal tract** (via vagal and sympathetic afferent pathways)
      (3) **Vestibular apparatus** (via cholinergic and histaminergic afferent pathways)
   b. The vomiting reflex is **developed in carnivores, primates,** and **swine.** Horses, ruminants, rodents, and rabbits do not possess this protective reflex and should never be administered emetics.

2. **Indications for emetics.** Emetics are used in conscious dogs and cats to induce elimination of noncorrosive poisons or prior to the induction of general anesthesia. They generally remove less than 80% of the stomach contents.

B. Centrally acting emetics

1. **Apomorphine**
   a. **Mechanism of action.** Apomorphine induces vomiting by stimulating the chemoreceptor trigger zone. It is not effective in swine.
   b. **Administration**

    (1) Intravenous administration of a low dose (e.g., 20 μg/lb) **induces vomiting in dogs within 1 minute.** If vomiting does not occur, a **second dose should not be given,** because the vomiting center is depressed following the initial stimulation of the chemoreceptor trigger zone.

    (2) Intramuscular, subcutaneous, or **conjunctival administration** is also effective.

  c. Adverse effects. Apomorphine produces **excitement in cats** and should not be used in this species.

2. Xylazine (see Chapter 9 II B) is an α_2-adrenergic agonist that induces vomiting in cats following intravenous or intramuscular administration. Vomiting occurs within 2–5 minutes and may be followed by mild sedation for 30–90 minutes.

C. **Peripherally acting emetics**

1. Preparations
  a. Sodium chloride is administered as crystals or a saturated solution.
  b. Syrup of ipecac contains emetine alkaloid.
  c. Copper sulfate (1%), zinc sulfate (1%), and **hydrogen peroxide (3%)** are infrequently used.

2. Mechanism of action. Peripherally acting emetics stimulate sympathetic and vagal afferent receptors in the pharynx and stomach.

3. Therapeutic uses
  a. Sodium chloride is commonly used by pet owners to induce vomiting in dogs following ingestion of poisons.
  b. Syrup of ipecac may induce vomiting within 15–30 minutes, but its action is more reliable in humans than in dogs and cats.

4. Administration. Peripherally acting emetics are administered **orally as a single dose,** which should not be repeated even if vomiting does not occur.

VI. ANTIEMETICS

A. **General considerations**

1. Prolonged vomiting leads to electrolyte and acid–base imbalances and dehydration.

2. Diagnosis and treatment of the primary cause of vomiting should precede administration of the antiemetic. The most frequent causes of prolonged vomiting are:
  a. Inflammation, distention, or the presence of chemicals or drugs in the gastrointestinal tract
  b. Labyrinthine disease or motion sickness
  c. Inflammation, edema, or tumors of the CNS
  d. Stimulation of the chemoreceptor trigger zone by drugs, bacterial endotoxins, or toxic endogenous metabolites (e.g., urea)

B. **Antidopaminergic agents**

1. Phenothiazines (e.g., **acepromazine, chlorpromazine, promazine, prochlorperazine**)
  a. Mechanisms of action
    (1) Phenothiazines **block dopamine receptors in the chemoreceptor trigger zone.** At high doses, they **block dopamine receptors in the vomiting center** as well.
    (2) They have **weak anticholinergic and antihistaminic actions.**
  b. Pharmacokinetics
    (1) Absorption. Phenothiazines are well absorbed orally. They undergo significant first-pass metabolism.

(2) Fate. Phenothiazines are widely distributed to the tissues. They are metabolized by the liver, primarily to glucuronide or sulfate conjugates.

(3) Excretion. Phenothiazines are excreted by the kidneys.

c. Therapeutic uses. Phenothiazines are broad-spectrum antiemetics used in dogs and cats; however, their effectiveness is limited in arresting vomiting caused by severe inflammation of the gastrointestinal tract or the inner ear.

d. Administration. Phenothiazines are administered orally or intramuscularly every 6 hours.

e. Adverse effects

(1) Hypotension and **bradycardia** result from α-adrenergic blockade. α-Adrenergic agonists (e.g., norepinephrine, phenylephrine) may be used to counteract these effects, but epinephrine should not be used because of the possibility of epinephrine reversal.

(2) Mild sedation may occur.

2. Metoclopramide

a. Mechanism of action

(1) Central action results from blockade of dopamine receptors in the chemoreceptor trigger zone.

(2) Peripheral action results from stimulation of stomach and duodenum motility via increased smooth muscle sensitivity to acetylcholine (ACh). Motility prevents the gastric atony required for vomiting.

b. Pharmacokinetics

(1) Absorption by the gastrointestinal tract is rapid. Peak plasma levels are reached within 2 hours.

(2) Fate. First-pass metabolism results in 50%–70% bioavailability. The drug is widely distributed to the tissues, including those of the CNS.

(3) Excretion. Unchanged drug (25%) and conjugated metabolites (75%) are excreted in the urine.

c. Therapeutic uses

(1) Metoclopramide is used to control **severe vomiting in dogs and cats.**

(2) It is used in the treatment of **gastric motility disorders** and **esophageal reflux** in **dogs, cats,** and **foals.**

d. Administration

(1) As an antiemetic, metoclopramide is administered orally, subcutaneously, or intramuscularly every 8 hours. It can also be administered by slow intravenous infusion.

(2) In the treatment of gastric motility disorders and esophageal reflux, it should be administered 30 minutes prior to feeding.

e. Adverse effects

(1) Gastric hemorrhage or perforation may occur in animals with gastric outlet obstruction.

(2) Behavioral changes (e.g., excitement, disorientation) may occur in dogs and cats.

3. Butyrophenones (e.g., **droperidol, haloperidol**). These agents are neuroleptic drugs with centrally acting antiemetic effects.

a. Mechanism of action. Butyrophenones create a long-acting blockade of dopaminergic neurons in the chemoreceptor trigger zone.

b. Therapeutic uses. Butyrophenones are used to control vomiting resulting from cancer chemotherapy.

c. Administration. The butyrophenones are given orally or intramuscularly every 2–4 days.

d. Adverse effects. Butyrophenones may produce mild sedation and tranquilization.

C. **Antihistamines** (e.g., **dimenhydrinate, diphenhydramine, promethazine**)

1. Mechanism of action. Antihistamines block histaminergic and cholinergic afferent pathways from the vestibular organs to the vomiting center.

2. **Pharmacokinetics**
   a. **Absorption.** Antihistamines are well absorbed by the gastrointestinal tract.
   b. **Fate.** Their distribution has not been studied in animals.

3. **Therapeutic uses.** Antihistamines are used to prevent motion sickness in dogs.

4. **Administration.** Antihistamines are administered orally every 8 hours.

5. **Adverse effects.** Mild sedation may be observed.

D. **Anticholinergic agents** [e.g., **aminopentamide, propantheline, isopropamide, Darbazine** (isopropamide plus prochlorperazine)]

1. **Mechanism of action.** Anticholinergic drugs block cholinergic afferent pathways from the gastrointestinal tract to the vomiting center.

2. **Therapeutic uses.** Anticholinergics are used in dogs and cats to treat vomiting and diarrhea (see VIII C).
   a. Alone, anticholinergics are less effective than other antiemetics in the treatment of vomiting.
   b. Anticholinergics combined with phenothiazines (e.g., Darbazine) control vomiting resulting from severe gastroenteritis.

3. **Administration** to dogs and cats is as follows.
   a. **Aminopentamide** is administered orally, intramuscularly, or subcutaneously every 8–12 hours.
   b. **Propantheline** is administered orally every 8 hours.
   c. **Isopropamide** is administered orally every 12 hours.

4. **Adverse effects** include **xerostomia, xerophthalmia, loss of visual accommodation, tachycardia, urine retention, paralytic ileus,** and **constipation.**

5. **Contraindications.** Anticholinergics are contraindicated in patients with **glaucoma.**

E. **Miscellaneous antiemetics**

1. **Intestinal protectants and adsorbents** (e.g., **kaolin, pectin, bismuth salts**) may reduce vomiting caused by mild gastritis.

2. **Locally acting gastric antacids** (e.g., magnesium hydroxide, magnesium silicate, aluminum hydroxide, aluminum silicate) may reduce vomiting caused by gastric hyperacidity.

VII. LAXATIVES AND CATHARTICS

A. **General considerations.** Laxatives and cathartics are used for:

1. Relief of acute nondietary constipation

2. Removal of poisons from the gastrointestinal tract

3. Prevention of tenesmus in advanced pregnancy or prolapse

4. Evacuation of the bowel prior to surgery or radiography

B. **Osmotic cathartics**

1. **Preparations**
   a. Magnesium sulfate (Epsom salt), magnesium oxide
   b. Sodium sulfate (Glauber's salt)
   c. Polyethylene glycol electrolyte solutions (Golytely, Colyte), isotonic mixtures of polyethylene glycol, sodium sulfate, sodium bicarbonate, sodium chloride, and potassium chloride
   d. Sodium phosphate and sodium tartrate mixtures (Fleet enemas)

2. Mechanism of action. Osmotic cathartics are nonabsorbable or poorly absorbable salts or polymers that osmotically retain water in the intestinal lumen. They have a rapid onset of action that begins in the small intestine.

3. Therapeutic use. Osmotic cathartics are the cathartics of choice for **elimination of poisons.**

4. Administration
   a. Magnesium sulfate and **magnesium oxide** are administered orally.
   b. Sodium sulfate is administered orally or via a stomach tube as a 6% solution.
   c. Polyethylene glycol–electrolyte solutions are administered orally prior to colonoscopy.
   d. Sodium phosphate and sodium tartrate mixtures are administered rectally to dogs. In cats, they produce hyperphosphatemia and should not be used.

C. Irritant cathartics (e.g., **castor oil, aloe, senna, cascara sagrada**)

1. Chemistry. Irritant cathartics are plant derivatives.

2. Mechanisms of action
   a. Castor oil is cleaved by pancreatic lipases in the small intestine to **yield irritant ricinoleates,** which stimulate peristalsis and reduce fluid absorption.
   b. Aloe, senna, and **cascara sagrada** contain glycosides that are hydrolyzed in the large intestine to **yield irritant anthraquinones.** The anthraquinones stimulate smooth muscle and increase colonic motility. Because they act in the large intestine, their onset of action is slow.

3. Therapeutic use. Irritant cathartics are administered orally to relieve acute constipation in small and large animals.

D. Bulk laxatives (e.g., **methylcellulose, agar, psyllium, wheat bran**)

1. Mechanism of action. Bulk laxatives contain hydrophilic colloids, which absorb water and increase bulk. Bulk stimulates large bowel peristalsis.

2. Administration is oral; wheat bran is added to the diet. The laxative effect occurs within 1–3 days.

E. Lubricants. **Mineral oil (liquid petrolatum)** and **white petrolatum** lubricate and soften feces.

F. Surfactants. **Docusate** is an anionic surfactant that acts in the large bowel to hydrate and soften feces by an emulsifying action.

VIII. ANTIDIARRHEAL DRUGS

A. General considerations

1. Indications. Acute diarrhea may respond to symptomatic therapy with antidiarrheal drugs, but chronic diarrhea requires a definitive diagnosis and specific therapy.

2. Oral rehydration therapy represents a significant advance in treating diarrhea in the absence of vomiting.
   a. In addition to **glucose** or **amino acids,** or both, these solutions contain **sodium chloride, potassium chloride, sodium bicarbonate,** and **potassium phosphate.**
   b. Sodium–glucose- and **sodium–amino acid-linked absorption** by the enterocyte remains intact even in the presence of moderate damage to the intestinal villi, providing the driving force for water and electrolyte absorption from the lumen to replace fecal losses.

B. **Opiates**

1. **Preparations**
   a. **Paregoric** is a camphorated tincture of opium.
   b. **Diphenoxylate** is a synthetic congener of meperidine. **Lomotil** is diphenoxylate plus atropine.
   c. **Loperamide** is a synthetic piperidine opioid.
   d. **Codeine**

2. **Mechanisms of action**
   a. Opiates **inhibit ACh release.** The resultant increased gastrointestinal rhythmic segmentation and decreased propulsive motility slow the transit time of luminal contents and increase absorption.
   b. In addition, opiates **directly stimulate absorption of fluid and electrolytes** via μ-opiate receptors in the CNS and intestinal mucosa.

3. **Therapeutic use.** Opiates are effective in the symptomatic treatment of acute diarrhea.

4. **Administration**
   a. **Paregoric** is administered orally 2–3 times daily to dogs and cats, once daily to calves and foals.
   b. **Diphenoxylate** is administered orally 2–3 times daily to dogs and cats.
   c. **Loperamide** is administered orally 1–2 times daily to dogs and cats.
   d. **Codeine** is administered orally 2–3 times daily to dogs and cats.

5. **Adverse effects**
   a. **Bacterial overgrowth** in the intestinal lumen of animals with infectious diarrhea may result from slowed intestinal transit time.
   b. **In cats, excitatory reactions** render opiate use controversial.

C. **Anticholinergic agents. Methscopolamine** is used, as well as **aminopentamide, propantheline,** and **isopropamide,** which are also effective as antiemetics (see VI D).

1. **Mechanism of action.** Anticholinergic agents inhibit propulsive and nonpropulsive gastrointestinal motility. They also inhibit normal, cholinergically mediated basal secretions of the gastrointestinal tract.

2. **Therapeutic uses**
   a. Anticholinergic agents may be used to treat **diarrhea;** however, they are of **questionable benefit** in this capacity because diarrhea is more commonly associated with hypomotility than hypermotility.
   b. Anticholinergic agents may be used to treat **gastrointestinal spasm.**

3. **Administration**
   a. **Methscopolamine** is administered orally to dogs every 8–12 hours.
   b. Administration of **isopropamide, aminopentamide,** and **propantheline** is discussed in VI D 3.

4. **Adverse effects** are discussed in VI D 4.

D. **Protectant and adsorbent agents**

1. **Preparations**
   a. **Kaolin-pectin suspensions** [20% kaolin (hydrated aluminum silicate) and 1% pectin (a polygalacturonic acid carbohydrate polymer)]
   b. **Bismuth subsalicylate**

2. **Mechanisms of action**
   a. Protectives and adsorbents adsorb toxins and provide a protective coating on inflamed mucosa.

    b. Bismuth subsalicylate has an anti-PG action in addition to its adsorbent properties.

3. Therapeutic use. Protectants and adsorbents are used for the symptomatic therapy of acute diarrhea. Adsorbents may decrease fluidity of feces without actually decreasing fecal water loss, thereby limiting their usefulness.

4. Administration
    a. Kaolin-pectin suspensions are administered orally every 4–6 hours. Kaolin-pectin is effective in dogs, cats, birds, horses, cattle, sheep, and swine.
    b. Bismuth subsalicylate is administered orally every 6–8 hours. Bismuth subsalicylate is approved for use in dogs, horses, cattle, and swine. **Salicylates should not be administered to cats.**

5. Adverse effects. Bismuth subsalicylate may produce dark feces, which should not be confused with melena.

IX. AGENTS USED IN THE TREATMENT OF INFLAMMATORY BOWEL DISEASE

A. Sulfasalazine

1. Chemistry. Sulfasalazine is an enteric sulfonamide that consists of sulfapyridine and 5-aminosalicylic acid (5-ASA) linked by a diazo bond.

2. Mechanism of action. Sulfasalazine is cleaved by bacteria in the large bowel to release sulfapyridine and salicylate.
    a. Salicylates have anti-inflammatory effects on the bowel mucosa.
    b. Salicylates may inhibit PG synthesis in colonic mucosa.

3. Pharmacokinetics. Absorption of sulfapyridine and salicylate is minimal (less than 30% and 10%, respectively), allowing most of the dose to reach the colon.

4. Therapeutic uses. Sulfasalazine is used to treat **chronic inflammatory bowel disease** and **colitis** in **dogs and cats.**

5. Administration. Sulfasalazine is administered orally 2–3 times daily.

6. Adverse effects are rare, but long-term use may cause **sulfapyridine toxicity,** especially keratoconjunctivitis sicca. **Salicylate toxicity** may occur **in cats.**

B. Olsalazine

1. Chemistry. Olsalazine consists of two molecules of 5-ASA linked by a diazo bond. Olsalazine is less toxic than sulfasalazine because it lacks the sulfonamide moiety.

2. Mechanism of action. After cleavage of the diazo bond by colonic bacteria, salicylates are released.

3. Pharmacokinetics. Oral absorption of olsalazine is minimal, with over 98% of the dose reaching the colon.

4. Therapeutic uses. Olsalazine is used for **chronic inflammatory bowel disease** in **dogs and cats.**

5. Administration. Olsalazine is administered orally 2–3 times daily.

6. Adverse effects. Salicylate toxicity can occur in cats receiving long-term olsalazine therapy.

C. Tylosin

1. Chemistry. Tylosin is a macrolide antibiotic structurally related to erythromycin (see Chapter 11). Macrolides are organic bases that form salts with acids such as phosphate or tartrate.

2. Mechanism of action. Tylosin inhibits protein synthesis in susceptible bacteria by binding to the 50S ribosome and blocking long-chain peptide synthesis. Its bacteriostatic action suppresses bacterial overgrowth in chronic intestinal disease.

3. Pharmacokinetics
   a. Absorption and fate. Tylosin is absorbed from the intestine and widely distributed to tissues except those of the CNS.
   b. Excretion. Tylosin is excreted unchanged in bile and urine.

4. Therapeutic use. Tylosin is used to treat **chronic colitis** in **dogs and cats.**

5. Administration. Tylosin is administered orally 2–3 times daily with food.

6. Adverse effects. Tylosin may cause mild gastrointestinal disturbances (e.g., vomiting, diarrhea).

D. Metronidazole

1. Mechanism of action
   a. Metronidazole is an antiprotozoan nitroimidazole (see Chapter 13) and an antibacterial. It is especially effective against anaerobes.
   b. Metronidazole suppresses cell-mediated immune reactions.

2. Pharmacokinetics
   a. Absorption and fate. Metronidazole is well absorbed by the gastrointestinal tract and widely distributed.
   b. Excretion. Hepatic metabolites and unchanged drug are excreted in urine and feces.

3. Therapeutic use. Metronidazole is used to treat **colitis in dogs.**

4. Administration. Metronidazole is administered orally 2–3 times daily.

5. Adverse effects are infrequent, but high or prolonged doses may produce neurotoxicity, including tremors and ataxia.

6. Contraindications. Metronidazole should not be used in pregnant animals.

X. DRUGS FOR TREATMENT OF RUMINANT GASTROINTESTINAL DISORDERS

A. General considerations

1. Development of rumen function begins at 3–6 weeks of age and is complete by 9–13 weeks of age. In order to administer oral medication to lambs and calves, the nonfunctional ruminoreticulum must be bypassed by inducing closure of the esophageal (ruminoreticular) groove (see X B).

2. The **normal intraruminal pH range** is 5.5–7.

3. Innervation
   a. Extrinsic contractions of the ruminoreticulum are controlled by vagal efferents from the dorsal vagal nucleus in the CNS.
   b. Intrinsic contractions are controlled by intramural plexuses.

4. Rumen microflora function depends on proper nutrient intake and normal ruminoreticular motor activity.

B. Agents for inducing closure of the esophageal groove. When stimulated, buccal and pharyngeal receptors activate a vagal reflex that closes the groove within 2–5 seconds; effects last for 60 seconds. **Milk, sodium bicarbonate** (10% to calves), or **copper sulfate (5% to calves, 2% to lambs)** may be used to induce esophageal groove closure. Water is not effective.

C. **Ruminotorics**

1. **Bitters** (e.g., **nux vomica, ginger, capsicum**) stimulate salivation, which may enhance rumen function; however, the efficacy of bitters is minimal. Bitters are administered orally.

2. **Cholinergics** (e.g., **neostigmine, bethanechol**) transiently increase the frequency, but not the strength, of contractions in rumen atony. Cholinergics are administered subcutaneously.

3. **Opiate antagonists** (e.g., **naloxone**) stimulate extrinsic contractions when administered parenterally. Opiate antagonists are useful for the treatment of endotoxin-induced rumen stasis.

4. **Rumen fluid transfer.** Oral inoculation of viable rumen bacteria and protozoa is the most effective means of restoring rumen function following correction of the primary cause of stasis.

D. **Rumen antacids** (e.g., **magnesium oxide, magnesium carbonate, aluminum hydroxide, calcium carbonate, ammonium carbonate**)

1. **Therapeutic use.** Antacids treat mild cases of **lactic acidosis resulting from carbohydrate engorgement.**

2. **Administration.** These agents are administered orally every 8–12 hours.

3. **Adverse effects.** Systemic alkalosis may result from overdose, especially of magnesium oxide.

E. **Rumen acidifiers** (e.g., **vinegar, 4%–5% acetic acid**)

1. **Therapeutic uses**
   a. Rumen acidifiers may be used to treat **simple indigestion,** in which a constant inflow of bicarbonate-rich saliva raises the pH of the rumen.
   b. They are used in the treatment of **acute urea poisoning,** because they decrease ammonia absorption via formation of ammonium ion and inhibit urease activity of rumen microflora.

2. **Administration.** Rumen acidifiers are mixed with several liters of cold water and administered via a stomach tube every 6–8 hours.

F. **Viscosity-altering (antibloat) agents**

1. **Preparations** include **poloxalene, polymerized methyl silicone, mineral oil,** and **vegetable** (e.g., **soybean, peanut, sunflower**) oil.

2. **Mechanisms of action.** Viscosity-altering agents alter the surface tension of froth and break up the gas bubbles.

3. **Therapeutic use. Frothy (not free-gas) bloat** requires viscosity-altering drug therapy.

4. **Administration.** Antibloat agents are administered via drench or stomach tube.

STUDY QUESTIONS

DIRECTIONS: Each of the numbered items or incomplete statements in this section is followed by answers or by completions of the statement. Select the **one** numbered answer or completion that is **best** in each case.

1. Which one of the following drugs inhibits the proton pump in gastric parietal cells?

(1) Cimetidine
(2) Ranitidine
(3) Omeprazole
(4) Diazepam

2. Which one of the following is an antihistamine used to treat vomiting resulting from motion sickness or vestibular disease?

(1) Propantheline
(2) Metoclopramide
(3) Chlorpromazine
(4) Dimenhydrinate

3. Which cathartic is used to hasten the elimination of poisons from the gastrointestinal tract?

(1) Senna
(2) Methylcellulose
(3) Sodium sulfate
(4) Docusate

4. Retention of urine may be observed as an adverse effect of:

(1) chlorpromazine.
(2) isopropamide.
(3) droperidol.
(4) diphenoxylate.

5. Which of the following statements regarding gastrointestinal antacids, protectives, and adsorbents is correct?

(1) Rebound hydrochloric acid secretion is more likely with aluminum hydoxide than with magnesium oxide.
(2) Kaolin is a hydrated aluminum silicate.
(3) Bismuth subsalicylate tends to produce an osmotic laxative effect unless dosage is carefully controlled.
(4) The antidiarrheal action of pectin results from its rapid breakdown to galactose in the small intestine.

6. Anaerobic bacteria in the large bowel may release antigens that stimulate inflammation of the colonic mucosa in canine inflammatory bowel disease. Bactericidal activity against anaerobes and suppression of mucosal immune reactions characterize the action of which one of the following drugs?

(1) Olsalazine
(2) Tylosin
(3) Metronidazole
(4) Aminopentamide

7. How does the oral administration of vinegar (acetic acid) alleviate acute urea poisoning in cattle?

(1) It reduces ketonemia by providing acetate as an energy source.
(2) It stimulates bacterial urease to increase urea breakdown in the rumen.
(3) It slows rumen fermentation to allow regrowth of favorable bacteria.
(4) It reduces ammonia absorption into the systemic circulation.

8. Antiprostaglandin (anti-PG) activity and protective and adsorbent properties characterize the antidiarrheal action of:

(1) kaolin.
(2) sucralfate.
(3) magnesium trisilicate.
(4) bismuth subsalicylate.

9. In which condition is nutritional support with medium-chain triglycerides indicated?

(1) Gluten enteropathy
(2) Intestinal lymphangiectasia
(3) Lactose intolerance
(4) Acute colitis

Questions 10–13

(5) Oxazepam

10. A 15-year-old male cat that is depressed, uremic, and vomiting is brought to the veterinary clinic. Treatment might include all of the following *except:*

(1) oral administration of cimetidine.
(2) oral administration of sucralfate (2 hours prior to or after oral administration of other drugs).
(3) oral administration of metoclopramide.
(4) intravenous administration of glucose and electrolytes.
(5) administration of a sodium phosphate enema.

11. The cat is stabilized, but after 3 days in the hospital, he is still not eating. Which drug may be administered to increase the cat's appetite?

(1) Terpin hydrate
(2) Methscopolamine
(3) Chlorpromazine
(4) Ranitidine

12. The cat's appetite returns, but he develops diarrhea. Which opiate analog with an action limited to the gut should be administered?

(1) Loperamide
(2) Butorphanol
(3) Domperidone
(4) Meperidine
(5) Propantheline

13. The cat is sent home. Two days later, the owner thinks the cat has a fever, and he administers two acetaminophen tablets. He has second thoughts about this and calls the veterinarian 15 minutes later, who advises him to bring the cat in immediately for induction of vomiting. Which emetic should be used?

(1) Apomorphine
(2) Ammonium chloride
(3) Nux vomica
(4) Xylazine
(5) Bismuth subsalicylate

DIRECTIONS: The numbered item or incomplete statement in this section is negatively phrased, as indicated by an italicized word such as *not, least,* or *except.* Select the **one** numbered answer or completion that is **best**.

---

14. Increased segmentation, slowed transit, and stimulation of electrolyte absorption by gut mucosa characterize the antidiarrheal action of all of the following agents *except:*

(1) paregoric.
(2) methscopolamine.
(3) diphenoxylate.
(4) loperamide.
(5) codeine.

ANSWERS AND EXPLANATIONS

1. The answer is 3 [III A 2].
Inhibitors of gastric acid secretion are used in small animals to treat gastritis, gastric ulcers, and liver disease. Omeprazole decreases gastric acid secretion by inhibiting hydrogen ion generation by parietal cell adenosine triphosphatase (ATPase). Cimetidine and ranitidine are histamine$_2$ (H$_2$)-receptor antagonists. Diazepam is a benzodiazepine used for short-term stimulation of appetite.

2. The answer is 4 [VI C].
Dimenhydrinate prevents vomiting via blockade of histaminergic afferent pathways originating in the vestibular organs. Propantheline is an anticholinergic that blocks the afferent pathway from the gastrointestinal tract to the vomiting center. Metoclopramide and chlorpromazine are antidopaminergics with little or no antihistaminic action.

3. The answer is 3 [VII B 1, 3].
Osmotic cathartics such as sodium sulfate act in the small intestine and thus have a rapid onset of action. Therefore, they are the cathartics of choice for the elimination of poisons. Senna, methylcellulose, and docusate exert their laxative effect in the large intestine.

4. The answer is 2 [VI D 4].
Anticholinergic agents (e.g., isopropamide) may produce urine retention by inhibiting bladder contractility and tone. Chlorpromazine and droperidol are dopamine antagonists, and diphenoxylate is an opiate agonist.

5. The answer is 2 [III B 4 a; VIII D 1].
Kaolin is a hydrated, aluminum silicate with protective and adsorbent properties. Magnesium salts are more likely than aluminum salts to produce rebound hydrochloric acid secretion. Bismuth subsalicylate has antidiarrheal effects. Pectin is polymerized galacturonic acid, which is not readily hydrolyzed in the gastrointestinal tract.

6. The answer is 3 [IX D 1].
Metronidazole is bactericidal for anaerobes, and it suppresses cell-mediated immunity. Olsalazine is a salicylate dimer, which is

cleaved in the large bowel to release two molecules of 5-aminosalicylate (5-ASA), which inhibit prostaglandin (PG) synthesis. Tylosin suppresses colonic bacterial growth but has no effect on mucosal immune reactions. Aminopentamide is an anticholinergic used to control vomiting and diarrhea.

7. The answer is 4 [X E].
Acidification of the rumen shifts the equilibrium from ammonia to ammonium ion, which slows absorption of ammonia into the systemic circulation. Urease activity is also decreased at a lower rumen pH, resulting in a slower rate of ammonia formation. Ketonemia and excessive rumen fermentation are not related to urea poisoning.

8. The answer is 4 [VIII D 2 b].
The antidiarrheal action of bismuth subsalicylate results in part from inhibition of prostaglandin (PG) synthesis in the gut mucosa. Kaolin, magnesium trisilicate, and sucralfate are mucosal protectives that have no effect on PG synthesis.

9. The answer is 2 [I D].
Lymphatic absorption of lipids is impaired in lymphangiectasia. Because medium-chain triglycerides are absorbed via portal blood vessels, not lymphatics, they are able to provide calories in this malabsorptive condition. Gluten enteropathy and lactose intolerance require diets free of cereal or dairy products, respectively. Nondietary therapy is employed for acute colitis.

10–13. The answers are 10-5 [VII B 4 d], **11-5** [II C], **12-1** [VIII B], **13-4** [V B 2].
Sodium phosphate laxatives or enemas should not be used in cats because they produce hyperphosphatemia in this species. Inhibition of gastric acid secretion with cimetidine, protective coating of possible uremia-induced ulcers with sucralfate, prevention of vomiting with metoclopramide, and restoration of fluid and electrolyte balance are rational therapeutic measures.

Oxazepam, which increases γ-aminobutyric acid (GABA) and inhibits serotonin, may stimulate appetite by suppressing the satiety center in the hypothalamus. Terpin hydrate is an anti-tussive, methscopolamine is an anticholinergic, and chlorpromazine is a phenothiazine tran-quilizer and centrally acting antiemetic. Ranitid-ine is a histamine$_2$ (H$_2$)-receptor antagonist that inhibits gastric acid secretion.

Loperamide is a synthetic opiate antidiar-rheal with action limited to the gut. Butorpha-nol and meperidine are opiates that have both central and peripheral actions. Domperidone is a peripherally acting antidopaminergic that stimulates gastric motility. Propantheline is an anticholinergic agent.

Xylazine is the centrally acting emetic of choice in cats. Apomorphine should not be used in cats because of the potential for cen-tral nervous system (CNS) excitement. Ammo-nium chloride, nux vomica, and bismuth salts are not emetics.

14. The answer is 2 [VIII B, C].
Opiates increase gastrointestinal rhythmic seg-mentation, slow the transit time of luminal contents, and stimulate electrolyte absorption by the gut mucosa. Paregoric, diphenoxylate, loperamide, and codeine are opiates. Methsco-polamine is an anticholinergic that does not increase segmentation.

Chapter 11

Antimicrobial Drugs

Franklin A. Ahrens

I. INTRODUCTION

A. Antimicrobial therapy is **based on the selective toxicity of a drug for invading organisms rather than mammalian cells.** Final eradication of organisms generally requires host immune responses (e.g., phagocytosis), particularly with bacteriostatic antimicrobial drugs.

B. Principles of antimicrobial therapy

1. The organism must be sensitive to the drug, and effective tissue concentrations of the drug [e.g., five times the minimal inhibitory concentration (MIC)] should be maintained until the organism is eliminated.
   a. Culture and identification of the organism and antibiotic sensitivity testing may be necessary to facilitate antibiotic selection.
   b. Dosage regimens and routes of administration should be selected to ensure maintenance of therapeutic drug levels in affected tissues.

2. Effective antimicrobial therapy requires consideration of the total clinical problem. Treatment may necessitate drainage of abscesses or hematomas, debridement of devitalized tissue, or removal of foreign bodies and irrigation of cavities.

3. Prophylactic use of antimicrobials should be employed only when the identity of the invading organism can be reasonably surmised. For example, staphylococcal infections of bone following orthopedic surgery are prevented by administration of cephalosporins before or during surgery.

4. A single, narrow-spectrum antibiotic is usually more desirable than a less specific, broad-spectrum agent.

C. Resistance to antimicrobials

1. **Mechanisms of bacterial resistance**
   a. **Enzyme production.** Organisms may produce enzymes (via constitutive or inducible processes) that inactivate the drug.
   b. **Decreased cell wall permeability.** Cell wall permeability to the drug may be decreased, limiting uptake by the organism.
   c. **Active transport** of the drug out of the cell may be increased.
   d. **Alteration of the drug receptor** or binding site may result in reduced drug affinity.
   e. **Development of alternative pathways.** The organism may develop alternate metabolic or synthetic pathways to bypass or repair the effects of the antimicrobial agent.

2. **Development of resistance**
   a. **Mutation.** Bacterial chromosomal mutations may confer resistance either slowly (in a stepwise fashion with each succeeding generation of the mutant more resistant) or rapidly (in a single step in which the bacterium is resistant after the initial mutation). Mutation is a random event. Antimicrobials do not induce mutations but may promote resistant strains of bacteria by suppressing susceptible bacteria.
   b. **Conjugation.** Conjugation is a type of reproduction in which genetic material is transferred from cell to cell via a **pilus,** which is encoded by a **resistance transfer factor (RTF)** on a **plasmid.**
      (1) **Infectious (transferable) drug resistance** occurs when resistance factors

(R factors) from plasmid deoxyribonucleic acid (DNA), chromosomal DNA, or both encode for resistance to multiple drugs and are rapidly transferred to the bacterial population.

(2) **Conjugation,** which occurs in certain Gram-negative bacteria, has been observed clinically in enteric infections with *Salmonella* species, *Shigella* species, and *Escherichia coli.*

c. **Transduction.** The transference of drug-resistant genes by bacteriophages may be important in the development of resistant strains of *Staphylococcus aureus.*

d. **Transformation.** DNA-carrying genes for drug resistance may be incorporated by bacteria after its secretion or release following lysis of resistant organisms. Acquisition of resistance by transformation is relatively infrequent.

II. SULFONAMIDES

A. Chemistry

1. **Structure** (Figure 11-1). The sulfonamides are derivatives of *p*-aminobenzene sulfonic acid and are structurally similar to *p*-aminobenzoic acid (PABA), an intermediate in the bacterial synthesis of folic acid.

2. **Characteristics.** The sulfonamides behave as weak organic acids, which are **poorly water-soluble unless prepared as sodium salts.**
   a. Concentrated solutions of the sodium salts of most sulfonamides are alkaline and may be corrosive.
   b. According to the **law of independent solubility,** the solubility of a sulfonamide is not influenced by the presence of other sulfonamides in the solution; thus, **sulfonamide mixtures** are used to **increase solubility** and **reduce toxicity.**

B. Mechanism of action (Figure 11-2). Sulfonamides competitively **inhibit dihydropteroate synthetase,** the enzyme that catalyzes the incorporation of PABA into dihydrofolic acid.

1. Folic acid is required for purine and DNA synthesis; without it, bacterial growth is inhibited. Because they inhibit bacterial growth, sulfonamides are **bacteriostatic** agents.

2. Mammalian cells and bacteria that use preformed folic acid are not affected by sulfonamides.

C. Pharmacokinetics

1. **Absorption.** Sulfonamides are well absorbed orally and widely distributed to tissues.

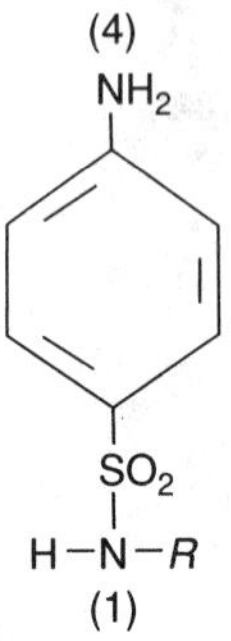

(4)
NH$_2$

SO$_2$
H—N—R
(1)

FIGURE 11-1. General structure of the sulfonamides. The *p*-amino group at position *4* must be free for antimicrobial activity to occur. Substitution with a heterocyclic ring (e.g., thiazole, pyrimidine, pyridine) at the *R* position on position *1* distinguishes the various sulfonamides. Replacement of the hydrogen with sodium at position *1* greatly increases the water solubility of the sulfonamide.

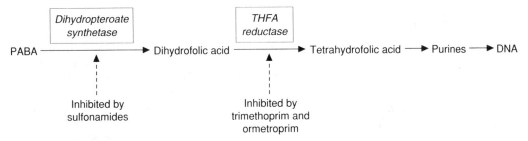

FIGURE 11-2. Mechanism of action of sulfonamides. Sulfonamides block dihydrofolic acid synthesis by competing with *p*-aminobenzoic acid *(PABA)* for binding sites on dihydropteroate synthetase. Dihydrofolic acid is necessary for the synthesis of tetrahydrofolic acid, and, ultimately, purines and deoxyribonucleic acid *(DNA)*. Trimethoprim and ormetoprim inhibit tetrahydrofolic acid reductase *(THFA reductase)*, which is necessary for tetrahydrofolic acid synthesis. Therefore, potentiated sulfonamides (i.e., those combined with trimethoprim or ormetoprim) block the second step of protein synthesis (i.e., tetrahydrofolic acid synthesis) as well as the first step.

2. Fate

a. Distribution. Transcellular fluid concentrations of the drug are 80% of the plasma concentration. Binding to plasma albumin varies with each sulfonamide but generally accounts for 50%–75% of the dose.

b. Metabolism. The type and extent of metabolism vary with the sulfonamide and the animal species.

(1) Metabolism by acetylation at the *p*-amino group and glucuronide conjugation occurs in most species; however, acetylation does not occur in dogs.

(2) Oxidation of the benzene and heterocyclic rings to quinone derivatives also occurs, especially in dogs.

3. Excretion. Renal excretion of the unchanged drug and metabolites is via glomerular filtration, active secretion, and passive tubular reabsorption. Reabsorption is pH–pK$_a$ dependent.

D. **Preparations and therapeutic uses.** Sulfonamides are widely used in the prevention and treatment of local and systemic infections in all species. They are **broad-spectrum** agents, even exhibiting antiprotozoal activity.

1. Sulfamethazine is used in cattle, sheep, and swine in the control of respiratory and gastrointestinal infections and to promote growth in swine. It is slowly excreted, and therapeutic levels are maintained in plasma for 24 hours with a single dose.

2. Sulfadimethoxine is a long-acting sulfonamide used in all species for the treatment of systemic and soft tissue infections and coccidiosis. Sulfadimethoxine is more soluble and less toxic than sulfamethazine. The plasma half-life is 10–15 hours.

3. Sulfathiazole is a rapidly excreted sulfonamide used in swine and poultry as a feed or water additive to treat respiratory and enteric diseases. In addition, sulfathiazole, along with sulfamethazine and sulfapyridine, is used to treat acute infections in food-producing animals.

4. Sulfachlorpyridazine is a rapidly absorbed and rapidly excreted sulfonamide used in cattle and swine for the therapy of respiratory and enteric infections, especially colibacillosis.

5. Sulfisoxazole and **sulfamethoxazole** are used to treat urinary tract infections in small animals. They are rapidly excreted and very soluble; thus, high concentrations may be attained in urine with minimal danger of renal crystalluria.

6. **Sulfacetamide** is the only sulfonamide that can be prepared as a sodium salt at a neutral pH and thus can be used in ophthalmic preparations.

7. **Sulfasalazine** is used for the therapy of enteric diseases (e.g., colitis and inflammatory bowel disease) in dogs and cats (see Chapter 10 IX A). It is cleaved by intestinal bacteria to sulfapyridine and 5-aminosalicylic acid (5-ASA), which have antibacterial and anti-inflammatory actions, respectively.

8. **Potentiated sulfonamides** are combinations of a sulfonamide with trimethoprim or ormetoprim. This combination results in a synergistic action via sequential blockade of folate synthesis (see Figure 11-2). Trimethoprim and ormetoprim inhibit dihydrofolate reductase in bacteria (but not mammalian cells) and thus block the formation of tetrahydrofolic acid, essential for purine and DNA synthesis.

   a. Potentiated sulfonamides have a broader spectrum of action and a reduced rate of development of bacterial resistance. They are used in the treatment of susceptible infections in all species.

   b. Preparations include sulfadiazine plus trimethoprim, sulfamethoxazole plus trimethoprim, and sulfadimethoxine plus ormetoprim.

E. Administration

1. **Oral administration.** Sulfonamides are generally administered orally because absorption is rapid. Slow-release boluses of sulfamethazine and sulfadimethoxine are available for ruminants. These preparations provide blood levels for 48–72 hours with a single dose.

2. **Intravenous administration** is used for initial treatment of severe, acute infections.

3. **Frequency of dosing** varies with the individual sulfonamides.

F. **Bacterial resistance.** Bacteria that are resistant to one sulfonamide are resistant to all. Mechanisms include:

1. Increased PABA production

2. Decreased affinity of the sulfonamide for dihydropteroate synthetase

3. Bacterial metabolism of sulfonamide

G. Adverse effects

1. **Renal crystalluria,** the result of precipitation of sulfonamides in neutral or acidic urine, may occur with large or prolonged doses or inadequate water intake, especially with the older, less soluble sulfonamides (e.g., sulfathiazole). Sulfonamide therapy generally should not extend beyond 5 days.

2. **Keratoconjunctivitis sicca** may be observed in dogs treated with sulfonamides such as sulfadiazine, which contain the pyrimidine nucleus. The mechanism of the toxic effect on lacrimal acinar cells is unknown.

3. **Hypoprothrombinemia, thrombocytopenia,** and **anemia** occur rarely and are probably immune-mediated reactions. Sulfonamides should not be used in animals with preexisting bleeding disorders.

III. FLUOROQUINOLONES (e.g., ENROFLOXACIN, CIPROFLOXACIN)

A. Chemistry

1. **Structure.** The fluoroquinolones consist of a carboxyl group, fluorine atom, and piperazine ring attached to a quinoline ring.

2. **Characteristics.** Fluoroquinolones are weak acids and are lipophilic. Water-soluble salts are used in parenteral preparations.

B. **Mechanism of action.** The fluoroquinolones **inhibit bacterial DNA gyrase,** an enzyme that controls DNA supercoiling as the replicating strands separate.

1. Inhibition of gyrase results in degradation of chromosomal DNA at the replicating fork.

2. Fluoroquinolones are **bactericidal.**

C. **Pharmacokinetics**

1. **Absorption.** Oral absorption of fluoroquinolones is rapid; for example, dogs achieve peak plasma concentrations 1 hour after administration.

2. **Fate**
    a. **Distribution** is wide and includes the central nervous system (CNS), bone, and prostate. The plasma half-life is 3 hours in dogs and 4 hours in cats.
    b. **Metabolism.** Some hepatic metabolism occurs.

3. **Excretion.** Both the parent drug and metabolites are excreted in urine and bile. Renal tubular active secretion results in high urinary concentrations.

D. **Spectrum of activity.** Although fluoroquinolones have broad-spectrum activity, anaerobes tend to be resistant.

E. **Preparations and therapeutic uses.** Enrofloxacin and ciprofloxacin are used in the treatment of dermal, respiratory, and urinary tract infections (including prostatitis) in dogs and cats.

F. **Administration.** Enrofloxacin and ciprofloxacin are administered orally twice daily. Intramuscular administration is acceptable in dogs, but not in cats.

G. **Bacterial resistance.** Development of bacterial resistance is relatively rare. Extended exposure to subtherapeutic dosages may lead to the appearance of mutants that resist fluoroquinolone binding to DNA gyrase.

H. **Adverse effects** include **erosion of articular cartilage in young dogs.** Fluoroquinolones should not be administered to small and medium breeds for the first 8 months of life or to large breeds for the first 18 months of life.

IV. PENICILLINS

A. **Chemistry** (Figure 11-3). Penicillins comprise a beta-lactam ring and a thiazolidone ring.

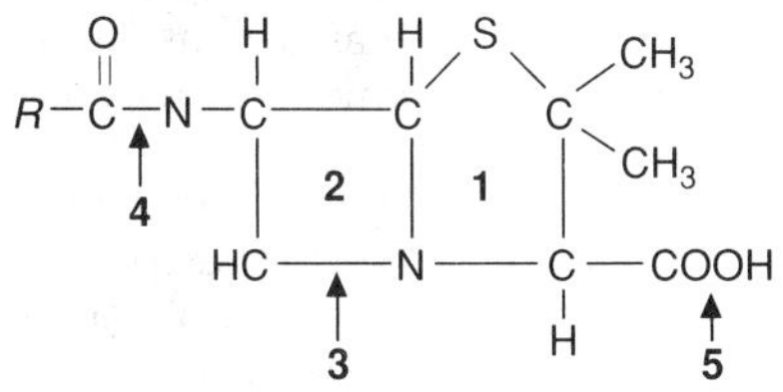

FIGURE 11-3. General structure of penicillins. Substituents at *R* distinguish the various penicillins. *(1)* Thiazolidone ring. *(2)* Beta-lactam ring. *(3)* Site of action of beta-lactamases (penicillinases). *(4)* Site of amidase cleavage to yield 6-aminopenicillanic acid (6-APA) nucleus for semisynthetic penicillins. *(5)* Site of salt formation (e.g., sodium, procaine).

1. Cleavage of the beta-lactam ring destroys antibiotic activity; some resistant bacteria produce beta-lactamases (penicillinases).

2. Amidase cleavage of the amide bond side chain yields the 6-aminopenicillanic acid (6-APA) nucleus used in producing semisynthetic penicillins.

3. The carboxyl group attached to the thiazolidone ring is the site of salt formation (e.g., sodium, potassium, procaine). Conversion to salt esters stabilizes the penicillins and affects solubility and absorption rates.

B. **Mechanism of action**

1. Penicillins bind to and **inhibit the transpeptidase involved in the cross-linking of the bacterial cell wall,** the third and final step in cell wall synthesis. The weakened cell wall ruptures, resulting in cell death.

2. Penicillins also inhibit other peptidases (penicillin-binding proteins) involved in cell wall synthesis and **block inhibition of autolysins.**

3. Rapidly growing bacteria are most susceptible to the **bactericidal** effect of penicillin.

C. **Pharmacokinetics**

1. **Absorption**
   a. Many penicillins (e.g., penicillin G, methicillin, ticarcillin) are degraded by gastric hydrochloric acid; therefore, they are poorly absorbed orally.
   b. Acid-stable penicillins (e.g., penicillin V, ampicillin, amoxicillin, hetacillin, oxacillin, cloxacillin, dicloxacillin, indanyl salt of carbenicillin) are well absorbed orally.

2. **Fate.** Penicillins are widely distributed to tissues and transcellular fluids, except those of the CNS and the eye.

3. **Excretion.** More than 90% of an administered dose is excreted unchanged in the urine by glomerular filtration and active tubular secretion. The remainder is metabolized by the liver to penicilloic acid derivatives, which may act as antigenic determinants in penicillin hypersensitivity.

D. **Spectrum of activity.** The penicillins are primarily effective against Gram-positive aerobes and anaerobes. The broad-spectrum, semisynthetic penicillins are effective against some gram-negative pathogens.

E. **Preparations and therapeutic uses**

1. **Natural penicillins**
   a. **Penicillin G (benzylpenicillin)** is used in all species for the treatment of infections caused by Gram-positive, non-penicillinase–producing pathogens. Penicillin G is the most potent penicillin against these organisms.
   b. **Penicillin V** is administered orally for long-term therapy of infections caused by Gram-positive organisms in dogs, cats, and horses.

2. **Penicillinase-stable penicillins** (e.g., **methicillin, oxacillin, cloxacillin, dicloxacillin)** are reserved for severe staphylococcal infections caused by beta-lactamase–producing organisms.

3. **Broad-spectrum penicillins**
   a. **Ampicillin, amoxicillin,** and **hetacillin** are active against many Gram-negative aerobes (e.g., *E. coli, Proteus* species, *Haemophilus* species) as well as Gram-positive pathogens. They are used in all species for the treatment of susceptible infections. They are acid-stable, but not penicillinase-stable.
   b. **Carbenicillin** and **ticarcillin** are used alone or in combination with gentamicin or tobramycin in the treatment of infections caused by *Pseudomonas* species.
   c. **Azlocillin, mezlocillin,** and **piperacillin** have an extended spectrum of activity against Gram-negative organisms, including *Pseudomonas, Enterobacter,* and

Klebsiella species. Their high cost limits their use to the treatment of severe Gram-negative infections in dogs and cats.

4. Potentiated penicillins are used in small animals to extend the spectrum of antimicrobial action.

  a. Clavulanic acid has minimal antibacterial action, but it inhibits many of the beta-lactamases produced by penicillin-resistant organisms. It is combined with amoxicillin or ticarcillin in commercial preparations.

  b. Sulbactam has an action similar to clavulanic acid and is combined with ampicillin.

F. | **Administration.** Penicillins are generally administered intramuscularly or, if they are acid-stable, orally 2–3 times per day.

  1. Procaine penicillin G is slowly absorbed from intramuscular injection sites and may provide therapeutic levels for 24 hours with a single dose.

  2. Benzathine penicillin G is even more slowly absorbed over 48–72 hours, but blood levels attained are relatively low.

  3. Sodium or potassium salts of penicillin G may be administered intravenously or intramuscularly every 4–6 hours.

G. | **Bacterial resistance**

  1. Inactivation of penicillins by bacterial production of beta-lactamases is the most common mechanism of resistance.

  2. Alterations in the structure of penicillin-binding proteins result in failure of the drug to bind.

H. | **Adverse effects**

  1. Allergic reactions to penicillin may occur in animals, especially cattle. Signs include skin eruptions, angioedema, and anaphylaxis. Procaine salts of penicillin should not be used in birds, snakes, turtles, guinea pigs, or chinchillas because these species are sensitive to procaine.

  2. Hyperkalemia and **cardiac arrhythmias** may result from intravenous administration of potassium penicillin.

V. **CEPHALOSPORINS**

A. | **Chemistry**

  1. Structure. Cephalosporins are beta-lactam antibiotics that have a 7-aminocephalosporanic acid nucleus analogous to the 6-APA nucleus of penicillins.

  2. Characteristics. Cephalosporins are weak acids that may be administered as a sodium salt, monohydrate, or free base.

B. | **Mechanism of action.** Like the penicillins, the cephalosporins inhibit the third stage of bacterial cell wall synthesis (i.e., the cross-linking of the peptidoglycan chain). Cephalosporins are **bactericidal.**

C. | **Pharmacokinetics**

  1. Absorption. Most cephalosporins are unstable in gastric acid and must be administered parenterally. Cephalexin and cefadroxil are acid-stable and are well absorbed orally.

2. Fate

a. Distribution. Cephalosporins are widely distributed, with excellent penetration of all body tissues except cerebrospinal fluid.

b. Metabolism is minimal. Some cephalosporins (e.g., cephalothin, cefotaxime) are deacetylated by the liver.

3. Excretion. Renal excretion is by glomerular filtration and active tubular secretion.

D. **Preparations and therapeutic uses**

1. **First-generation cephalosporins** (e.g., cephalexin, cefadroxil, cephapirin, cephalothin, cefazolin) are the first alternative to penicillins for treating infections caused by **Gram-positive aerobes.**
   a. They are used in all species for the treatment of **bone** and **soft tissue infections.**
   b. First-generation cephalosporins are frequently employed for antibiotic **prophylaxis** because of their ability to penetrate tissues and body fluids.

2. **Second-generation cephalosporins** (e.g., cefaclor, cefoxitin). These agents have a spectrum of activity that is broader than that of first-generation cephalosporins and includes **some Gram-negative pathogens.** Second-generation cephalosporins are not widely used in veterinary medicine.

3. **Third-generation cephalosporins** (e.g., ceftiofur, moxalactam) have an extended spectrum of activity against Gram-negative organisms, are resistant to beta-lactamases (cephalosporinases), and penetrate the blood–brain barrier.
   a. They are used in the treatment of **Gram-negative meningitis** in small animals.
   b. Ceftiofur is used in the treatment of **respiratory disease in cattle.**

E. **Administration.** Most cephalosporins are administered every 8 hours.

F. **Bacterial resistance.** Bacterial beta-lactamase production may confer resistance, although cephalosporins tend to be less susceptible than the penicillins.

G. **Adverse effects**

1. **Nephrotoxicity** may develop with prolonged administration; dosages should be adjusted in the presence of renal disease.

2. **Hypersensitivity** and **allergic reactions** may occur. Cephalosporins may be used in penicillin-intolerant patients; however, caution should be exercised because cross-reactivity can occur.

VI. AMINOGLYCOSIDES

A. **Chemistry**

1. **Structure.** Aminoglycosides consist of two or three amino sugars joined to aminocyclitol, a hexose, by glycosidic bonds.

2. **Characteristics**
   a. Numerous amino groups contribute to the **highly polar** and **basic** character of the aminoglycosides.
   b. **Sulfate salts** are **water-soluble.**

B. **Mechanism of action.** The aminoglycosides bind to the 30S ribosome and inhibit the rate of protein synthesis and the fidelity of messenger ribonucleic acid (mRNA) translation, resulting in the synthesis of abnormal proteins.

1. Aminoglycoside uptake by bacteria involves an energy-dependent step (EDP_1) that is oxygen-linked. Uptake is inhibited by an anaerobic or acidic environment and by calcium or magnesium ions.

2. Aminoglycosides are **bactericidal.**

C. **Pharmacokinetics**

   1. **Absorption.** Aminoglycosides are not absorbed from the gastrointestinal tract.

   2. **Fate.** Aminoglycosides are distributed to the extracellular fluid volume and to transcellular fluids (e.g., pleural and peritoneal fluids).
      a. Penetration of the CNS and ocular tissue is minimal.
      b. Aminoglycosides tend to accumulate in the renal cortex and otic endolymph, predisposing these tissues to toxicity.

   3. **Excretion.** Aminoglycosides are excreted unchanged in the urine by glomerular filtration. Plasma half-lives are 1–3 hours in most species.

D. **Spectrum of activity.** The aminoglycosides are used in the treatment of infections caused by **Gram-negative aerobes** in all species.

E. **Preparations and therapeutic uses**

   1. **Streptomycin** and **dihydrostreptomycin** are the oldest members of this class of antibiotics. Their use has declined with the advent of broader spectrum aminoglycosides, such as gentamicin and amikacin.

   2. **Neomycin** is administered orally to treat enteric infections and topically to treat skin, ear, and eye infections.

   3. **Extended-spectrum aminoglycosides**
      a. **Gentamicin** and **amikacin** are effective against *Pseudomonas, Proteus, Staphylococcus,* and *Corynebacterium* species, as well as Gram-negative aerobes. They are used in all species for the treatment of septicemia and all susceptible infections of the skin, respiratory tract, ear, eye, and urinary tract.
      b. **Tobramycin** is similar to gentamicin but has more potent antipseudomonal activity.
      c. **Kanamycin** has a spectrum of activity similar to that of gentamicin, except it is not effective against *Pseudomonas* species. Kanamycin is used in dogs and cats to treat Gram-negative infections of the skin and soft tissue, urinary tract, and respiratory tract.

F. **Administration**

   1. For **systemic infections,** aminoglycosides are administered **intramuscularly** or **subcutaneously** every 8–12 hours.

   2. For **enteric infections,** aminoglycosides are administered **orally** once or twice per day.

G. **Bacterial resistance** may be plasmid-mediated and may develop quickly. Inactivation of aminoglycosides by bacterial enzymes is the most common form of resistance.

   1. The numerous amino and hydroxyl side groups are sites of attack by acetylases, phosphorylases, and adenylases.

   2. Amikacin is more resistant to enzymatic degradation than other members of this class.

H. **Adverse effects.** The aminoglycosides are relatively more toxic than other classes of antimicrobials. Toxicity is reversible if treatment is stopped early. Aminoglycosides should not be used with other ototoxic or nephrotoxic drugs (e.g., furosemide, amphotericin B).

   1. **Ototoxicity** results from progressive damage to cochlear sensory cells (causing deafness), vestibular cells (causing ataxia), or both.

   2. **Nephrotoxicity** is caused by damage of the membranes of proximal tubular cells, resulting in a loss of brush border enzymes, impaired absorption, proteinuria, and

decreased glomerular filtration rate. Dosages must be adjusted for animals with decreased renal function.

3. **Neuromuscular blockade** is a relatively rare adverse effect of aminoglycosides. It is caused by prejunctional blockade of acetylcholine (ACh) release and decreased postsynaptic sensitivity to ACh. Muscle paralysis and apnea are treated with calcium gluconate.

VII. TETRACYCLINES

A. **Chemistry.** The tetracyclines are polycyclic compounds that are amphoteric and that fluoresce when exposed to ultraviolet light. Most are prepared as the hydrochloride salt. They form insoluble chelates with cations such as calcium, magnesium, iron, and aluminum.

B. **Mechanism of action.** Tetracyclines, which are **bacteriostatic, inhibit bacterial protein synthesis** by binding to the 30S ribosome and preventing attachment of aminoacyl transfer ribonucleic acid (tRNA) to the mRNA–ribosome complex. They block the addition of amino acids to the growing peptide chain.

C. **Pharmacokinetics**

1. **Absorption.** Oral absorption of tetracyclines ranges from 60%–90% of the administered dose except for chlortetracycline, which is only 35% absorbed. Divalent or trivalent cations impair absorption; thus, milk, antacids, or iron salts should be avoided 3 hours before and after oral administration.

2. **Fate**
   a. **Distribution** is wide and includes all tissues except those of the CNS. Doxycycline is more lipid-soluble than tetracycline, chlortetracycline, and oxytetracycline; it penetrates the CNS, eye, and prostate at therapeutic concentrations.
   b. **Metabolism** is minimal in domestic animals. Plasma half-lives range from 6–12 hours for most tetracyclines.

3. **Excretion.** Renal excretion by glomerular filtration is the major route of elimination for most tetracyclines, but small amounts are excreted into feces via bile or diffusion from the blood into the intestine. Doxycycline is unique in that intestinal excretion is the major route of elimination (75%).

D. **Spectrum of activity.** The antimicrobial spectrum of tetracyclines includes Gram-positive and Gram-negative aerobes and anaerobes, rickettsiae, spirochetes, chlamydiae, mycoplasmae, and some protozoa such as *Anaplasma* species and *Haemobartonella* species.

E. **Preparations and therapeutic uses**

1. **Tetracycline, chlortetracycline,** and **oxytetracycline** are used in the treatment of local and systemic bacterial, chlamydial, rickettsial, and protozoal infections in cattle, sheep, horses, and swine. These agents are also used as feed additives and growth promoters in cattle and swine.

2. **Doxycycline** and **tetracycline** are used in the treatment of respiratory and urinary tract infections in dogs and cats and as specific therapy for infections caused by *Borrelia* (Lyme disease), *Brucella*, *Haemobartonella*, and *Ehrlichia* species. These agents are also effective in the treatment of psittacosis in birds.

F. **Administration**

1. Tetracyclines are administered orally or intravenously every 8–12 hours. Oral doses should be avoided in adult ruminants and used with caution in horses.

2. If administered intramuscularly, special buffered solutions should be used to avoid pain and local irritation.

G. **Bacterial resistance** may be plasmid-mediated and usually involves decreased drug uptake or active transport of the tetracycline out of the bacterial cell.

H. Adverse effects

1. The tetracyclines (except for doxycycline) are **potentially nephrotoxic** and should be avoided if renal function is impaired. They should not be used with methoxyflurane anesthesia because acute renal failure may result.

2. **Permanent staining of unerupted teeth** may occur in young animals. Formation of a tetracycline–calcium phosphate complex in enamel and dentine is the probable cause.

3. **Suprainfections** of fungi, yeast, or resistant bacteria may occur in the gastrointestinal tract with prolonged administration of broad-spectrum antibiotics such as the tetracyclines.

4. **Phototoxicity** and **hepatotoxicity** are rare side effects in animals.

5. Oral therapeutic doses **may disrupt ruminal microflora** in adult ruminants **or colonic microflora** in horses.

VIII. CHLORAMPHENICOL

A. **Chemistry.** Chloramphenicol is an unusual natural compound because it contains dichloracetate and nitrobenzene moieties as part of its structure.

1. Palmitate salts are water-insoluble and are administered orally.

2. Chloramphenicol sodium succinate is water-soluble for parenteral use.

B. **Mechanism of action.** Chloramphenicol, a **bacteriostatic** agent, binds to the bacterial 50S ribosome unit to **inhibit peptide bond formation and protein synthesis.**

C. Pharmacokinetics

1. Absorption. Chloramphenicol is rapidly absorbed from the gastrointestinal tract.

2. Fate
  a. Distribution. Chloramphenicol is widely distributed to all tissues, including those of the CNS and eye.
  b. Metabolism is hepatic, via **glucuronide conjugation.** In cats, 75% of the dose is metabolized, and in dogs, 90% of the administered drug is metabolized.

3. Excretion. The elimination half-life is 1–1.5 hours in dogs and horses and 4–5 hours in cats.

D. **Spectrum of activity.** Chloramphenicol, a broad-spectrum antibiotic, is effective against most anaerobic bacteria.

E. **Therapeutic uses.** Chloramphenicol is used in dogs, cats, horses, and birds for local and systemic infections, inducing respiratory, CNS, and ocular infections, and infections caused by anaerobes and *Salmonella* species.

F. **Administration.** Chloramphenicol is administered orally every 6–8 hours to dogs, birds, and horses, and every 12 hours to cats.

G. **Bacterial resistance.** Resistant bacteria inactivate chloramphenicol by producing acetyltransferase and other metabolizing enzymes.

H. **Adverse effects**

1. **Anemia**

   a. **Dose-related anemia** may occur in animals and humans. Chloramphenicol may inhibit the uptake of iron by erythrocytes and slow their rate of maturation in bone marrow.

   b. **Non–dose-related** anemia may occur in humans. It is rare, but the resulting aplastic anemia is often fatal. Because of the potential for residue-induced aplastic anemia in humans, use of chloramphenicol is banned in food-producing animals.

2. **Anorexia** and **diarrhea** may occur with high or prolonged dosages, especially in cats.

IX. MACROLIDES

A. **Chemistry.** The macrolide antibiotics are basic, lipid-soluble compounds consisting of deoxy sugars attached to a lactone ring. They are prepared as sulfate salts or as esterified salts of stearate, tartrate, estolate, or lactobionate.

B. **Mechanism of action.** Macrolides **inhibit bacterial protein synthesis by** binding to the 50S ribosome, preventing translocation of amino acids to the growing peptide chain. Macrolides are **bacteriostatic.**

C. **Pharmacokinetics**

1. **Absorption.** Enteric-coated preparations protect the antibiotic from gastric acid destruction, allowing oral absorption. Oral absorption is also possible when the stable, esterified salts are used.

2. **Fate.** Macrolide antibiotics are widely distributed to all tissues except those of the CNS. Tilmicosin is concentrated in lung tissue at levels sixty times higher than serum levels.

3. **Excretion**

   a. Erythromycin is metabolized by the liver and excreted in bile.

   b. Tylosin and tilmicosin are excreted unchanged in bile and urine.

D. **Spectrum of activity.** The antimicrobial activity of macrolides is primarily against Gram-positive aerobes and anaerobes and *Mycoplasma* species.

E. **Preparations and therapeutic uses**

1. **Erythromycin**

   a. Erythromycin is an alternative to penicillin for the treatment of infections caused by Gram-positive aerobes and anaerobes in dogs, cats, and horses.

   b. It is the **drug of choice** for the treatment of **enteritis** caused by *Campylobacter jejuni* in dogs and foals and for *Rhodococcus equi* **pneumonia** in foals.

2. **Tylosin**

   a. Tylosin is used in cattle, sheep, and swine for the treatment of local and systemic infections caused by **mycoplasma, Gram-positive bacteria,** and some **Gram-negative pathogens** (e.g., *Pasteurella, Haemophilus*). It is also used as a **growth promoter** in these species.

   b. Tylosin is used in dogs and cats for the treatment of **chronic colitis.**

3. **Tilmicosin** is used only in **cattle** for the treatment of **respiratory disease caused by** *Pasteurella* **species.**

F. **Administration**

1. **Erythromycin** is administered orally or intramuscularly three times daily to dogs, cats, and foals.

2. **Tylosin** is administered intramuscularly or orally once or twice daily to swine, calves, lambs, dogs, and cats.

3. **Tilmicosin** is administered subcutaneously to cattle every 72 hours.

G. **Bacterial resistance** to macrolide antibiotics may be chromosomal or plasmid-mediated and results from decreased drug binding by the 50S ribosome.

H. **Adverse effects**

1. **Erythromycin** and **tylosin** have relatively few side effects.
   a. **Mild gastrointestinal upset** may result from oral doses.
   b. **Pain** and **irritation at intramuscular injection sites** may occur.
   c. **Edema of the rectal mucosa** with **mild anal prolapse** may be seen in swine following intramuscular administration of tylosin.
   d. **Severe diarrhea** may occur if erythromycin is administered orally to adult ruminants or if tylosin is administered orally or parenterally to adult horses.

2. **Tilmicosin** produces **cardiovascular toxicity** in species other than cattle.

X. LINCOSAMIDES (e.g., LINCOMYCIN, CLINDAMYCIN)

A. **Chemistry.** Lincomycin and clindamycin are derivatives of a sulfur-containing octose with an amino acid–like side chain. They are prepared as hydrochloride or phosphate salts, which are water-soluble, or clindamycin palmitate for oral administration.

B. **Mechanism of action.** The lincosamides, which are **bacteriostatic,** bind to the bacterial 50S ribosome to **inhibit protein synthesis.** Because this is the same binding site of chloramphenicol and the macrolides, combination therapy should be avoided.

C. **Pharmacokinetics**

1. **Absorption.** Oral absorption is 50% for lincomycin and 90% for clindamycin.

2. **Fate**
   a. **Distribution** is wide, with excellent penetration of bone and soft tissues, including tendon sheaths. CNS levels are low unless the meninges are inflamed.
   b. **Metabolism.** Lincosamides are metabolized by the liver (60%, lincomycin; 90%, clindamycin).

3. **Excretion.** Unchanged drug and metabolites are excreted in the urine, bile, and feces. Elimination half-lives are 3–5 hours in dogs and cats.

D. **Spectrum of activity.** The lincosamides are active against Gram-positive aerobes and anaerobes, *Toxoplasma* species, and *Mycoplasma* species. The antibacterial activity of clindamycin is greater than that of lincomycin, especially against anaerobes.

E. **Therapeutic uses**

1. **Lincomycin** is used in swine for the control and treatment of **swine dysentery** and the treatment of **staphylococcal, streptococcal,** and **mycoplasmal infections.**

2. **Clindamycin** is used in dogs and cats for **periodontal disease, osteomyelitis, dermatitis,** and **deep soft tissue infections** caused by Gram-positive organisms. It is used for treating **toxoplasmosis** in dogs and cats.

F. **Administration**

1. **Lincomycin** is administered intramuscularly to swine once daily or added to the drinking water.

2. **Clindamycin** is administered orally or intramuscularly twice daily to dogs and cats.

G. **Bacterial resistance.** Altered drug binding by bacterial ribosomes is the usual form of resistance. Cross-resistance between lincosamides and macrolides is common.

H. **Adverse effects**

1. In **horses, rabbits, hamsters,** and **guinea pigs,** lincosamides are contraindicated because they may produce a **severe, often fatal, diarrhea** caused by altered gastrointestinal flora.

2. In **dogs, cats,** and **swine,** side effects are rare. **Neuromuscular blockade** may occur at high doses or when lincosamides are administered with anesthetics.

XI. MISCELLANEOUS ANTIBACTERIALS

A. **Aminocyclitols (spectinomycin, apramycin)**

1. **Chemistry.** Aminocyclitols are chemically related to the aminoglycosides.

2. **Mechanism of action.** Aminocyclitols bind to the 30S ribosome and **inhibit protein synthesis.** Unlike the aminoglycosides, aminocyclitols are **bacteriostatic.**

3. **Pharmacokinetics.** The pharmacokinetics of aminocyclitols are similar to those of the aminoglycosides.
   a. **Absorption.** Less than 10% of the dose is absorbed orally.
   b. **Fate.** Parenterally administered spectinomycin distributes to the extracellular fluid (ECF).
   c. **Excretion.** Aminocyclitols are excreted unchanged by the kidney.

4. **Spectrum of activity.** Aminocyclitols are effective primarily against Gram-negative aerobes and *Mycoplasma* species.

5. **Preparations and therapeutic uses**
   a. **Spectinomycin** is used in dogs, cats, horses, swine, and poultry for the treatment of **enteric** and **respiratory disease.**
   b. **Apramycin** is used in swine and calves for the treatment of enteric diseases, especially **colibacillosis.**

6. **Bacterial resistance.** Resistant mutants fail to bind aminocyclitols to the 30S ribosome. Plasmid-mediated resistance, manifested as the production of degrading enzymes, is less common.

7. **Adverse effects.** No significant toxicity is associated with clinical use of spectinomycin or apramycin.

B. **Metronidazole**

1. **Mechanism of action.** Metronidazole is taken up by anaerobic bacteria and protozoa and reduced to a cytotoxic metabolite that disrupts DNA.

2. **Pharmacokinetics**
   a. **Absorption.** Metronidazole is well absorbed orally.
   b. **Fate**
      (1) **Distribution.** Metronidazole is widely distributed and penetrates the CNS.
      (2) **Metabolism.** One-third to one-half of the administered drug is metabolized by oxidation and conjugation in the liver.

    c. Excretion. Metabolites and the unchanged drug are excreted in the urine and feces.

    3. Spectrum of activity. Metronidazole is bactericidal against most obligate anaerobes and is active against protozoa, including *Giardia* and *Trichomonas* species.

    4. Therapeutic uses. Metronidazole is used in dogs, cats, and horses for the treatment of severe infections caused by anaerobic pathogens, especially pelvic, genitourinary, and respiratory tract infections and brain abscesses.

    5. Adverse effects. High or prolonged dosages may produce **neurotoxicity** (i.e., nystagmus, ataxia, seizures).

C. Rifampin

    1. Mechanism of action. Rifampin inhibits DNA-dependent RNA polymerase, preventing initiation of RNA synthesis. It is **bactericidal.**

    2. Pharmacokinetics
      a. Absorption. Rifampin is absorbed orally.
      b. Fate. It is rapidly distributed to cells and tissues. Its distribution to cells makes it effective against intracellular infections.
      c. Excretion. Rifampin is metabolized by the liver and excreted primarily in bile. Metabolites may impart a red color to the urine, feces, and saliva.

    3. Spectrum of activity. Rifampin is bactericidal for mycobacteria and Gram-positive pathogens.

    4. Therapeutic uses. Rifampin is combined with erythromycin in the treatment of *R. equi* infections in foals.

    5. Bacterial resistance may develop quickly. Alterations in the structure of DNA-dependent RNA polymerase prevent rifampin from binding to the organism.

    6. Adverse effects are rare. Hepatotoxicity may occur in animals with preexisting liver disease.

D. Tiamulin

    1. Mechanism of action. Tiamulin binds to the 50S bacterial ribosome to inhibit protein synthesis. Its mechanism of action and spectrum of activity are similar to those of the macrolides such as tylosin.

    2. Pharmacokinetics
      a. Absorption. Tiamulin is well absorbed orally.
      b. Fate. It is widely distributed and metabolized by the liver.
      c. Excretion. Elimination of metabolites occurs via the feces (70%) and urine (30%).

    3. Spectrum of activity. Tiamulin is active against Gram-positive cocci, mycoplasmae, spirochetes, and certain Gram-negative pathogens (e.g., *Haemophilus* species).

    4. Therapeutic uses. Tiamulin is used in **swine** for the control and treatment of ***Haemophilus* pneumonia** and **swine dysentery.**

    5. Adverse effects. Irritant metabolites in the urine may cause **dermatitis** with erythema and pruritus in pigs confined in overcrowded areas.

E. Vancomycin

    1. Mechanism of action. Vancomycin blocks the second step of bacterial cell wall synthesis by inhibiting polymer release from the cell membrane. It is **bactericidal.**

    2. Pharmacokinetics
      a. Absorption. Vancomycin is not absorbed orally.
      b. Fate. It is distributed to the ECF and transcellular fluids.
      c. Excretion. It is excreted unchanged by glomerular filtration.

3. **Spectrum of activity.** Vancomycin is effective against Gram-positive organisms.

4. **Therapeutic uses.** Vancomycin is a reserve antibiotic used intravenously for **methicillin-resistant staphylococcal infections of bone and soft tissue** in dogs and cats.

5. **Adverse effects. Ototoxicity** and **nephrotoxicity** occur with large dosages or prolonged administration.

F. **Bacitracin**

1. **Mechanism of action.** Bacitracin inhibits the second step of cell wall synthesis and is **bactericidal.**

2. **Pharmacokinetics.** Bacitracin is not absorbed orally. It is too nephrotoxic for systemic use.

3. **Spectrum of activity.** Bacitracin is effective against Gram-positive bacteria and spirochetes.

4. **Therapeutic uses**
   a. Bacitracin is used in ointments and solutions and is frequently combined with polymyxin B or neomycin or both to treat topical infections.
   b. It is also added to swine and poultry rations to **prevent and treat clostridial enteritis** and to **promote growth.**

G. **Polymyxin B**

1. **Mechanism of action.** Polymyxin B interacts with phospholipids in the bacterial cell membrane to produce a detergent-like effect and membrane disruption. It is rapidly bactericidal for Gram-negative organisms.

2. **Pharmacokinetics.** Polymyxin B is not absorbed orally and is too nephrotoxic for systemic use.

3. **Therapeutic uses**
   a. Polymyxin B is used topically to treat **Gram-negative infections of the skin, eye,** and **ear** in all species. It is usually combined with bacitracin for broad-spectrum antibacterial effects.
   b. Polymyxin B is administered orally to cattle and swine for the treatment of **Gram-negative enteric infections.**

4. **Adverse effects.** Polymyxin B does not produce systemic toxicity when administered topically or orally.

H. **Nitrofurans** (e.g., **nitrofurantoin, nitrofurazone**)

1. **Mechanism of action.** Nitrofurans are reduced by bacteria to reactive intermediates that inhibit the enzyme systems of carbohydrate metabolism. They may also block mRNA translation. Nitrofurans are **broad-spectrum** and **bacteriostatic.**

2. **Pharmacokinetics**
   a. **Absorption.** Nitrofurantoin is absorbed orally.
   b. **Excretion.** It is rapidly excreted by glomerular filtration and active secretion. Peak urine levels are achieved less than 1 hour after administration.

3. **Therapeutic uses**
   a. **Nitrofurantoin** is occasionally used in the treatment of **lower urinary tract infections** in dogs and cats. It is most effective in an acid urine.
   b. **Nitrofurazone** is used topically as an **antibacterial ointment, powder,** and **water-soluble wound dressing** in all species.

4. **Adverse effects** are rare.
   a. **Nausea, vomiting,** and **diarrhea** may occur in dogs and cats following oral administration.
   b. Oral administration of nitrofurans is contraindicated in food-producing animals because nitrofurans have been shown to be **potential carcinogens in laboratory animals.**

XII. ANTIFUNGAL AGENTS

A. Griseofulvin

1. **Chemistry.** Griseofulvin is a cyclohexane benzofuran antibiotic derived from *Penicillium griseofulvum*. It is insoluble in water.

2. **Mechanism of action.** Griseofulvin is actively taken up by growing dermatophytes (ringworm). It binds to microtubules to inhibit spindle formation and mitosis. Griseofulvin is **fungistatic** and its action is slow—infected cells must be shed and replaced with uninfected cells.

3. **Pharmacokinetics**
   a. **Absorption.** Oral absorption is increased by high-fat foods and by preparations consisting of microsized particles.
   b. **Fate.** Griseofulvin distributes to the keratin precursor cells of the skin, hair shafts, and nails.
   c. **Excretion.** It is metabolized by the liver by demethylation and glucuronide conjugation and excreted in urine.

4. **Spectrum of activity.** Griseofulvin is effective against dermatophytes such as *Microsporum* species and *Trichophyton* species.

5. **Therapeutic uses.** Griseofulvin is used in dogs, cats, and horses for multifocal dermatophyte infections.

6. **Administration.** Griseofulvin is administered orally twice per day to dogs and cats and once daily to horses for 4–6 weeks.

7. **Adverse effects** are rare. Leukopenia and anemia may occur as an idiosyncratic reaction in kittens.

B. Ketoconazole

1. **Chemistry.** Ketoconazole is an **imidazole antifungal** for systemic use. Other imidazoles used only topically for dermatophyte or yeast infections include miconazole and clotrimazole.

2. **Mechanism of action.** Ketoconazole inhibits the synthesis of ergosterol in fungal cytoplasmic membranes by blocking cytochrome P-450 enzymes. It is **fungistatic.**

3. **Pharmacokinetics**
   a. **Absorption.** Ketoconazole is absorbed orally.
   b. **Fate.** It is widely distributed, except to the CNS.
   c. **Excretion.** It is metabolized by the liver and excreted in bile.

4. **Spectrum of activity.** Ketoconazole is effective against **most pathogenic fungi responsible for systemic infections** (e.g., *Blastomyces, Coccidioides, Cryptococcus,* and *Histoplasma* species). It is also effective against **candidiasis** (yeast infections) and **griseofulvin-resistant dermatophytes.**

5. **Therapeutic uses**
   a. In dogs, cats, horses, and birds, ketoconazole is used to treat **systemic mycoses** and **severe yeast infections.**
   b. In dogs and cats, high dosages are used to treat **hyperadrenocorticism.**

6. **Administration.** To treat systemic mycotic infections, ketoconazole is administered orally, twice per day for 3–6 months.

7. **Adverse effects**
   a. **Anorexia, vomiting,** and **diarrhea** may occur.
   b. **Suppression of adrenal or gonadal steroids** may also occur, but the effects are transient at dosages employed in antifungal therapy.

C. Amphotericin B

1. **Chemistry.** Amphotericin B is a polyene macrolide that is stabilized with sodium desoxycholate as a colloidal suspension.

2. **Mechanism of action.** Amphotericin B binds to the ergosterol of fungal cell membranes to form pores or channels, which results in leakage of cell contents. Amphotericin B is **fungicidal.**

3. **Pharmacokinetics**
   a. **Absorption.** Amphotericin B is not absorbed from the gastrointestinal tract.
   b. **Fate.** After intravenous administration, it is slowly distributed to most tissues, except those of the CNS, eye, and bone.
   c. **Excretion.** Elimination is biphasic, with serum half-lives of 24–48 hours and 1–2 weeks. Less than 5% of the unchanged drug is excreted in the urine.

4. **Spectrum of activity.** Amphotericin B is effective against most organisms causing systemic mycoses (e.g., *Aspergilli, Blastomyces, Coccidioides, Cryptococcus, Histoplasma* species).

5. **Therapeutic uses**
   a. Amphotericin B is used to treat **systemic fungal infections** in dogs, cats, horses, and birds. Combination with ketoconazole reduces toxicity.
   b. Amphotericin B is used with flucytosine in the treatment of CNS, bone, and ocular infections.

6. **Administration.** Amphotericin B is diluted in 5% dextrose and administered intravenously. Treatment frequency and duration vary with the type of infection.

7. **Adverse effects. Renal toxicity** is a serious side effect.
   a. Amphotericin B produces renal vasoconstriction, decreased glomerular filtration, and damage to tubular epithelium.
   b. Renal function must be monitored weekly during therapy [e.g., by evaluating blood urea nitrogen (BUN) levels].

D. **Flucytosine**

1. **Chemistry.** Flucytosine is a fluorinated pyrimidine that is deaminated by fungi (not mammalian cells) to 5-fluorouracil (5-FU), a potent antimetabolite.

2. **Mechanism of action.** Flucytosine, which is fungicidal, inhibits thymidylate synthetase, thereby inhibiting DNA and RNA synthesis in susceptible fungi.

3. **Pharmacokinetics**
   a. **Absorption.** Flucytosine is well absorbed orally.
   b. **Fate.** It is widely distributed, including to the CNS.
   c. **Excretion.** It is excreted unchanged in urine.

4. **Spectrum of activity.** Flucytosine is effective against *Cryptococcus, Candida,* and *Aspergilli* species.

5. **Therapeutic uses**
   a. Flucytosine is combined with amphotericin B for synergistic action in the treatment of **cryptococcosis (especially meningeal** cryptococcosis) in dogs and cats.
   b. It is used alone in treating **aspergillosis** and **candidiasis** in psittacine birds.

6. **Administration.** Flucytosine is administered orally 3–4 times a day for a minimum of 4 weeks.

7. **Adverse effects.** Toxicity is low. Mild gastrointestinal disturbances and, more rarely, bone marrow suppression have been reported.

STUDY QUESTIONS

DIRECTIONS: Each of the numbered items or incomplete statements in this section is followed by answers or by completions of the statement. Select the **one** numbered answer or completion that is **best** in each case.

1. Infectious (transferable) drug resistance, which involves transfer of multiple-drug resistant genes via pili, has been observed clinically in Gram-negative infections of which organ system?

(1) Urinary
(2) Gastrointestinal
(3) Respiratory
(4) Integumentary

2. The primary reason for using mixtures of sulfonamides to treat cattle is:

(1) to decrease the likelihood of bacterial resistance, because most organisms would be sensitive to one of the sulfonamides in the mixture even if resistant to the others.
(2) to decrease the rate of acetylation, because each sulfonamide competes for enzyme.
(3) to provide a broader spectrum of antimicrobial action.
(4) to reduce renal toxicity based on the law of independent solubility.
(5) to allow the formulation of neutral solutions.

3. Which one of the following statements is true of the fluoroquinolones enrofloxacin and ciprofloxacin?

(1) They have an antibacterial spectrum that is limited to Gram-negative pathogens, especially anaerobes.
(2) They are used primarily for enteric infections because they are not absorbed from the gut.
(3) They are useful for respiratory, skin, and urinary tract infections in puppies.
(4) They are bactericidal via inhibition of deoxyribonucleic acid (DNA) gyrase.

4. Which one of the following tetracyclines may be safely administered to an aged cat with hemobartonellosis and impaired renal function?

(1) Chlortetracycline
(2) Doxycycline
(3) Oxytetracycline
(4) Tetracycline

5. Which one of the following statements regarding the aminoglycoside antibiotics (e.g., streptomycin, gentamicin) is true?

(1) They are lipid-soluble and widely distributed to tissues, including the central nervous system (CNS).
(2) They are not effective against Gram-negative anaerobes because their uptake by bacteria is oxygen-linked.
(3) They are bacteriostatic at therapeutic concentrations.
(4) They are well absorbed orally if they are enteric-coated to protect them from gastric acid.

6. Which one of the following statements regarding clindamycin is true?

(1) It is primarily active against Gram-negative pathogens.
(2) It is used in equine enteric infections because it is a poorly absorbed "enteric" macrolide.
(3) Its distribution is generally limited to the extracellular fluid (ECF).
(4) It is frequently effective in staphylococcal osteomyelitis.

7. Which one of the following antibiotics is combined with erythromycin for treating *Rhodococcus equi* infections in foals?

(1) Spectinomycin
(2) Vancomycin
(3) Rifampin
(4) Tylosin

8. Which one of the following pairs of penicillins is effective against *Pseudomonas* species?

(1) Methicillin and ampicillin
(2) Ampicillin and hetacillin
(3) Hetacillin and carbenicillin
(4) Carbenicillin and ticarcillin
(5) Ticarcillin and oxacillin

DIRECTIONS: Each of the numbered items or incomplete statements in this section is negatively phrased, as indicated by an italicized word such as *not, least,* or *except.* Select the **one** numbered answer or completion that is **best** in each case.

---

9. All of the following antibiotics are susceptible to bacterial resistance caused by the secretion of drug-inactivating enzymes *except*:

(1) penicillin G.
(2) ampicillin.
(3) gentamicin.
(4) tetracycline.
(5) cephalexin.

10. All of the following statements concerning penicillin G and the first-generation cephalosporins are true *except*:

(1) they inhibit peptidoglycan cross-linking in the third stage of bacterial cell wall synthesis.
(2) bacterial resistance is most commonly due to beta-lactamase production.
(3) tissue penetration of cephalosporins is superior to penicillin G; and thus, they are preferred for antibiotic prophylaxis in surgery.
(4) they are eliminated primarily by hepatic metabolism and biliary excretion of conjugated drug.
(5) nephrotoxicity is more likely to occur with high dosages of or prolonged therapy with cephalosporins.

11. Adverse reactions to the aminoglycoside antibiotics include all of the following *except*:

(1) neuromuscular blockade.
(2) myelosuppression and anemia.
(3) nephrotoxicity.
(4) auditory ototoxicity.
(5) vestibular ototoxicity.

12. All of the following statements concerning ketoconazole are true *except*:

(1) it is more effective than flucytosine for meningeal cryptococcosis.
(2) it inhibits ergosterol synthesis in both systemic mycotic infections and yeast infections.
(3) cortisol and testosterone synthesis in mammals is inhibited at high doses.
(4) it must be administered for 3–6 months to treat systemic mycoses.

ANSWERS AND EXPLANATIONS

1. The answer is 2 [I C 2 b (2)].
Infectious (transferable) drug resistance has been observed clinically in enteric infections caused by Gram-negative organisms such as *Salmonella, Shigella,* and *Escherichia coli.* Infectious drug resistance is mediated by conjugation (i.e., the transfer of genetic material from cell to cell via a pilus).

2. The answer is 4 [II A 2].
Renal toxicity results from the precipitation of sulfonamides in neutral or acid urine. According to the law of independent solubility, the solubility of one sulfonamide is not affected by the presence of other sulfonamides in the solution. Therefore, because of their independent solubility, mixtures of sulfonamides are more soluble for a given concentration and less likely to cause renal toxicity. Bacterial resistance, metabolism, spectrum of activity, and neutrality of solutions are minimally affected by mixtures.

3. The answer is 4 [III B, D, H].
The fluoroquinolones are bactericidal; they inhibit bacterial deoxyribonucleic acid (DNA) gyrase, which results in degradation of replicating DNA. They are broad-spectrum antimicrobials, but anaerobes tend to be resistant. They are absorbed orally. They should not be administered to puppies because they may produce erosion of articular cartilage in growing dogs.

4. The answer is 2 [VII E 2, H 1].
Tetracyclines are effective in treating hemobartonellosis, but they are excreted by the kidney and are nephrotoxic in the presence of preexisting renal disease. Doxycycline, however, is excreted primarily by the intestine and could be safely administered to this animal.

5. The answer is 2 [VI B, C].
The uptake of aminoglycosides by bacteria includes an energy-dependent step (EDP$_1$) that is oxygen-linked. Because anaerobes do not use oxygen, uptake of aminoglycosides by these bacteria is minimal. Aminoglycosides are highly polar and poorly lipid-soluble. They are bactericidal and are not absorbed orally.

6. The answer is 4 [X E 2, H].
Clindamycin is active against Gram-positive aerobes and anaerobes and has excellent penetration of soft tissues and bones, which renders it effective in staphylococcal osteomyelitis. It is contraindicated in horses because it suppresses colonic flora and produces a severe, often fatal, diarrhea.

7. The answer is 3 [XI C 4].
Rifampin is bactericidal for mycobacteria and Gram-positive pathogens. It is combined with erythromycin to treat *Rhodococcus equi* infections in foals. Spectinomycin is an aminocyclitol used for enteric and respiratory diseases. Vancomycin is used to treat methicillin-resistant staphylococcal infections. Tylosin is a macrolide similar to erythromycin.

8. The answer is 4 [IV E 3 b].
Carbenicillin and ticarcillin are antipseudomonal penicillins used alone or in combination with gentamicin or tobramycin in severe infections caused by *Pseudomonas* species. Methicillin and oxacillin are used to treat severe staphylococcal infections caused by beta-lactamase–producing organisms. Ampicillin and hetacillin are broad-spectrum antimicrobials, but they are not effective against *Pseudomonas* species.

9. The answer is 4 [VII G].
Bacterial resistance to tetracyclines usually results from decreased uptake or active transport of the drug out of the bacterial cell. Resistance to penicillin G, ampicillin, and cephalexin is through beta-lactamase production. Gentamicin is enzymatically inactivated by resistant bacteria, which acetylate, phosphorylate, or adenylate the drug.

10. The answer is 4 [IV C 3, V C 3].
Penicillins and cephalosporins are eliminated by renal mechanisms (i.e., glomerular filtration, active tubular secretion). Their mechanism of action and inactivation by resistant bacteria are similar. Tissue penetration and nephrotoxicity are greater for the cephalosporins.

11. The answer is 2 [VI H].
Aminoglycosides do not produce myelosuppression. Nephrotoxicity and ototoxicity are most likely in patients with impaired renal function. Neuromuscular blockade occurs rarely and is reversed by administration of calcium gluconate.

12. The answer is 1 [XII B 2, 4, 7 b, D 5 a].
Flucytosine is the only antifungal that penetrates the central nervous system (CNS) and cerebrospinal fluid well. It is used with amphotericin B in the treatment of meningeal cryptococcosis. Ketoconazole inhibits ergosterol synthesis in fungi and yeast and, at high doses, steroid synthesis in mammals. Long-term therapy is required for the treatment of systemic mycotic infections with ketoconazole.

Chapter 12

Antineoplastic Drugs

Franklin A. Ahrens

I. INTRODUCTION

A. Cancer treatment objectives

1. **Cure, remission, or palliation.** The type and clinical stage of neoplasia (cancer) determine the degree of treatment response.

2. **Total cell kill.** Every neoplastic cell should be targeted.
   a. A single malignant cell may multiply to a lethal stage of neoplasia.
   b. **First order kinetics.** A constant percentage, rather than a constant number, of cells is killed by antineoplastic drugs. Thus, small tumors are more susceptible than large tumors to chemotherapy.

B. Cancer treatment considerations

1. **Dosage calculations.** Body surface area, rather than body weight, is used to calculate dosages of antineoplastic drugs because of their narrow therapeutic index.

2. **Duration of treatment.** Treatment should continue beyond cessation of clinical signs to achieve total cell kill. Treatment should be temporarily suspended if the white blood cell count falls below $3000/mm^3$ or the platelet count is less than $50,000/mm^3$.

3. **Combination therapy.** A combination of drugs with different mechanisms of action reduces drug toxicity, decreases cell resistance, and kills more neoplastic cells than one drug alone.

4. **Adjunct therapy.** Antineoplastic drugs are often used as an adjunct to surgery, radiation therapy, or both.

5. **Resistance.** Neoplastic cells develop resistance mechanisms, such as:
   a. Decreased cellular permeability or uptake of drug
   b. Increased production of enzymes that degrade the drug
   c. Increased capacity to repair or bypass the effects of the drug
   d. Decreased binding of drug to receptors or target enzymes

C. Cancer treatment adverse effects include **hair loss, gastrointestinal upset,** and **myelosuppression.** Because antineoplastic drugs act on rapidly multiplying and growing cells, normal and neoplastic, the integument, gastrointestinal tract, and bone marrow are susceptible.

D. Cell cycle (Figure 12-1). Some antineoplastic agents act only on cells in specific phases of the cell cycle.

1. **G_1 phase. Protein and ribonucleic acid (RNA) synthesis** lasts hours to days, depending on the cell type.

2. **S phase. Deoxyribonucleic acid (DNA) synthesis** lasts 2–4 hours. Many drugs act on cells in this phase.

3. **G_2 phase. Protein and RNA synthesis** lasts 3–8 hours.

4. **M phase. Mitosis** lasts 1 hour.

5. **G_0 phase. Resting** lasts hours to weeks, depending on the cell type. Nonproliferating cells in this stage are resistant to antineoplastic drugs.

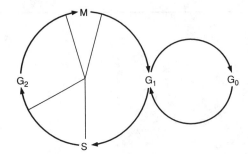

FIGURE 12-1. The cell cycle. Mitosis (*M*) is followed by the first growth phase (*G₁*), or by a resting phase (*G₀*). During the *S* phase, deoxyribonucleic acid (DNA) synthesis takes place. The *S* phase is followed by a second growth phase (*G₂*). (Modified and redrawn from Jacob L: *NMS Pharmacology*, 3rd ed. Baltimore, Williams & Wilkins, 1992, p 234.)

II. ALKYLATING AGENTS

A. **Chemistry** (Figure 12-2). Alkylating agents contain at least one alkyl group, but most contain two and are termed bifunctional because each alkyl group reacts with a DNA base in the double helix to form a cross-link.

B. **Mechanism of action. Alkylation** is the substitution of an alkyl group for an active hydrogen atom in an organic compound.

1. Alkylation cross-links DNA, inhibits its replication, and increases its breakdown.

2. Alkylation of proteins and RNA may also occur to inhibit transcription.

3. Alkylating agents are not cell-cycle specific.

C. **Preparations**

1. **Nitrogen mustards**
   a. **Cyclophosphamide** is the most commonly used alkylating agent in veterinary medicine.
      (1) **Pharmacokinetics**
         (a) **Absorption.** Cyclophosphamide is well absorbed from the gastrointestinal tract.
         (b) **Fate.** Cyclophosphamide in widely distributed to all tissues except those of the central nervous system (CNS). Cyclophosphamide is hydroxylated in the liver as the first step in its conversion to the **active metabolites phosphoramide mustard** and **acrolein.**
         (c) **Excretion.** Cyclophosphamide and its metabolites are excreted by the kidneys within 48–72 hours.
      (2) **Therapeutic uses.** Cyclophosphamide is used in dogs and cats to treat:
         (a) Lymphoreticular neoplasia
         (b) Carcinomas
         (c) Sarcomas
         (d) Multiple myelomas
         (e) Mast cell tumors
      (3) **Administration**

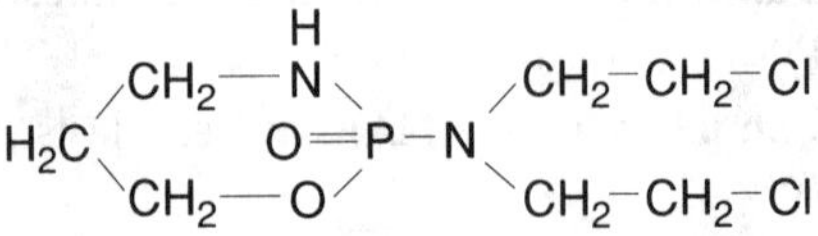

$$H_2C \begin{array}{c} \nearrow CH_2 - \overset{\overset{\displaystyle H}{|}}{N} \searrow \\ \searrow CH_2 - O \nearrow \end{array} O = P - N \begin{array}{c} \nearrow CH_2 - CH_2 - Cl \\ \searrow CH_2 - CH_2 - Cl \end{array}$$

FIGURE 12-2. Cyclophosphamide. Alkylating agents contain one or more alkyl groups ($R\text{-}CH_2\text{-}CH_2\text{-}X$) that are converted to reactive intermediates to form covalent bonds with compounds containing hydroxyl, amino, phosphate, sulfhydryl, or other nucleophilic groups. The alkyl radical ($R\text{-}CH_2\text{-}CH_2^+$) replaces a hydrogen atom on these groups.

      (a) Cyclophosphamide is administered **orally or intravenously.** Intralesion injection is ineffective because of the required liver metabolism.

      (b) Cyclophosphamide is used alone or in combination protocols.

      (c) Cyclophosphamide is commonly administered 4 consecutive mornings a week, but dosage intervals vary with the type of tumor and the protocol employed.

      (d) Diuresis should be encouraged (via diuretics and increased water intake) to reduce bladder irritation.

    (4) Adverse effects include nausea, vomiting, diarrhea, myelosuppression, alopecia, and sterile hemorrhagic cystitis (caused by acrolein, which can irritate the bladder).

  b. Chlorambucil is a slow-acting nitrogen mustard. It is not very effective in rapidly growing tumors.

    (1) Therapeutic uses. Chlorambucil is used in dogs and cats to treat:

      (a) Lymphatic leukemia

      (b) Lymphosarcoma

      (c) Macroglobulinemia

      (d) Polycythemia vera

    (2) Administration. Chlorambucil is well tolerated when administered orally every 2 days.

    (3) Adverse effects of chlorambucil are more readily controlled than those of faster-acting alkylating agents. **Myelosuppression** may occur after several weeks of treatment but reverses rapidly after treatment is stopped.

  c. Melphalan

    (1) Therapeutic use. Melphalan is used to treat multiple myelomas in dogs and cats.

    (2) Administration. Melphalan is administered orally 3 times weekly.

    (3) Adverse effects. Myelosuppression is the most common adverse effect.

2. Thiotepa, carmustine, lomustine, and **busulfan** are used infrequently in veterinary medicine.

  a. Thiotepa is an **ethylenimine,** effective against carcinomas. It is administered intravenously or injected directly into solid tumors.

  b. Carmustine and **lomustine,** which are **nitrosoureas,** are lipid-soluble and cross the blood–brain barrier. They are administered orally to treat adenocarcinomas and malignant melanomas. Delayed but severe myelosuppression limits their usefulness.

  c. Busulfan is an **alkylsulfonate,** administered orally for chronic granulocytic leukemia.

III. ANTIMETABOLITES

A. **Chemistry.** Antimetabolites are structurally similar to folic acid, pyrimidines, or purines.

B. **Mechanism of action**

  1. Antimetabolites act through competitive inhibition to impair DNA synthesis.

  2. They are most effective during the S phase of the cell cycle.

C. **Preparations**

  1. Methotrexate

    a. Chemistry. Methotrexate is a **folic acid analog.**

    b. Mechanism of action. Methotrexate inhibits dihydrofolate reductase, an enzyme necessary for purine and pyrimidine synthesis.

    c. Pharmacokinetics

(1) **Absorption.** Methotrexate is well absorbed from the gastrointestinal tract.

(2) **Fate.** Methotrexate is distributed to all tissues except those of the CNS.

(3) **Excretion.** Renal excretion occurs by glomerular filtration and active secretion.

d. **Therapeutic uses.** Methotrexate is used in dogs and cats to treat:

(1) Lymphomas

(2) Carcinomas

(3) Sarcomas

(4) Transmissible venereal tumors (TVTs)

e. **Administration**

(1) Methotrexate is administered intravenously, intramuscularly, or orally.

(2) It is administered alone or in combination protocols.

f. **Adverse effects** include nausea, vomiting, diarrhea, and myelosuppression. **Folinic acid (leucovorin)** may reverse the adverse effects of methotrexate.

2. **5-Fluorouracil (5-FU)**

a. **Chemistry.** 5-FU is a **pyrimidine analog.**

b. **Mechanism of action.** 5-FU is phosphorylated in cells to 5-fluoro-2′-deoxyuridine-5′-monophosphate (F-dUMP), which blocks thymidylate synthetase reactions, thereby inhibiting DNA synthesis. In addition, 5-FU is incorporated into RNA and DNA.

c. **Pharmacokinetics**

(1) **Absorption.** Gastrointestinal absorption is unpredictable.

(2) **Fate.** 5-FU is widely distributed to tissues, including cerebrospinal fluid. 5-FU is metabolized by the liver.

d. **Therapeutic uses.** 5-FU is used to treat canine carcinomas of the gastrointestinal tract, mammary glands, liver, or lungs.

e. **Administration.** 5-FU is administered intravenously once weekly.

f. **Adverse effects** include nausea, vomiting, myelosuppression, and CNS toxicity (e.g., excitement, ataxia, tremors, and convulsions). **In cats, CNS toxicity is so severe as to render 5-FU unsuitable for use.**

3. **Cytosine arabinoside**

a. **Chemistry.** Cytosine arabinoside is a **pyrimidine analog.**

b. **Mechanism of action.** Cytosine arabinoside is phosphorylated in cells to a nucleotide (ara-CTP) that inhibits DNA synthesis.

c. **Therapeutic uses.** Cytosine arabinoside is used in dogs and cats to treat:

(1) Lymphoreticular neoplasms

(2) Myeloproliferative disease

(3) CNS lymphoma

d. **Administration.** Cytosine arabinoside is administered intravenously or subcutaneously once daily.

e. **Adverse effects.** Myelosuppression results in leukopenia (most common), anemia, and thrombocytopenia.

4. **6-Mercaptopurine (6-MP)**

a. **Chemistry.** 6-MP is a **purine analog.**

b. **Mechanism of action.** 6-MP is phosphorylated in cells and inhibits multiple steps of DNA and RNA synthesis.

c. **Therapeutic uses.** 6-MP is used in dogs and cats to treat:

(1) Acute lymphocytic leukemia

(2) Granulocytic leukemia

(3) Lymphosarcoma

d. **Administration.** 6-MP is administered orally once daily.

e. **Adverse effects.** Leukopenia and thrombocytopenia are the most common adverse effects.

5. **6-Thioguanine (6-TG)**

a. **Chemistry.** 6-TG is a **purine analog.**

b. **Mechanism of action.** 6-TG has a similar mechanism of action to that of 6-MP.

c. **Therapeutic use.** 6-TG is used to treat acute leukemia in dogs and cats.

d. Administration. 6-TG is administered orally once daily.

e. Adverse effects. Leukopenia and thrombocytopenia are the most common adverse effects.

IV. MITOSIS INHIBITORS

A. **Chemistry.** These drugs are **vinca alkyloids,** the most common agents being **vincristine** and **vinblastine.**

B. **Mechanism of action**

1. The vinca alkaloids bind to tubulin protein in the mitotic spindle and block its polymerization into microtubules, thus preventing cell division during metaphase.

2. They act during the M phase of the cell cycle.

C. **Pharmacokinetics**

1. **Absorption.** Vinca alkaloids are not absorbed from the gastrointestinal tract, making intravenous administration necessary.

2. **Fate.** They are rapidly distributed to all tissues except the CNS. Approximately 75% are bound to tissue proteins. Vinca alkyloids are metabolized by the liver.

3. **Excretion.** They are excreted in the bile.

D. **Therapeutic uses.** The vinca alkaloids are suitable for use in dogs and cats.

1. **Vincristine** is more commonly used than vinblastine. It is effective for treating:
   (a) Lymphoreticular neoplasms
   (b) Carcinomas
   (c) Sarcomas
   (d) TVTs

2. **Vinblastine** is used to treat lymphomas and mastocytomas.

E. **Administration.** Vinca alkaloids are administered intravenously every 7–14 days, usually in combination protocols. TVTs require a different protocol.

F. **Adverse effects**

1. **Peripheral neurotoxicity** may occur because neural tissue has a high concentration of tubulin. Vinca alkaloid neurotoxicity is manifested as **neuromuscular weakness** and **constipation.**

2. **Myelosuppression** may occur, but it is less severe than that produced by other antineoplastic drugs.

3. **Severe local blistering** may occur if the drug is injected perivascularly.

V. ANTIBIOTICS

A. **Doxorubicin**

1. **Chemistry.** Doxorubicin is an anthracycline antibiotic.

2. **Mechanism of action**
   a. Doxorubicin intercalates with DNA to inhibit DNA replication, cleaves DNA chains, and induces formation of free radicals, which damage cell membranes.

b. Doxorubicin's action is not specific for any one phase of the cell cycle, but it is most effective against cells in the S phase.

3. Pharmacokinetics
   a. Absorption. Doxorubicin is not absorbed from the gastrointestinal tract.
   b. Fate. It is rapidly and widely distributed to all tissues except those of the CNS, and it is metabolized by the liver.
   c. Excretion. Doxorubicin is excreted in bile and feces.

4. Therapeutic uses. Doxorubicin is used in dogs and cats to treat carcinomas and sarcomas (especially lymphosarcomas and osteosarcomas).

5. Administration
   a. Doxorubicin is administered intravenously every 21 days as part of a combination drug protocol.
   b. Pretreatment with glucocorticoids or antihistamines prevents urticarial reactions.

6. Adverse effects
   a. In **dogs,** doxorubicin may cause myelosuppression, gastroenteritis, cardiomyopathy (via free radical damage to myocardial membranes), and urticaria.
   b. In **cats,** it may cause nephropathy, leukopenia, thrombocytopenia, vomiting, and urticaria.
   c. Severe tissue damage results from perivascular injection.

B. Bleomycin

1. Chemistry. Bleomycin is a mixture of glycopeptide antibiotics.

2. Mechanism of action
   a. Bleomycin glycopeptides generate free radicals, which cleave and fragment DNA.
   b. Bleomycin is specific for cells in the G_2 phase of the cell cycle.

3. Pharmacokinetics
   a. Absorption. Bleomycin is not absorbed from the gastrointestinal tract.
   b. Fate. Bleomycin is widely distributed, with high concentrations in the skin and lungs. It does not cross the blood–brain barrier.
   c. Excretion. Bleomycin is excreted by the kidneys.

4. Therapeutic uses. Bleomycin is used in dogs and cats to treat:
   a. Testicular tumors
   b. Squamous cell carcinoma
   c. Lymphoma

5. Administration. Bleomycin is commonly administered intravenously or subcutaneously once daily for 3–4 days, then once weekly.

6. Adverse effects include nausea, pulmonary fibrosis, skin ulcers, and minimal myelosuppression.

C. Actinomycin D

1. Chemistry. Actinomycin D is a chromopeptide antibiotic.

2. Mechanism of action
   a. Actinomycin D intercalates with the DNA helix and blocks transcription by RNA polymerase.
   b. It is not cell-cycle specific.

3. Pharmacokinetics
   a. Absorption. Actinomycin D is not well absorbed from the gastrointestinal tract.
   b. Fate. Actinomycin D does not reach the CNS.
   c. Excretion. Actinomycin D is excreted unchanged in urine and bile.

4. Therapeutic uses. Actinomycin D is used in dogs and cats to treat:
   a. Lymphoreticular neoplasms
   b. Rhabdomyosarcomas
   c. Choriocarcinomas

5. Administration. Actinomycin D is administered intravenously once weekly.

6. Adverse effects include nausea, vomiting, and leukopenia.

VI. HORMONES

A. Glucocorticoids (prednisone, prednisolone, dexamethasone)

1. Mechanism of action
   a. Glucocorticoids decrease the number of circulating lymphocytes (by suppressing mitosis) and increase the number of circulating red blood cells.
   b. They are not cell-cycle specific.

2. Pharmacokinetics
   a. Absorption. Glucocorticoids are absorbed from the gastrointestinal tract.
   b. Fate. Glucocorticoids are widely distributed to all tissues, including the CNS. Metabolism takes place in hepatic and extrahepatic sites.
   c. Excretion. Glucocorticoids are excreted by the kidneys.

3. Therapeutic use
   a. Glucocorticoids are used in dogs and cats to treat lymphoreticular neoplasms (including CNS lymphomas and mast cell tumors).
   b. They are frequently employed in cancer therapy with other drugs for their ability to stimulate appetite and a sense of well-being.

4. Administration. Glucocorticoids are administered orally or intravenously.

5. Adverse effects include immunosuppression, peptic ulcers, glucose intolerance, and Cushing syndrome.

B. Estrogens [diethylstilbestrol (DES), estradiol cypionate (ECP)]

1. Mechanism of action. Estrogens inhibit gonadotropin secretion in the male, thereby decreasing androgen levels and effects.

2. Pharmacokinetics
   a. Absorption. Estrogens are absorbed through the gastrointestinal tract.
   b. Fate. They are metabolized by the liver.
   c. Excretion. They are excreted by the kidneys.

3. Therapeutic uses. Estrogens are used in dogs to treat prostatic hypertrophy and perianal adenomas.

4. Administration
   a. DES is administered orally once daily.
   b. ECP is administered intramuscularly once weekly.

5. Adverse effects include aplastic anemia and thrombocytopenia.

VII. MISCELLANEOUS AGENTS

A. Cisplatin

1. Chemistry (Figure 12-3). Cisplatin is *cis* diaminodichloroplatinum (CDDP), an inorganic platinum complex.

2. Mechanism of action. Although cisplatin is not a true alkylating agent, its action is similar in that it cross-links DNA and prevents replication of DNA strands.

3. Pharmacokinetics
   a. Absorption. Cisplatin is not absorbed from the gastrointestinal tract.

FIGURE 12-3. Cisplatin is activated within cells when chloride atoms (Cl^-) are removed by binding to nucleophiles such as thiols. The platinum (Pt^{2+}) complex then cross-links deoxyribonucleic acid (*DNA*) by binding to guanosine (*G*) bases.

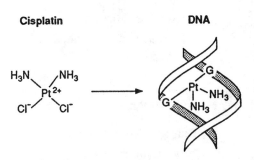

b. Fate. Cisplatin accumulates in the kidneys, liver, and gastrointestinal tract.

c. Excretion. Free platinum is excreted through the kidneys.

4. Therapeutic uses

  a. In **cats,** cisplatin is **contraindicated** because it causes severe pulmonary toxicity.

  b. In **dogs,** cisplatin is used to treat carcinomas and sarcomas.

  c. In **horses,** cisplatin is used to treat sarcoids, squamous cell carcinomas, papillomas, and melanomas.

5. Administration

  a. In **dogs,** cisplatin is administered intravenously once every 3 weeks, alone or in combination protocols. Intravenous saline administered for 4 hours before and 2 hours after intravenous cisplatin reduces renal toxicity.

  b. In **horses,** cisplatin in sesame oil is injected into solid tumors once every 2 weeks. Aluminum needles inactivate cisplatin and should not be used.

6. Adverse effects include:

  a. Nausea and vomiting

  b. Renal toxicity (caused by platinum accumulation)

  c. Myelosuppression (less severe than that caused by alkylating agents)

  d. Ototoxicity (rare)

  e. Neurotoxicity (rare)

B. **L-Asparaginase**

1. Mechanism of action

  a. L-Asparaginase is an enzyme that hydrolyzes the amino acid L-asparagine, thereby depleting circulating levels. Unlike normal cells, certain neoplastic cells cannot synthesize L-asparagine and thus require an exogenous source for survival.

  b. L-Asparaginase is specific for cells in the G_1 phase of the cell cycle.

2. Therapeutic uses. L-Asparaginase is used in dogs and cats to treat lymphoid neoplasia (especially lymphoblastic lymphosarcoma).

3. Administration

  a. L-Asparaginase is administered intravenously, intramuscularly, or intraperitoneally once weekly.

  b. Combination protocols are commonly used.

4. Adverse effects include allergic or anaphylactic reactions and pancreatitis.

C. **Mitotane**

1. Chemistry. Mitotane is a chlorinated hydrocarbon (o, p'-DDD).

2. Mechanism of action. Mitotane selectively destroys cells of the adrenal cortex, but its mechanism of action is unknown.

3. **Therapeutic uses.** Mitotane is used in dogs and cats to treat adrenocortical hyperplasia and as palliation therapy for inoperable tumors of the adrenal cortex.

4. **Administration.** Mitotane is administered orally once daily until post-adrenocorticotropic hormone cortisol levels are low to normal, and then administration is reduced to once weekly.

5. **Adverse effects** include vomiting, anorexia, and lethargy.

STUDY QUESTIONS

DIRECTIONS Each of the numbered items or incomplete statements in this section is followed by answers or by completions of the statement. Select the **one** numbered answer or completion that is **best** in each case.

1. If a plasma concentration of 1 mg/ml maintained for 6 hours kills 99% of tumor cells, how long must this same concentration be maintained to kill 99.99% of tumor cells (under ideal conditions)?

(1) 9 hours
(2) 12 hours
(3) 18 hours
(4) 24 hours

2. Which of the following general principles of antineoplastic drug therapy is correct?

(1) Large tumors are more susceptible to antineoplastic drugs than small tumors because they have a higher percentage of actively dividing cells.
(2) When clinical signs of malignant disease cease, antineoplastic drug therapy should be discontinued.
(3) Cells in the G_0 phase are killed by antimetabolites but are resistant to alkylating agents.
(4) Development of resistant cells is reduced in combination drug therapy.

3. Which of the following statements regarding cyclophosphamide is true?

(1) Cyclophosphamide tends to produce less myelosuppression than other antineoplastic drugs.
(2) Cyclophosphamide is usually injected directly into body cavities or tumor masses.
(3) Cyclophosphamide readily crosses the blood–brain barrier.
(4) Cyclophosphamide cross-links deoxyribonucleic acid (DNA), interfering with its ability to act as a template.
(5) Cyclophosphamide is excreted by the liver.

4. Which of the following statements is true regarding chlorambucil?

(1) Chlorambucil is a fast-acting nitrogen mustard.
(2) Adverse effects such as myelosuppression are more easily controlled than those of cyclophosphamide.
(3) Chlorambucil is more effective than cyclophosphamide in rapidly growing tumors.
(4) Chlorambucil is not absorbed when administered orally.

5. Folinic acid (leucovorin) may ameliorate myelosuppression caused by which antineoplastic drug?

(1) Cyclophosphamide
(2) L-Asparaginase
(3) Melphalan
(4) Doxorubicin
(5) Methotrexate

6. Which agent arrests lymphosarcoma cells in metaphase?

(1) Vincristine
(2) 6-Mercaptopurine (6-MP)
(3) Chlorambucil
(4) Doxorubicin
(5) Cisplatin

7. Which one of the following is an alkylating agent used in solid and disseminated tumors in dogs?

(1) 5-Fluorouracil (5-FU)
(2) Methotrexate
(3) Vincristine
(4) Doxorubicin
(5) Cyclophosphamide

8. Pretreatment with glucocorticoids or antihistamines is necessary to reduce urticarial reactions following intravenous administration of:

(1) doxorubicin.
(2) cytosine arabinoside.
(3) cisplatin.
(4) cyclophosphamide.

9. Which agent is phosphorylated in cells to a derivative that blocks thymidylate synthetase?

(1) 5-Fluorouracil (5-FU)
(2) Actinomycin D
(3) Carmustine
(4) Bleomycin

10. Which of the following statements regarding prednisolone is true?

(1) Its lympholytic action extends to lymphomas of the central nervous system (CNS).
(2) It is specific for the M phase of the cell cycle.
(3) It requires parenteral administration because gastrointestinal absorption is poor.
(4) Anemia is a major adverse effect.

11. Which of the following statements regarding diethylstilbestrol (DES) is true?

(1) Its only significant side effect is feminization.
(2) It is not effective orally because it is rapidly metabolized by the intestinal mucosa.
(3) It decreases androgen levels in canine prostatic hypertrophy.
(4) It is curative for transmissible venereal tumors (TVTs).

12. Cardiomyopathy may accompany myelosuppression and gastroenteritis in dogs treated with:

(1) 6-mercaptopurine (6-MP).
(2) vincristine.
(3) doxorubicin.
(4) thiotepa.

13. Intravenous saline infusions prior to and following drug administration are necessary to reduce the renal toxicity of:

(1) melphalan.
(2) vinblastine.
(3) methotrexate.
(4) cisplatin.

14. Which antineoplastic drug requires concurrent administration of furosemide and stimulation of water intake and of urine voiding to reduce the hemorrhagic cystitis associated with it?

(1) Prednisone
(2) Methotrexate
(3) Actinomycin D
(4) Cyclophosphamide

15. Hyperplasia of the adrenal cortex or adrenocortical tumors responds to treatment with:

(1) actinomycin D.
(2) glucocorticoids.
(3) mitotane.
(4) methotrexate.

ANSWERS AND EXPLANATIONS

1. The answer is 2 [I A 2 b].
Because cell kill kinetics are first order, a constant percentage of cells is killed. If 99% of the cells are killed in six hours, 99% of the remaining cells (a total of 99.99%) would be killed in 12 hours.

2. The answer is 4 [I A 2 b, B 2–3].
A major objective for combination antineoplastic drug therapy is to reduce the rate of development of resistant cells. Antimetabolites are most effective during the S phase of the cell cycle. Alkylating agents are not cell-cycle specific; however, rapidly dividing cells, susceptible to antineoplastic drugs, are limited in the G_0 phase and in large tumors that may have reached maximal growth. Therapy with antineoplastic drugs is extended beyond cessation of clinical signs as part of the total cell kill concept of treatment.

3. The answer is 4 [II B 1, C 1 a].
Cyclophosphamide is a bifunctional alkylating agent that cross-links deoxyribonecleic acid (DNA). It is activated by the liver and excreted by the kidneys. It does not enter the central nervous system (CNS). Myelosuppression is its major adverse effect. Administration is oral or intravenous to facilitate the conversion of cyclophosphamide into active metabolites by the liver.

4. The answer is 2 [II C 1 b].
The alkylating action of chlorambucil is slower than other agents; therefore, it is less effective against rapidly growing tumors, but its adverse effects are more easily controlled. It is absorbed when administered orally.

5. The answer is 5 [III C 1 f].
The cytotoxic effects of methotrexate result from inhibition of folic acid synthesis. Its toxicity is reversed by folinic acid, which is administered as a "rescue" agent if severe toxicity develops. It is the only antineoplastic drug for which a "rescue" agent is available.

6. The answer is 1 [IV B 1, D 1].
The vinca alkaloid vincristine blocks cell division in metaphase by binding to tubulin in the mitotic spindle. 6-Mercaptopurine (6-MP) is an antimetabolite that acts during the S

phase of the cell cycle. Chlorambucil and cisplatin cross-link deoxyribonucleic acid (DNA). Doxorubicin is an antineoplastic antibiotic that intercalates with DNA and induces formation of free radicals.

7. The answer is 5 [II C 1 a (2)].
Cyclophosphamide is the most common alkylating agent used in dogs. Methotrexate and 5-fluorouracil (5-FU) are antimetabolites. Doxorubicin is an antibiotic. Vincristine is a mitosis inhibitor.

8. The answer is 1 [V A 5 b].
Doxorubicin may produce severe urticarial reactions when administered intravenously. This effect may be prevented by pretreatment with glucocorticoids or antihistamines. Urticarial reactions are not a significant adverse effect of cytosine arabinoside, cisplatin, or cyclophosphamide.

9. The answer is 1 [III C 2 b].
Purine and pyrimidine analogs are phosphorylated to active derivatives in cells. 5-Fluorouracil (5-FU) a pyrimidine analog, is converted to 5-fluoro-2′-deoxyuridine-5′-monophosphate (F-dUMP), which blocks thymidylate synthetase reactions in neoplastic cells. Actinomycin D and bleomycin are antibiotics that inhibit deoxyribonucleic acid (DNA) replication. Carmustine is a nitrosourea alkylating agent that cross-links DNA.

10. The answer is 1 [VI A 2 b, 3].
The lympholytic action of prednisolone, a glucocorticoid, extends to the central nervous system (CNS) because prednisolone readily diffuses into the brain. Its action is not cell-cycle specific, and it is well absorbed when administered orally. Glucocorticoids increase the number of circulating red blood cells.

11. The answer is 3 [VI B 3].
Diethylstilbestrol (DES) inhibits gonadotropin secretion and testosterone levels; therefore, it reduces prostatic hypertrophy. It is well absorbed when administered orally. Aplastic anemia may be observed as an adverse effect. It is not effective against transmissible venereal tumors (TVTs).

12. The answer is 3 [V A 6 a].
Doxorubicin may produce cardiomyopathy in dogs via the formation of free radicals, which damage myocardial membranes. 6-Mercaptopurine (6-MP), vincristine, and thiotepa do not cause cardiomyopathy.

13. The answer is 4 [VII A 5 a].
The renal toxicity of cisplatin, an inorganic platinum complex, is reduced by intravenous saline infusions prior to and following drug administration. Saline-induced diuresis reduces the accumulation of platinum in renal tubules. Renal toxicity is not a significant side effect of melphalan, methotrexate, or vincristine.

14. The answer is 4 [II C 1 a (3) (d)].
Hemorrhagic cystitis caused by the irritant effects of the cyclophosphamide metabolite acrolein is reduced by increasing urine volume with furosemide and stimulating water intake and urine voiding. Prednisone, methotrexate, and actinomycin D do not cause cystitis.

15. The answer is 3 [VII C 3].
The chlorinated hydrocarbon mitotane is selectively toxic to cells of the adrenal cortex and is used to treat hyperplasia or inoperable neoplasia of the adrenal cortex. Methotrexate, glucocorticoids, and actinomycin D are not selectively cytotoxic to adrenal cortical cells.

Chapter 13

Antiparasitic Agents

Walter H. Hsu

I. **INTRODUCTION.** Antiparasitics are drugs that reduce parasite burdens to a tolerable level by killing parasites or inhibiting their growth. The ideal antiparasitic has a wide therapeutic index (i.e., the toxic dose is at least three times the therapeutic dose), is effective after only one dose, is easy to administer, is inexpensive, and does not leave residues (an important consideration for use in food-producing animals).

A. Mechanisms of action

1. **Paralysis of parasites** by stimulating or inhibiting the release or action of putative neurotransmitters (Table 13-1)

2. **Alteration of metabolic processes**
   a. Inhibition of fumarate reductase
   b. Inhibition of folic acid synthesis or metabolism
   c. Inhibition of thiamine utilization
   d. Uncoupling of oxidative phosphorylation
   e. Inhibition of chitin formation in arthropods
   f. Simulation of insect juvenile hormones

3. **Alteration of parasite reproduction**
   a. Inhibition of replication in protozoans
   b. Inhibition of egg production in nematodes

B. **Disadvantages** of antiparasitics include:

1. Expense

2. Development of resistant strains

3. Inhibition of host immunity

C. **Current trends** include the use of broad-spectrum drugs or combination therapy to increase efficiency.

II. **EXTERNAL ANTIPARASITICS (INSECTICIDES)**

A. Introduction

1. **Uses.** Insecticides are used on animals to control mites, fleas, ticks, and flies, in the environment to control flies and other insects, and on feedstuffs.

2. **Toxicity.** Individual animals vary in response to insecticides.
   a. **Age.** Young animals are most susceptible.
   b. **Health.** Healthy animals are least likely to experience adverse effects.
   c. **Stress** (e.g., extremely hot or humid weather) can increase susceptibility to insecticide toxicity.
   d. **Species.** Some species are especially sensitive to insecticides.
      (1) **Horses** tend to develop urticaria and hyperemia following application of insecticides.
      (2) **Cats** are very susceptible to cholinergic stimulants.

3. **Formulations** influence the degree of toxicity, the duration of action, and the convenience of application.
   a. **Sprays, dips,** and **shampoos** are suitable when conditions are above freezing.

TABLE 13-1. Putative Neurotransmitters of Various Parasites

| Parasite | Neurotransmitters | |
	Excitatory	Inhibitory
Nematodes	ACh	GABA, histamine
Cestodes	5-HT	ACh
Trematodes	5-HT	ACh, DA, NE
Arthropods	ACh	GABA, octopamine

ACh = acetylcholine; DA = dopamine; GABA = γ-aminobutyric acid;
5-HT = serotonin; NE = norepinephrine.

    b. Pour-ons and **dusts** can be used when conditions are below freezing.
    c. Oil sprays should be applied to the haircoat but not the skin, in order to avoid systemic absorption.
    d. Feed additives that are absorbed are effective against bloodsucking parasites. Whether they are absorbed or not, they are effective against both the larval and pupal stages of ectoparasites in the feces.
    e. Collars and **ear tags** are available.

B. **Organophosphates.** Hundreds of organophosphates are available as insecticides. The withdrawal of chlorinated hydrocarbons from the market is increasing the importance of these agents.

    1. Preparations
        a. Thio compounds include **coumaphos, cythioate, fenthion, chlorpyrifos, diazinon, famphur, phosmet,** and **pirimifos.**
        b. Oxy compounds include **dichlorvos, tetrachlorvinphos,** and **trichlorfon.**

    2. Mechanism of action. The organophosphate insecticides inhibit acetylcholine (ACh) breakdown by inhibiting acetylcholinesterase (AChE) irreversibly (see Chapter 2 V A). The thio compounds must be metabolized to oxy compounds in order to inhibit AChE.

    3. Pharmacokinetics
        a. Absorption. Organophosphates are lipid-soluble; thus, they are well absorbed through the skin and gastrointestinal tract.
        b. Excretion. The organophosphates pose no residue problems.

    4. Administration. Organophosphates are applied to animals topically or administered orally.

    5. Adverse effects
        a. Toxicity (see Chapter 15 III I)
            (1) Acute toxicity
                (a) Clinical signs include **SLUD (s**alivation, **l**acrimation, **u**rination, and **d**efecation), dyspnea, fasciculation, ataxia, and convulsions.
                (b) Treatment involves decontamination and administration of atropine sulfate. Pyridine aldoxime methiodide (2-PAM, an AChE reactivator) may be administered along with atropine (see Chapter 15 III I 4). 2-PAM should not be used alone to treat organophosphate overdose.
            (2) Chronic toxicity. Some organophosphates (e.g., chlorpyrifos, dichlorvos) can cause severe peripheral nerve damage by inducing demyelination.
        b. Drug interactions may occur with drugs that activate cholinergic receptors, skeletal muscle relaxants, and chlorinated hydrocarbons.

C. **Carbamates**

    1. Preparations. Frequently used carbamates include **carbaryl** and **propoxur.**

    2. Mechanism of action. Carbamates inhibit AChE via carbamylation. Their effects are more reversible than those of the organophosphates.

3. **Pharmacokinetics.** The pharmacokinetics of the carbamate insecticides are not well understood.

4. **Adverse effects** include **toxicity.** Carbamate poisoning is similar to acute organo-phosphate poisoning. Atropine sulfate is an effective antidote. 2-PAM should not be used to treat carbamate poisoning for two reasons:
   a. Carbamate binding to AChE is reversible.
   b. 2-PAM itself inhibits cholinesterase.

D. **Chlorinated hydrocarbons**

1. **Chlorinated ethane derivatives** (e.g., **DDT, methoxychlor**) are very effective synthetic insecticides. However, because of the environmental hazard posed by DDT residues, DDT has been banned by the Environmental Protection Agency (EPA) since 1972.
   a. Mechanism of action. These insecticides increase cytosolic calcium (Ca^{2+}) concentrations via two mechanisms.
      (1) They prevent the closure of sodium (Na^+) channels, leading to an increase in intracellular Na^+ concentrations. Subsequently, the intracellular Ca^{2+} concentration is increased through the action of the Na^+-Ca^{2+} antiporter (exchanger).
      (2) They block Ca^{2+}-ATPase to inhibit sequestration of Ca^{2+}.
   b. Pharmacokinetics
      (1) Absorption. Both DDT and methoxychlor are highly lipid soluble. Fat in feed promotes absorption (and, therefore, increases toxicity); however, obese animals are more resistant to insecticide toxicity.
      (2) Fate
         (a) DDT is metabolized into DDD and DDE.
            (i) DDD is further metabolized into DDA, which is water soluble and is excreted in the urine.
            (ii) DDE is lipid soluble and cannot be further metabolized. DDE is permanently stored in the adipose tissue of animals, causing residue problems.
         (b) Methoxychlor is a biodegradable derivative of DDT that does not cause the severe residue problems associated with DDT.
   c. Adverse effects
      (1) Toxicity. Acute toxicity in animals is rare; however, overdoses (e.g., 10 mg/kg DDT) can cause CNS excitation that may lead to **convulsions.**
         (a) Detoxification. Activated charcoal should be administered to remove the toxicant from the gastrointestinal tract.
         (b) Symptomatic therapy
            (i) Anticonvulsants can be administered for seizures. Phenobarbital, in addition to controlling seizures, induces microsomal enzymes, increasing the metabolism of chlorinated hydrocarbons.
            (ii) Artificial respiration may be needed in cases of asphyxia.
      (2) Drug resistance in arthropods may be a significant problem.
      (3) Environmental concerns. DDT and methoxychlor present little risk of acute toxicity in animals; however, DDT poses a hazard to the environment by persisting in the food chain.
         (a) Eggshell thinning results from the ability of DDT to block the estrogen receptors that mediate the deposition of Ca^{2+} into the eggshell.
         (b) Toxicity to aquatic life

2. **Hexachlorocyclohexanes** [e.g., **lindane (r-BHC)**] are used primarily to control screwworm and ear tick infestations in cattle, horses, swine, sheep, and goats.
   a. Mechanism of action. Lindane antagonizes γ-aminobutyric acid (GABA) receptors.
   b. Pharmacokinetics. The pharmacokinetics of the hexachlorocyclohexanes are not clear.
   c. Adverse effects. Lindane is one and one half times more toxic than DDT. Young animals, especially calves, are extremely sensitive to **lindane poisoning.**

(1) **Signs** of toxicity are similar to those produced by DDT (e.g., tremors, ataxia, convulsions, prostration, tachypnea).

(2) **Treatment** of poisoning is nonspecific.

E. **Insect growth regulators (juvenile hormone analogs)**

1. **Preparations** include **cyromazine, fenoxycarb,** and **methoprene.**

2. **Mechanism of action.** Insect growth regulators mimic the actions of the juvenile hormones of insects. These preparations maintain the larvae in an immature stage and interfere with reproductive organ differentiation.

3. **Pharmacokinetics.** The pharmacokinetics of these agents are not well understood.

4. **Therapeutic uses and administration**
   a. **Fecal maggot control in poultry.** Cyromazine is administered orally to control fecal maggots in poultry.
   b. **Flea control**
      (1) Fenoxycarb and methoprene are sprayed in households and on animals to prevent eggs, pupae, and larvae from developing into adult fleas. These drugs are effective for at least 21 weeks. Methoprene is also available as a flea collar for dogs.
      (2) Fenoxycarb and methoprene are mixed with pyrethroids to kill adult fleas.

5. **Adverse effects.** These products are safe when used as directed.

F. **Botanicals**

1. **Rotenone**
   a. **Chemistry.** Rotenone is an alkaloid derived from the root of the *derris* plant.
   b. **Mechanism of action.** Rotenone inhibits cellular respiratory metabolism by blocking electron generation from reduced nicotinamide adenine dinucleotide (NADH). As a result, oxidation of lactate, glutamate, and other substances is reduced and nerve conduction is adversely affected.
   c. **Therapeutic uses**
      (1) Rotenone is used to kill **fleas, lice, ticks,** and **mites.** It has fast "knockdown" action on all arthropods, with little persistence.
      (2) Rotenone is also used to kill unwanted fish in ponds and lakes.
   d. **Adverse effects** include local irritation and CNS disturbances (e.g., excitation, convulsions, depression).

2. **Pyrethroids**
   a. **Preparations** include **pyrethrins, allethrin, cypermethrin, lambdacyhalothrin,** and **permethrin.**
   b. **Chemistry**
      (1) Pyrethrins are alkaloids of pyrethrum, which is one of the oldest insecticides known to man.
      (2) The other pyrethroids, which are synthetic, are more resistant to breakdown.
   c. **Mechanism of action**
      (1) Pyrethroids block nicotinic receptors.
      (2) Pyrethroids increase GABA release.
   d. **Pharmacokinetics.** The pharmacokinetics of the pyrethroids are not well understood.
   e. **Therapeutic uses.** Pyrethroids exert a rapid "knockdown" effect but have little residual activity. The "knockdown" effect may or may not be fatal; therefore, these agents are **usually combined with other insecticides or a synergist** (e.g., piperonyl butoxide) to increase insecticidal activity. Synergists inhibit induction of the microsomal enzymes that degrade pyrethroids.
   f. **Adverse effects.** Pyrethroids are generally safe, but may cause allergy, nausea and vomiting, and headache.

G. **Other insecticides**

1. **Amitraz** is a formamidine insecticide cleared for use on dogs, pigs, and cattle.
    a. **Mechanism of action.** Amitraz activates octopamine receptors in arthropods.
    b. **Pharmacokinetics.** The pharmacokinetics of amitraz are not well understood.
    c. **Therapeutic uses**
        (1) Amitraz is used to eliminate **mites, lice,** and **ticks** in dogs, swine, and cattle. No preslaughter withdrawal period is necessary in cattle, and it can be used on lactating dairy cattle without incurring a withdrawal period for milk following application.
        (2) Three to six biweekly treatments may be used to control **demodectic mange.**
    d. **Adverse effects.** In animals, amitraz activates α_2-adrenergic receptors. Therefore, the adverse effects of amitraz are similar to the pharmacological effects of xylazine (e.g., sedation, bradycardia, hyperglycemia, gastrointestinal stasis). α_2-Adrenergic antagonists can be used as an antidote.
    e. **Contraindications**
        (1) Amitraz should not be applied to swine within 3 days of slaughter.
        (2) Amitraz may cause fatal colon impaction in horses.

2. **Lufenuron (Program)**
    a. **Mechanism of action.** Lufenuron inhibits chitin synthesis. (Chitin is an essential constituent of flea eggshells and the exoskeleton of immature fleas.)
    b. **Pharmacokinetics.** Following oral dosing, lufenuron is distributed to the adipose tissues and then back into the blood stream, reaching therapeutic concentrations in 6–12 hours. Therapeutic blood levels are maintained for over 32 days.
    c. **Therapeutic uses.** Lufenuron is used in dogs and cats older than 6 weeks of age to control fleas. It is effective against eggs and immature fleas, but has no proven effect on adult fleas.
    d. **Administration.** Lufenuron is administered orally once monthly. Doses should be given with or immediately following the meal.
    e. **Adverse effects.** At recommended doses, lufenuron has no side effects or contraindications. It is safe in young animals (i.e., those older than 6 weeks of age), in reproducing and lactating dogs and cats and their offspring, and when used in conjunction with other insecticides.

III. **ANTINEMATODAL AGENTS (NEMATOCIDES)** may be **broad spectrum** or **narrow spectrum** (Table 13-2).

A. **Benzimidazoles**

1. **Thiabendazole** (Figure 13-1) is the prototypical agent. It is approved for use in ruminants and horses.
    a. **Mechanism of action.** Thiabendazole inhibits fumarate reductase, which catalyzes the formation of succinate from fumarate. Interference with succinate formation leads to the inhibition of adenosine triphosphate (ATP) formation.

TABLE 13-2. Classification of Antinematodal Agents

Broad Spectrum	Narrow Spectrum
Benzimidazoles	Phenothiazine
Nicotine-like compounds	Piperazine
Organophosphates	Toluene
Antibiotics	Thenium closylate

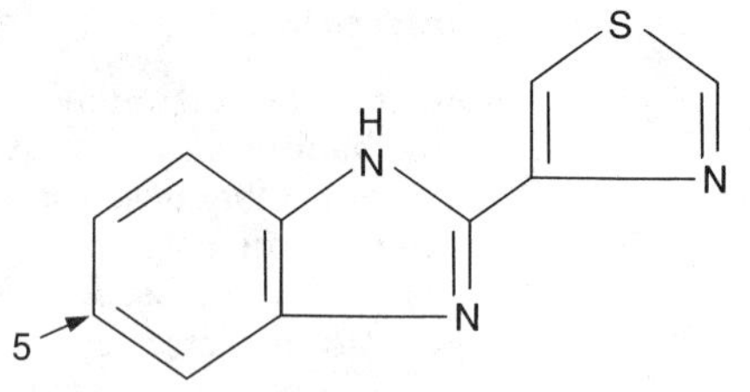

FIGURE 13-1. Thiabendazole, the prototypical benzimidazole. Metabolism occurs via hydroxylation at position 5. The other benzimidazoles are more potent than thiabendazole because they have a side chain that prevents hydroxylation at position 5.

  b. Pharmacokinetics
    (1) Absorption. Thiabendazole is lipid soluble. As a result of poor dissolution in digestive fluids, thiabendazole may be poorly or erratically absorbed from the gastrointestinal tract.
    (2) Metabolism and excretion. Hydroxylation on position 5 (see Figure 13-1) is followed by conjugation. The 5-hydroxy metabolites are excreted as urinary glucuronide and sulfate. In cattle, excretion is complete within 3 days.
  c. Therapeutic uses
    (1) Ruminants. Thiabendazole is effective against **major gastrointestinal nematodes.** It is not effective against whipworms, lungworms, or filariae.
    (2) Horses
      (a) Thiabendazole is effective against **strongyles,** but large doses are needed to kill *Strongylus vulgaris.* It is not effective against immature strongyles.
      (b) Thiabendazole is used to treat **intestinal threadworms** and **pinworms.**
      (c) Thiabendazole has some degree of **larvicidal and ovicidal activity;** however, it is not effective against bots.
  d. Adverse effects. Because fumarate reductase does not exist in mammals, thiabendazole is one of the safest antinematodal drugs.

 2. Other benzimidazoles
  a. Preparations include albendazole, fenbendazole, mebendazole, oxfendazole, oxibendazole, and febantel (a pro-benzimidazole that is converted to fenbendazole and oxfendazole in animals).
  b. Chemistry. All of these preparations, with the exception of febantel, have a side chain that prevents hydroxylation of position 5 (see Figure 13-1). Therefore, these compounds are more potent than thiabendazole, and dosages are usually less than those of thiabendazole.
  c. Pharmacokinetics
    (1) Absorption. Gastrointestinal absorption varies, depending on the water solubility of the compound.
    (2) Metabolism. The degree of metabolism is related to the 5C substitution (see Figure 13-1).
    (3) Excretion. The majority of benzimidazoles (except thiabendazole) are excreted unchanged in feces.
      (a) Drug residues persist for 1–3 weeks. They approach the low limit of detection in 2 days; however, residues in the liver are detectable for 2 weeks.
      (b) The **preslaughter withdrawal period in cattle** is 27 days for albendazole, 8 days for fenbendazole, and 7 days for oxfendazole.
  d. Therapeutic uses
    (1) Ruminants. Albendazole, fenbendazole, and oxfendazole are effective against **major gastrointestinal worms** (in both the adult and larval stages). In addition, they are effective against **lungworms.** However, they are ineffective against filariae.
    (2) Horses. Fenbendazole, mebendazole, oxfendazole, oxibendazole, and febantel have activity similar to that of thiabendazole. In addition, they are effective against **ascarids.**
      (a) Fenbendazole is effective against *Habronema.*

(b) Mebendazole is active against **lungworms** at dosages of 15–20 mg/kg/day for 5 consecutive days.

(3) Dogs and cats. Febendazole, mebendazole, oxibendazole, and febantel are effective against **ascarids, hookworms,** and **whipworms.**

(a) Febantel is the only agent approved for use in cats.

(b) Three to five consecutive daily dosages are usually necessary.

(4) Mebendazole is used for the treatment of **trichinosis,** particularly at the muscular stage of *Trichinella spiralis.*

(5) These agents have more **larvicidal** and **ovicidal activity** than thiabendazole.

e. Drug resistance. Cross-resistance occurs among all benzimidazoles.

f. Adverse effects. These agents are generally safe, although albendazole and oxfendazole may be teratogenic. Hepatotoxicity may occur in dogs (partially as a result of repeated administrations for 3–5 consecutive days).

B. **Nicotine-like nematocides**

1. Levamisole is approved for use in ruminants and pigs.

a. Mechanism of action. Levamisole paralyzes worms by causing depolarizing neuromuscular blockade.

b. Pharmacokinetics:

(1) Absorption is excellent following gastrointestinal, topical, or parenteral administration.

(2) Excretion. The plasma half-life is 4 hours, and the drug is eliminated from the body in 2 days.

(a) Forty percent of the dose is excreted in the urine within 12 hours.

(b) The **preslaughter clearance periods** in pigs and cattle are 3 days and 7 days, respectively.

c. Therapeutic uses

(1) Ruminants. Levamisole is effective against most **mature gastrointestinal worms** and **lungworms,** but it has marginal activity against *Strongyloides* and immature gastrointestinal worms.

(2) Pigs. It is effective against **ascarids, intestinal threadworms, lungworms, nodular worms,** and **kidney worms.**

(3) Dogs. The use of levamisole as a **microfilaricide for canine heartworms** is an extralabel use.

d. Adverse effects. Levamisole is one of the most toxic anthelmintics. It has a low safety margin, especially when given by injection.

(1) Signs of levamisole poisoning include parasympathetic stimulation, convulsions, CNS depression, and asphyxia, which is primarily the result of respiratory muscle paralysis.

(2) Atropine cannot counteract levamisole-induced depolarizing blockade of skeletal muscle; therefore, it is not an antidote for levamisole overdose.

(3) Coadministration of levamisole and pyrantel, another nicotine-like nematocide, increases toxicity.

2. Butamisole is a derivative of levamisole.

a. Therapeutic uses. Butamisole is an injectable used to treat **whipworms** and **hookworms** in dogs. Butamisole has **microfilaricidal activity against heartworms;** therefore, it may cause anaphylactic reactions when inadvertently used in microfilaremic animals.

b. Contraindications. Butamisole is contraindicated in severely debilitated animals or those with renal or hepatic disorders.

3. Pyrantel and morantel

a. Chemistry

(1) Pyrantel, which is inactivated in aqueous solution upon exposure to light, should be stored in tight, light-resistant containers. The drug should be used soon after preparation of a drench solution or suspension.

(2) Morantel, the methyl ester of pyrantel, forms stable solutions.

b. Preparations

(1) Pyrantel tartrate is approved for horses and pigs.

(2) Pyrantel pamoate is approved for horses and dogs.

(3) Morantel tartrate is approved for cattle.

c. Mechanism of action. Like levamisole, pyrantel and morantel paralyze worms by causing depolarizing neuromuscular blockade.

d. Pharmacokinetics

(1) Absorption

(a) Pyrantel tartrate is water soluble; therefore, gastrointestinal absorption is excellent following oral administration. Peak plasma concentrations occur 2–3 hours after dosing.

(b) Pyrantel pamoate is poorly soluble in water, limiting gastrointestinal absorption. Therefore, pyrantel pamoate is good for treatment of bowel worms (e.g., pinworms).

(c) Morantel tartrate is absorbed rapidly from the abomasum and small intestine. Peak plasma concentrations occur 4–6 hours after dosing.

(2) Metabolism and excretion. The absorbed pyrantel and morantel are rapidly metabolized and excreted, mostly via the feces, but also via urine. Preslaughter withdrawal requirements are 1 day for pyrantel tartrate in swine and 14 days for morantel in cattle.

e. Therapeutic uses

(1) Horses. Pyrantel is effective against strongyles, ascarids, and pinworms, but not against bots.

(2) Pigs. Pyrantel is effective against ascarids, nodular worms, and stomach worms.

(3) Dogs. Pyrantel is effective against all gastrointestinal nematodes, but its activity against whipworms is erratic.

(4) Ruminants. Morantel is effective against stomach worms, nodular worms, and other principal intestinal worms.

f. Adverse effects. At recommended doses, adverse effects are not common. Emesis may occur in dogs and pigs.

g. Contraindications. Because morantel and pyrantel have the same mechanism of action as levamisole, these agents should not be used concurrently.

C. Organophosphates

1. Preparations. Dichlorvos, trichlorfon, and coumaphos are widely used.

a. Dichlorvos and **trichlorfon** are approved for use in horses, pigs, and dogs. Dichlorvos is rather unsafe in cattle and poultry.

b. Coumaphos is approved for use in cattle.

2. Mechanism of action. The organophosphate nematocides inhibit ACh breakdown by irreversibly inhibiting AChE.

3. Pharmacokinetics

a. Dichlorvos is a lipophilic liquid that is incorporated into polyvinyl chloride resin pellets. As these pellets traverse the gastrointestinal tract, dichlorvos diffuses into the intestinal fluid, allowing the drug to come into contact with nematodes. The pellets release approximately 50% of the drug in 48 hours. When passed into the feces, the pellets still contain approximately 50% of the original dose of dichlorvos, enough to kill fecal fly larvae.

b. Trichlorfon is a white crystal with poor water solubility that must be converted to dichlorvos to be effective. Trichlorfon is metabolized rapidly after oral dosing and may inhibit AChE for 2–3 weeks.

c. Coumaphos. The pharmacokinetics of coumaphos are not well understood.

4. Therapeutic uses. Organophosphates are effective against the major gastrointestinal parasites.

a. Dichlorvos

(1) Pigs and dogs. Dichlorvos is effective against whipworms, nodular worms, *Strongyloides,* hookworms, and ascarids in pigs and dogs. It has little or no activity against migrating larvae of ascarids and hookworms.

(2) Horses. Dichlorvos is effective against bots, strongyles, ascarids, and pinworms.

Levamisole, pyrantel > Organophosphates > Benzimidazoles, antibiotics

FIGURE 13-2. Relative toxicity of antinematodal drugs. Organophosphates are of moderate toxicity.

  b. Trichlorfon is used mainly in horses. Its spectrum of activity is similar to that of dichlorvos. It is one of the safest organophosphates and thus can be used in fish ponds.

  c. Coumaphos is used in cattle to control stomach worms, whipworms, and *Cooperia.* To improve safety, the drug is given orally as a feed supplement at the rate of 2 mg/kg/day for 6 consecutive days.

5. Adverse effects

  a. Toxicity (Figure 13-2)

   (1) Acute. Stimulation of cholinergic receptors may induce the SLUD syndrome.

   (2) Chronic. Organophosphates may cause demyelination, inducing chronic neurotoxicity.

  b. Acute death may result from respiratory paralysis and cardiovascular arrest.

6. Contraindications. Organophosphate nematocides are not to be given to weak animals, those exposed to other anticholinesterase agents, or those with gastrointestinal disorders.

D. Antibiotics

1. Ivermectin is an antibiotic extracted from *Streptomyces avermitilis.*

  a. Mechanism of action. Ivermectin activates the $GABA_A$-receptor–chloride channel macromolecular complex, thus inhibiting neurotransmission in both arthropods and animals. It may also increase the release of GABA from nerve terminals.

  b. Pharmacokinetics

   (1) After administration, more than 95% of the dose is metabolized in the liver. The plasma half-life is 3 days in cattle.

   (2) Ivermectin remains in tissues with long persistency; one dose is usually effective for 2–4 weeks. Preslaughter clearance periods are 18 days in swine and 35 days in cattle. Ivermectin should not be administered to milking dairy cattle.

  c. Therapeutic uses and administration

   (1) Ruminants. Ivermectin is effective against **all major gastrointestinal worms** and **lungworms.** The standard dose is 0.2 mg/kg administered orally or subcutaneously.

   (2) Horses. It is effective against **bots, stomach worms, strongyles, pinworms,** and **ascarids.** The dose and route of administration are the same as for ruminants.

   (3) Pigs. Ivermectin is effective against **major gastrointestinal worms, lungworms,** and **kidney worms.** It is not effective against *Trichinella* during the muscular stage. The standard dose is 0.3 mg/kg administered subcutaneously.

   (4) Dogs

    (a) Ivermectin is effective against **ascarids, hookworms,** and **whipworms** at a dosage of 0.2 mg/kg. However, this dose may not be safe in some breeds (e.g., collies) and is therefore not approved for dogs.

    (b) It is effective as a **microfilaricide** (50 μg/kg) and **heartworm preventive** (6–12 μg/kg). The use of ivermectin as a microfilaricide is an extralabel use.

   (5) All species. Ivermectin is effective against all ectoparasites. It is used especially to control **mites.**

  d. Adverse effects. Ivermectin has a high safety margin in ruminants, horses, and swine, and is safe for use in pregnant animals and breeders.

   (1) Local irritation may occur following subcutaneous administration to swine.

   (2) CNS depression. At high doses, ivermectin may evoke CNS depression as evidenced by listlessness, mydriasis, ataxia, recumbency, and coma. Although ivermectin enhances the activity of the GABA system, the GABA receptor antagonist **picrotoxin does not work as an antidote.**

  2. **Milbemycin** is isolated from *Streptomyces hygroscopicus.*
   a. **Mechanism of action.** The mechanism of action is the same as that of ivermectin.
   b. **Pharmacokinetics.** Following oral administration, approximately 90% of the dose passes through the gastrointestinal tract unchanged. The remaining approximately 10% is absorbed and subsequently excreted in the bile. Therefore, nearly the entire dose is eliminated in the feces.
   c. **Therapeutic uses.** Milbemycin is approved for use in dogs only and is effective against the infective larvae of *Dirofilaria immitis,* **hookworms, whipworms,** and **ascarids.** Milbemycin at the recommended dose of 0.5 mg/kg can be used in all dog breeds, including collies, and is safe in pregnant dogs and breeders.
   d. **Adverse effects.** Milbemycin has a high safety margin in dogs; however, at high doses, milbemycin may evoke CNS depression as evidenced by pyrexia, ataxia, and recumbency.

E. | **Miscellaneous antinematodal drugs**
  1. **Phenothiazine,** the oldest antinematodal drug, was discovered in 1938.
   a. **Mechanism of action.** The mechanism of action is not well understood. Phenothiazine may inhibit the enzyme system involved in carbohydrate metabolism. Very high concentrations of phenothiazine may inhibit cholinesterase.
   b. **Pharmacokinetics**
    (1) **Absorption.** The gastrointestinal absorption of phenothiazine may be erratic; generally, up to 50% of the dose is absorbed.
    (2) **Metabolism and excretion.** Phenothiazine may be converted to phenothiazine sulfoxide in the intestinal epithelium. Phenothiazine and phenothiazine sulfoxide are further metabolized into two brown-red dyes, phenothiazone and thionol, which may be evident in urine and milk.
   c. **Therapeutic uses.** Phenothiazine has excellent efficacy against **small strongyles,** and at high doses, it has good efficacy against **large strongyles.** It is mixed with piperazine and trichlorfon as a tube formulation for use in horses.
   d. **Adverse effects.** Phenothiazine may evoke dullness, weakness, anorexia, oliguria, colic, constipation, fever, tachycardia, and signs of hemolysis (e.g., icterus, anemia, hemoglobinuria).
   e. **Contraindications.** Phenothiazine should not be used in pregnant, constipated, or weak animals.

  2. **Piperazine**
   a. **Preparations.** Piperazine is available in adipate, citrate, hydrochloride, tartrate, or phosphate form.
   b. **Chemistry.** Piperazine is inactivated by moisture, carbon dioxide, and light; therefore, containers should be tightly closed and protected from light.
   c. **Mechanism of action.** Piperazine is a GABA-receptor agonist that inhibits neurotransmission, resulting in paralysis of worms.
   d. **Pharmacokinetics**
    (1) **Absorption.** Piperazine salts are well absorbed from the gastrointestinal tract.
    (2) **Metabolism and excretion.** Some piperazine is metabolized in the liver and the remainder (30%–40%) is excreted in the urine. Urinary excretion of piperazine starts as early as 30 minutes after dosing, and is complete within 24 hours.
   e. **Therapeutic uses.** Piperazine is effective against **ascarids** and **nodular worms** in all species; however, its use is limited in ruminants, because ascarids are not a significant problem in this species. Thiabendazole is combined with piperazine to increase ascaricidal activity.
   f. **Adverse effects.** Piperazine is a very safe drug, but large doses may produce vomiting, diarrhea, and ataxia.

  3. **Toluene**
   a. **Chemistry.** Toluene is an organic liquid.
   b. **Pharmacokinetics**

(1) Absorption. Toluene is absorbed well from the gastrointestinal tract following oral administration.

(2) Metabolism and excretion. It is metabolized into benzoic acid within 24 hours of administration and is excreted in the urine.

  c. **Therapeutic uses and administration.** Toluene is approved for use in dogs and cats. Because it is irritating to the oral mucosa, toluene is administered in gelatin capsules.

    (1) It is effective against **ascarids** and has limited activity against **hookworms.** To enhance efficacy, toluene may be combined with n-butyl chloride (another mild drug effective against ascarids and hookworms).

    (2) Toluene is used in combination with dichlorophen (an anticestodal drug).

  d. **Adverse effects.** Toluene may cause anorexia, vomiting, diarrhea, tremors, and ataxia.

4. Thenium closylate (Canopar)

  a. **Chemistry.** Thenium closylate is a nicotine-like quaternary drug that is soluble in water.

  b. **Mechanism of action.** Like levamisole and pyrantel, thenium closylate paralyzes worms by causing depolarizing neuromuscular blockade.

  c. **Pharmacokinetics.** When administered orally, thenium closylate is poorly absorbed from the gastrointestinal tract because of its quaternary structure.

  d. **Therapeutic uses.** Thenium closylate is used strictly in dogs to control **hookworms.** It is effective against adult worms, immature worms, and fourth stage larvae. It has no activity against other worms.

  e. **Adverse effects.** Thenium closylate has a wide margin of safety because gastrointestinal absorption is limited.

    (1) Vomiting. Approximately 20% of dogs treated with the drug experience vomiting.

    (2) Rarely, **sudden death** may occur following dosing with thenium closylate.

IV. DRUGS FOR HEARTWORM PREVENTION AND THERAPY

A. Introduction. Treatment and prevention of heartworm involve three aspects:

1. Removal of adult heartworms requires an **adulticide.**

2. Interruption of the life cycle requires a **microfilaricide.** Treatment to eliminate microfilariae should be initiated 3–4 weeks after the adulticide treatment.

  a. Microfilaricidal treatment reduces the incidence of glomerulonephritis, which may be induced by masses of microfilariae.

  b. Microfilaricidal treatment reduces the possibility of an anaphylactic reaction to diethylcarbamazine (DEC) in microfilariae-positive dogs.

  c. Microfilaricidal treatment eliminates the source of heartworm infection (minor reason for eliminating microfilariae).

3. Prevention of infection requires a **larvicide.**

B. Adulticides eliminate both immature (L_5) and adult heartworms.

1. Thiacetarsamide (Caparsolate) is the only adulticide available commercially.

  a. **Chemistry.** Thiacetarsamide is a trivalent arsenic compound.

  b. **Mechanism of action:** Thiacetarsamide denatures enzymes by binding to the sulfhydryl groups of cysteine residues.

  c. **Pharmacokinetics**

    (1) Distribution. The drug is widely distributed in the body, but is concentrated in the liver and kidneys.

    (2) Metabolism and excretion. Thiacetarsamide is metabolized in the liver. Following intravenous injection, thiacetarsamide has an elimination half-life of approximately 45 minutes and a clearance rate of approximately 200 ml/kg/

min. After administration, 85% of the dose is eliminated within 48 hours, primarily in the feces (66%). Some of the dose is excreted in the urine as well.

d. **Administration.** The dosage is 2.2 mg/kg intravenously, twice daily for 2 days.

e. **Adverse reactions.** Thiacetarsamide has a narrow margin of safety; therefore, dosages must be accurately determined to avoid serious adverse effects. In case of overdose, dimercaprol (BAL) can be used as an antidote.

   (1) **Tissue sloughing** and **phlebitis** may occur if thiacetarsamide is injected into the perivascular space. Local injection of a glucocorticoid may inhibit the reaction.

   (2) **Vomiting.** Dogs may vomit after thiacetarsamide administration. Only persistent vomiting, which may be indicative of hepatotoxicity, warrants concern.

   (3) **Hepatotoxicity** affects approximately 20% of animals receiving thiacetarsamide. Should severe liver damage occur, thiacetarsamide should be discontinued and supportive treatment for liver disease should be instituted as needed.

   (4) **Renal toxicity** may occur after thiacetarsamide therapy. Renal casts alone are generally not an indication that thiacetarsamide treatment should be interrupted; however, blood urea nitrogen greater than 100 mg/dl and albuminuria are indications that treatment should be discontinued for at least 4 weeks.

   (5) **Thromboembolic pneumonia** may result as dead heartworms accumulate, usually in the caudal lung lobes. Adult heartworms begin to die within days of thiacetarsamide treatment and continue to die over a 3-week period. To minimize mortality, animals should be kept on strict rest, usually for 1 month following therapy.

      (a) **Signs** include coughing, dyspnea, hemoptysis, fever, anorexia, and lethargy.

      (b) **Treatment.** Aspirin and glucocorticoids may be used for 2 weeks to treat thromboembolic pneumonia. Antibiotics may be administered to prevent secondary bacterial infection.

2. **Melarsomine (Immiticide)**

   a. **Chemistry.** Melarsomine is also a trivalent arsenical compound.

   b. **Mechanism of action.** Its mechanism of action is the same as that of thiacetarsamide.

   c. **Pharmacokinetics**

      (1) **Absorption.** Following intramuscular injection, melarsomine has a mean absorption half-life of 2.6 minutes and a peak concentration in blood at 8 minutes.

      (2) **Distribution.** Melarsomine is found in both plasma and red blood cells, whereas thiacetarsamide is found only in red blood cells.

      (3) **Excretion.** Melarsomine is retained in the body five times longer than thiacetarsamide. The body clearance is approximately three times lower for melarsomine than thiacetarsamide.

   d. **Administration.** The advantage of melarsomine over thiacetarsamide is that melarsomine can be administered intramuscularly.

      (1) The usual dosage is 2.5 mg/kg once daily for 2 days.

         (a) The first injection should be administered in the right lumbar muscles and the second in the left.

         (b) This two-dose schedule completely eliminates all worms from 60%–81% of dogs. The regimen can be repeated in 4 months to increase the efficacy to 98%.

      (2) For dogs with severe infection, a single dose (2.5 mg/kg) is followed by the full two-dose treatment 1 month later. The initial single dose kills 88% of male and 17% of female worms, hence providing some relief of clinical signs while reducing the risk of complications from pulmonary embolism [see IV B 1 e (5)]. This regimen removes all worms from approximately 85% of dogs.

e. Adverse reactions
  (1) Mild localized edema may occur following intramuscular injection.
  (2) Hepatotoxicity and **renal toxicity** may be milder than thiacetarsamide.
  (3) Thromboembolic pneumonia may be as severe as that seen with thiacetarsamide treatment.
  (4) Overdose may result in distress, restlessness, pawing, salivation, vomiting, tachycardia, tachypnea, dyspnea, abdominal pain, hindlimb weakness, and recumbency. Severe cases terminate in circulatory collapse, orthopnea, coma, and death. Toxicity can be reversed by intramuscular injection of 3 mg/kg dimercaprol (BAL) within 3 hours of the onset of symptoms. However, dimercaprol may reduce the efficacy of melarsomine.

C. Microfilaricides

1. Agents. Microfilaricidal use is an extralabel use for **ivermectin** and **milbemycin;** however, these are the only two drugs that may be safely and effectively used for this purpose. These agents are discussed in detail in III D.

2. Administration
  a. Ivermectin. Therapy entails one dose (50 μg/kg) administered orally or subcutaneously. This drug is contraindicated in collies.
  b. Milbemycin. One dose (0.5 mg/kg) is administered orally; the treatment may be repeated in 2 weeks. This drug can be safely used in collies.

3. Adverse reactions. Transient weakness, pale membranes, intestinal hyperperistalsis, and tachypnea may be seen following administration of a microfilaricide, suggesting a mild cardiovascular shock resulting from reactions to dead microfilariae. The higher the microfilaria count, the greater the chance of encountering noticeable adverse effects.

D. Larvicides

1. Diethylcarbamazine (DEC) kills the L_3 larvae, thereby eliminating stages L_3–L_5 of the heartworm life cycle.
  a. Chemistry. DEC is a piperazine derivative.
  b. Mechanism of action. Like piperazine, DEC is a GABA-receptor agonist.
  c. Pharmacokinetics
    (1) After oral administration, plasma levels peak at 3 hours and fall to zero in 48 hours. The therapeutic level of DEC has to be maintained by daily dosing.
    (2) Ten to thirty percent of the dose is excreted as the unchanged drug in urine. The rest is excreted as metabolites.
  d. Administration. DEC citrate (2.5–3 mg/lb/day) is administered orally during and 2 months after the mosquito season.
  e. Adverse reactions
    (1) Adverse reactions are minimal if there are no microfilariae in the blood stream. DEC causes potentially fatal **anaphylactic reactions in microfilariae-positive dogs.** It has been suggested that DEC liberates substances from microfilariae that constrict the hepatic vein.
    (2) At high doses (i.e., greater than 50 mg/kg), DEC may induce **vomiting** and **gastric mucosa irritation.**

2. Ivermectin (Heartgard) is a larvicide that kills the L_4 larvae. It is administered orally at dosages of 6–12 μg/kg once monthly. The first dose is given within 1 month of the first exposure to mosquitoes. The last dose is given within 1 month following the last exposure to mosquitoes. Because it takes 2.5 months for L_4 larvae to develop into L_5 larvae, the elimination of larvae in the L_4 stage once monthly is effective.

3. Milbemycin (Interceptor). When used as a larvicide, milbemycin is administered orally once monthly (0.5 mg/kg) following the same principles as those for ivermectin administration.

V. ANTICESTODAL AGENTS

A. General information

1. These agents kill tapeworms, as opposed to arecoline, an obsolete taeniafuge that only paralyzes them.

2. Worms killed by these drugs may be digested by the host animal; therefore, they may not be evident in the feces.

3. Control of intermediate hosts (e.g., fleas for *Dipylidium* and rodents for *Taenia*) is necessary.

B. Dichlorophen

1. **Mechanism of action.** Dichlorophen causes uncoupling of oxidative phosphorylation to deplete ATP.

2. **Pharmacokinetics.** Gastrointestinal absorption of dichlorophen, a lipid-soluble drug, is greatly enhanced when it is combined with toluene (an organic solvent).

3. **Therapeutic uses.** Dichlorophen is used to treat *Taenia* infestations in dogs and cats. Its efficacy against *Echinococcus* and *Dipylidium* is variable.

4. **Administration.** Dichlorophen is best given orally after an overnight fast. As with all of the anticestodal agents, purgation is unnecessary.

5. **Adverse effects.** No side effects have been reported, other than salivation if the animal bites the gelatin capsule.

C. Benzimidazoles (see III A). Mebendazole, fenbendazole, oxfendazole, and albendazole are effective against mature *Taenia* and *Echinococcus* in dogs and cats, and *Moniezia* in ruminants. They may kill intermediate cysts of *Taenia* in infected sheep and cattle. These agents are not effective against *Dipylidium*. Mebendazole and albendazole are used to control hydatid cysts in humans.

D. Praziquantel (Droncit)

1. **Mechanism of action.** Praziquantel causes paralysis and digestion of tapeworms as well as irreversible focal vacuolization and disintegration of integument. The exact mechanism of action is unknown, but these activities may be mediated by an increase in intracellular Ca^{2+} concentration, attributable to increased Ca^{2+} influx.

2. **Pharmacokinetics**
   a. **Absorption.** Praziquantel is completely absorbed within 30–120 minutes of oral dosing.
   b. **Distribution.** It is distributed throughout the body, including the CNS.
   c. **Metabolism and excretion.** Praziquantel is metabolized to unknown compounds in the liver and excreted primarily in the urine. The elimination half-life is 3 hours in dogs.

3. **Therapeutic uses.** Praziquantel is effective against all species of tapeworms and kills both adults and juveniles. However, its activity against hydatid cysts is erratic.

4. **Administration**
   a. Praziquantel is approved for use in dogs and cats, and has been used in birds and other animals. Use in large animals may not be economically feasible.
   b. Praziquantel may be administered orally or subcutaneously. Fasting is not necessary.

5. **Adverse effects.** Praziquantel is the safest anticestodal drug available.
   a. Overdose induces anorexia, vomiting, salivation, diarrhea, and lethargy in less than 5% of animals receiving the drug.
   b. It exerts no teratogenic or embryotoxic effects.

E. **Epsiprantel (Cestex),** a praziquantel analog, is approved for use in dogs and cats. Epsiprantel is administered orally. Unlike praziquantel, epsiprantel is absorbed poorly after oral administration and most of the drug is eliminated in the feces (less than 0.1% of the drug is recovered in the urine after dosing).

VI. ANTITREMATODAL DRUGS

A. **Albendazole** (see III A 2) is approved for use against mature liver flukes (e.g., *Fasciola hepatica*) in cattle. Albendazole requires a 27-day preslaughter withdrawal period. Because albendazole is a teratogen, it cannot be used in pregnant cattle during the first 45 days of gestation or in female dairy cattle of breeding age.

B. **Praziquantel** (see V D) is effective against lung flukes in dogs. It is also effective against liver flukes; however, it is too expensive for use in ruminants.

C. **Clorsulon (Curatrem)**

1. **Mechanism of action.** Clorsulon inhibits 3-phosphoglycerate kinase and phosphoglyceromutase in the glycolytic pathway, depriving the flukes of a metabolic energy source.

2. **Pharmacokinetics.** Clorsulon is lipid soluble. After oral dosing, it is absorbed rapidly. Peak levels occur within 4 hours, and blood levels of clorsulon peak 8–12 hours after administration. The preslaughter withdrawal period is 8 days and the milk withdrawal period is 4 days.

3. **Therapeutic uses.** Clorsulon is the most effective drug against *F. hepatica,* killing both mature and immature flukes in cattle. However, its activity against *F. magna* is poor.

4. **Adverse effects.** When used as directed, adverse effects are rare. Clorsulon is safe in pregnant and breeding animals.

VII. ANTIPROTOZOAL DRUGS. This discussion focuses on anticoccidial drugs and metronidazole. With the exception of metronidazole, other antiprotozoal drugs are not safe for use in animals.

A. **Aniticoccidial drugs**

1. **Introduction**
   a. **Financial implications of coccidiosis.** Coccidiosis, a prevalent disease in calves, piglets, and poultry, costs the United States poultry industry more than 50 million dollars annually, despite expenditures of more than 85 million for anticoccidial drugs. These losses are caused primarily by impaired feed conversion, slow growth, and the poor quality of carcasses at processing.
   b. **Therapeutic approaches**
      (1) **Poultry.** Most of the anticoccidial drugs discussed in this section are used in chickens.
         (a) **Broilers** are not vaccinated against coccidia because latent infection may retard growth. Amprolium, the nonwithdrawal anticoccidial drug, is administered 1 week prior to slaughter.
         (b) **Layers** are vaccinated against coccidia. Outbreaks are usually treated with a sulfonamide on an as-needed basis.
      (2) **Mammals** can be treated with sulfonamides and ormetroprim, amprolium, decoquinate, or Na^+ ionophores.

    c. Resistance to anticoccidial drugs is minimized by using two or more drugs sequentially. Overemphasized switching may decrease immunity; therefore, it may be self-defeating.

        (1) Shuttle program. Different anticoccidial drugs are used in a single grow-out.

        (2) Rotation (switch) program. Different anticoccidials are used between two grow-outs.

    d. Life cycle of avian coccidia (Figure 13-3)

  2. Agents

    a. Decoquinate

        (1) Chemistry. Decoquinate is a quinolone.

        (2) Mechanism of action. Decoquinate may block DNA synthesis by inhibiting DNA gyrase.

        (3) Pharmacokinetics. The pharmacokinetics of decoquinate are not well understood. The preslaughter withdrawal period is 5 days when used in broilers.

        (4) Therapeutic uses

            (a) Decoquinate is approved for use in calves, young goats, and broilers for the **prevention of coccidiosis.** It is not effective for treating clinical coccidiosis.

            (b) It should be effective against all species of avian *Eimeria* on the first sporozoite stage. Use is limited because of its tendency to induce drug resistance (attributable to its action on such an early stage of the asexual cycle of the coccidia).

            (c) It is effective against bovine *Eimeria, E. bovis,* and *E. zuernii* and caprine *E. christenseni* and *E. ninakohlyakimovae.*

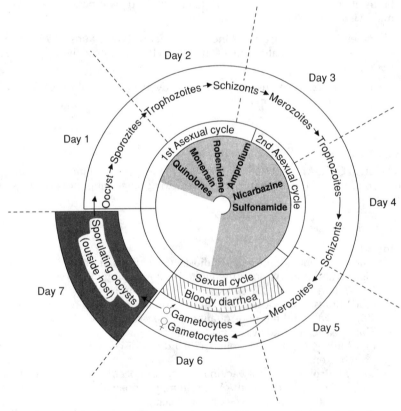

FIGURE 13-3. Life cycle of avian coccidia. All anticoccidial drugs are effective during the asexual cycle only. Second-generation schizonts seem to play an important role in the development of coccidial immunity. (Redrawn and modified with permission from Booth, McDonald: *Veterinary Pharmacology and Therapeutics,* 6th ed. Ames, Iowa State University Press, 1988, p 953.)

(5) Toxicity. No adverse effects are seen when the drug is used as directed.

b. Na$^+$ ionophores

(1) Preparations include **monensin, salinomycin,** and **lasalocid.** These antibiotics are used exclusively as anticoccidial drugs.

(2) Mechanism of action. Na$^+$ ionophores facilitate the transport of Na$^+$ into cells, elevating intracellular Na$^+$ concentrations. As a result, certain mitochondrial functions (e.g., substrate oxidations) and ATP hydrolysis are inhibited.

(3) Therapeutic uses

(a) Ionophores are effective against all *Eimeria* **species** in chickens, cattle, and sheep.

(i) Monensin is approved for use in cattle and sheep.

(ii) Lasalocid is approved for use in cattle, sheep, and chickens for prevention of coccidiosis. In chickens, it attacks the first generation of trophozoites and schizonts. The preslaughter withdrawal period for lasalocid is 5 days in chickens.

(iii) Salinomycin is approved for use in chickens only. The preslaughter withdrawal is not required.

(b) Ionophores are also used as **growth promoters.**

(4) Adverse effects. These drugs may cause **severe cardiovascular side effects.** In animal cells, intracellular Na$^+$ further exchanges for extracellular Ca^{2+}, thereby increasing intracellular Ca^{2+} concentrations. In addition, these drugs may directly facilitate Ca^{2+} transport into the cells. High intracellular Ca^{2+} levels in cardiac and skeletal muscle cells are responsible for the toxic effects of these drugs in animals.

(5) Contraindications. Horses and turkeys are very sensitive to Na$^+$ ionophores. Accidental consumption by these animals can be fatal.

c. Amprolium

(1) Chemistry. Amprolium is a quaternary compound.

(2) Mechanism of action. Amprolium prevents coccidia from utilizing thiamine by blocking thiamine receptors.

(3) Pharmacokinetics

(a) Amprolium is poorly absorbed after oral administration.

(b) No preslaughter withdrawal period is necessary.

(4) Therapeutic uses. Amprolium is the only anticoccidial agent that can be used in laying birds and cattle for both the prevention and treatment of outbreaks.

(a) It is effective against the first generation of trophozoites and schizonts.

(b) Amprolium is rarely used alone, because *E. maxima, E. mivati,* and other species are resistant; combination with sulfa drugs increases the efficacy of amprolium against these organisms in chickens.

(5) Adverse effects. Amprolium is a safe drug when used as directed. **Thiamine deficiency** may occur in the host following overdose.

d. Nicarbazin

(1) Chemistry. Nicarbazin is a mixture of 4,4'-dinitrocarbanilide (DNC) and 2-hydroxy-4,6-dimethylpyrimidine (HDP).

(2) Mechanism of action. Nicarbazin's mechanism of action is unknown.

(3) Pharmacokinetics

(a) Absorption. DNC and HDP are absorbed separately from the digestive tract. DNC is absorbed more rapidly but disappears more slowly from the tissues than HDP.

(b) A 4-day withdrawal period is required before broilers are marketed.

(4) Therapeutic uses. Nicarbazin is approved for use in chickens to **prevent coccidiosis outbreaks.**

(a) It is effective against all *Eimeria* species.

(b) Its peak activity is on second-generation trophozoites.

(5) Toxicity

(a) Nicarbazin may bleach brown-shelled eggs, cause mottled egg yolks and poor hatchability, and impair egg production.

(b) Medicated broilers may be more susceptible to heat stress.

    e. Robenidine
      (1) Pharmacokinetics. The pharmacokinetics of robenidine are not well understood.
      (2) Mechanism of action. The mechanism of action is undetermined. Its peak activity is on the first generation schizonts.
      (3) Therapeutic uses. Robenidine is approved for use in chickens to prevent outbreaks of coccidiosis. It is effective against all *Eimeria* species.
      (3) Adverse effects. Robenidine imparts an unpleasant taste to the flesh of broilers if therapy is not terminated 5 days before slaughter. The taste is imparted to eggs when birds are fed at dosages equal to or greater than 66 ppm. The ability of humans to taste robenidine is apparently genetically linked.

   f. Sulfonamides have the longest history of use as anticoccidial drugs. These agents are discussed in detail in Chapter 11 II.
      (1) Preparations. Sulfonamides used most frequently as anticoccidial agents include **sulfadimethoxine, sulfachloropyrazine, sulfaquinoxaline,** and **ethopabate** [not a sulfa drug, but also a *p*-aminobenzoic acid (PABA) antagonist].
      (2) Therapeutic uses. These drugs are used for both the prevention and treatment of coccidiosis outbreaks in all species.
         (a) They are more effective against the intestinal than cecal species of coccidia.
         (b) Their peak activity is against the second-generation schizonts.
         (c) Use of these drugs does not impair immunity development.

   g. Antifolate compounds
      (1) Preparations include **ormetoprim** and **pyrimethamine.** Pyrimethamine is not approved for food animal use.
      (2) Mechanism of action. These drugs block the conversion of dihydrofolate into tetrahydrofolate, thereby inhibiting thymidine synthesis in protozoans and bacteria.
      (3) Pharmacokinetics. After oral dosing, therapeutic levels of ormetoprim are maintained for over 24 hours.
      (4) Therapeutic uses. Ormetoprim and pyrimethamine are synergistic with sulfa drugs; when combined with a sulfonamide, they are used to treat **coccidiosis outbreaks** and **toxoplasmosis.** The preslaughter withdrawal period for sulfonamides plus ormetoprim is 5–10 days in chickens.

B. **Metronidazole**

   1. Chemistry. A nitroimidazole antiprotozoal and antibacterial agent, metronidazole is sparingly soluble in water.

   2. Mechanism of action. A ferredoxin-linked metabolite of metronidazole disrupts DNA synthesis in protozoans and bacteria.

   3. Pharmacokinetics
      a. Absorption. The oral bioavailability of metronidazole in animals varies from 50%–100%. If given with food, absorption is enhanced in dogs, attributable to increased bile secretion that helps dissolve metronidazole. Peak blood levels occur within approximately 1 hour of dosing.
      b. Distribution. Metronidazole is rapidly and widely distributed after oral absorption because it is highly lipid soluble.
      c. Metabolism and excretion. Metronidazole undergoes hydroxylation and conjugation in the liver. Both metabolites and unchanged drug are eliminated in the urine and feces in 24 hours. Elimination half-lives of metronidazole are 4–5 hours in dogs and 3–4.5 hours in horses.

   4. Therapeutic uses. Metronidazole is a broad-spectrum antiprotozoal drug that is effective against **giardiasis, histomoniasis, babesiosis, trichomoniasis,** and **amebiasis.** It is approved as a human drug and has been used largely in small animals.

   5. Toxicity. Metronidazole may induce lethargy, weakness, ataxia, rigidity, anorexia, vomiting, diarrhea, reversible leukopenia, and hepatotoxicity. Because metronidazole affects DNA synthesis, it may have teratogenic and carcinogenic effects.

STUDY QUESTIONS

DIRECTIONS: Each of the numbered items or incomplete statements in this section is followed by answers or by completions of the statement. Select the **one** numbered answer or completion that is **best** in each case.

1. Of the following drugs used in heartworm therapy or prevention, which one has the greatest potential for causing icterus and bilirubinuria?

(1) Diethylcarbamazine
(2) Ivermectin
(3) Milbemycin
(4) Thiacetarsamide

2. Which one of the following antinematodal drugs is effective against equine bots (*Gasterophilus*)?

(1) Fenbendazole
(2) Phenothiazine
(3) Piperazine
(4) Pyrantel
(5) Trichlorfon

3. Which one of the following insecticides may cause xylazine-like effects in animals?

(1) Amitraz
(2) DDT
(3) Lindane
(4) Permethrin
(5) Rotenone

4. Which one of the following anthelmintics requires the longest preslaughter withdrawal period when used in beef cattle?

(1) Albendazole
(2) Clorsulon
(3) Ivermectin
(4) Levamisole
(5) Thiabendazole

5. A 5-year-old Arabian mare is diagnosed with a *Strongylus vulgaris* infection. Repeated dosings with **febantel** have failed to improve the mare's condition, which suggests that the worms are resistant to the treatment. The veterinarian decides to use another nematocide to treat the mare for this condition. Under the circumstances, which one of the following drugs should be avoided?

(1) Mebendazole
(2) Ivermectin
(3) Pyrantel
(4) Trichlorfon

6. Clinical signs of a coccidiosis outbreak are detected in a flock of layers. Which one of the following anticoccidial drugs would be most appropriate?

(1) Sulfadimethoxine
(2) Lasalocid
(3) Decoquinate
(4) Amprolium

7. Which one of the following benzimidazole drugs is most easily metabolized by the liver and thus has the shortest plasma half-life and highest clinical dose?

(1) Fenbendazole
(2) Mebendazole
(3) Oxfendazole
(4) Thiabendazole

8. Which one of the following antinematodal drugs is effective during the muscular stage of *Trichinella spiralis*?

(1) Dichlorvos
(2) Ivermectin
(3) Levamisole
(4) Mebendazole
(5) Pyrantel

9. Which one of the following antitrematodal drugs is most effective against immature (i.e., less than 14 weeks old) *Fasciola hepatica* in cattle?

(1) Albendazole
(2) Clorsulon
(3) Praziquantel

DIRECTIONS: Each of the numbered items or incomplete statements in this section is negatively phrased, as indicated by an italicized word such as *not, least,* or *except.* Select the **one** numbered answer or completion that is **best** in each case.

---

10. Which one of the following antinematodal drugs does *not* have significant activity against hookworms in dogs?

(1) Butamisole
(2) Dichlorvos
(3) Milbemycin
(4) Piperazine
(5) Thenium closylate

11. All of the following anticoccidial drugs have shown good results in the control of mammalian coccidiosis *except:*

(1) amprolium.
(2) decoquinate.
(3) monensin.
(4) robenidine.
(5) sulfaquinoxaline.

12. All of the following are toxic effects of metronidazole *except:*

(1) convulsions.
(2) carcinogenicity.
(3) cardiac arrhythmia.
(4) diarrhea.
(5) reversible leukopenia.

ANSWERS AND EXPLANATIONS

1. The answer is 4 [IV B 5 c].
Thiacetarsamide is hepatotoxic. Signs of toxicity include persistent vomiting, bilirubinuria, hyperbilirubinemia, icterus, melena, stupor, and coma. Affected animals may show increased serum concentrations of alkaline phosphatase and alanine transaminase. Diethylcarbamazine, ivermectin, and milbemycin are not hepatotoxic.

2. The answer is 5 [III C 4 b].
Organophosphate compounds, such as trichlorfon, are effective against bots. Benzimidazoles, phenothiazine, piperazine, and pyrantel are not.

3. The answer is 1 [II G 1 d].
Like xylazine, amitraz is an α_2-adrenergic agonist. Therefore, it can cause sedation, bradycardia, and hyperglycemia in animals. Other insecticides do not have this activity.

4. The answer is 3 [III A 1 b (2), 2 c (3) (b), B 1 b (2) (b), D 1 b (2), VI C 2].
In cattle, the preslaughter withdrawal period for ivermectin (35 days) is longer than that for albendazole (27 days), clorsulon (8 days), levamisole (7 days), or thiabendazole (3 days).

5. The answer is 1 [III A 2 e].
Febantel is a pro-benzimidazole that is converted to fenbendazole and oxfendazole in the animal. Cross-resistance occurs among all benzimidazoles. Thus, if a nematode species becomes resistant to febantel, one should avoid using another benzimidazole as an alternative nematocide. Ivermectin, pyrantel, and trichlorfon are not benzimidazoles; thus, cross-resistance with febantel is not a problem.

6. The answer is 1 [VII A 1 b (1) (b), 2 c (4) (b), 2 f (2)].
Sulfa drugs and ormetoprim are the only drugs that are recommended for treatment of coccidial outbreaks in poultry. Lasalocid and decoquinate are used for prevention only. Amprolium can be used to treat the outbreaks of coccidiosis, but the development of resistance is a severe drawback.

7. The answer is 4 [III A 1 b (2), 2 b].
Benzimidazoles undergo hydroxylation at C-5. Because all of them except thiabendazole have a side chain at C-5 to protect them, they are more resistant to metabolism than thiabendazole.

8. The answer is 4 [III A 2 d (4)].
Mebendazole has good activity against *Trichinella spiralis*. Other nematocides, including ivermectin, do not have this activity.

9. The answer is 2 [VI C 3].
Clorsulon has excellent activity against both mature and immature *Fasciola hepatica*. Albendazole is used to kill mature *F. hepatica* only. Praziquantel has not been tested for activity against liver flukes in cattle for economic reasons.

10. The answer is 4 [III B 2 a, C 4 a (1), D 2 c, E 2 d, 4 d].
Piperazine is effective against ascarids and nodular worms in all species, but it has no activity against hookworms. Butamisole, dichlorvos, milbemycin, and thenium closylate are effective against hookworms.

11. The answer is 4 [VII A 1 b (2)].
Sulfonamides and ormetoprim, amprolium, decoquinate, monensin, and lasalocid are used as anticoccidial drugs in mammals. Robenidine is approved for use in birds only.

12. The answer is 3 [VII B 5].
Cardiac arrhythmia is not an adverse effect of metronidazole. However, metronidazole may induce lethargy, weakness, ataxia, rigidity, anorexia, vomiting, diarrhea, and, rarely, reversible leukopenia. Metronidazole may be hepatotoxic, teratogenic, and carcinogenic.

Chapter 14

Drug Interactions

Franklin A. Ahrens

I. **INTRODUCTION.** Altered pharmacologic response to one drug caused by the presence of a second drug is known as a **drug interaction.** The expected response may be increased or decreased as a result of the interaction.

A. **Pharmacokinetic interactions** are those in which plasma or tissue levels of a drug (or both) are altered by the presence of another drug.

B. **Pharmacodynamic interactions** are those in which the action or effect of one drug is altered by a second drug.

C. **Pharmaceutic interactions (drug incompatibilities)** result from chemical or physical reactions of drugs mixed *in vitro*.

II. **PHARMACOKINETIC INTERACTIONS**

A. **Interactions affecting absorption**

1. **Gastric emptying time**
   a. Drugs that increase gastric motility (e.g., metoclopramide) hasten delivery of the drug to the small intestine and increase the rate of absorption.
   b. Conversely, drugs that delay gastric emptying (e.g., anticholinergic drugs such as atropine) decrease the rate of intestinal absorption.

2. **Gastric pH.** Antacids and H_2-blockers reduce gastric acidity, slowing the absorption of salicylates and ketoconazole.

3. **Complex formation.** Tetracyclines chelate cations such as calcium, magnesium, and aluminum to form insoluble complexes that are poorly absorbed from the gastrointestinal tract. Therefore, milk and magnesium-containing antacids should be avoided during therapy with tetracyclines.

B. **Interactions affecting distribution**

1. **Plasma protein binding.** Many drugs (e.g., sulfonamides, salicylates, nonsteroidal anti-inflammatory drugs) are highly bound to plasma albumin. Displacement of bound drugs may occur when a second drug with greater binding affinity is administered concurrently. The resulting increase in free drug concentration may produce an exaggerated response.

2. **Tissue protein binding.** Competitive binding of drugs to tissue may also result in drug displacement and altered distribution.

C. **Interactions affecting drug metabolism**

1. **Inhibition of metabolism.** Drugs that inhibit hepatic microsomal enzymes include chloramphenicol, cimetidine, ketoconazole, phenothiazines, and organophosphate insecticides. These drugs may prolong the action of drugs that are normally inactivated by microsomal oxidation (type I) reactions (e.g., barbiturates, theophylline, digoxin).

2. **Increased rate of metabolism.** Drugs that induce hepatic microsomal enzymes include barbiturates (especially phenobarbital), phenylbutazone, rifampin, phenytoin, and halogenated hydrocarbon insecticides. These drugs diminish the efficacy and duration of action of drugs metabolized by the cytochrome P-450 system, such as corticosteroids, griseofulvin, digoxin, theophylline, and coumarin.

D. Interactions affecting renal excretion

  1. **Decreased active secretion.** Many acidic drugs (e.g., penicillins, cephalosporins, salicylates, methotrexate, probenecid) are actively secreted into urine by the renal tubular acid transport system. Competition for active transport between drugs may slow the rate of excretion. Prolonging penicillin blood levels by concomitant administration of probenecid is beneficial. However, methotrexate toxicity is increased by salicylates.

  2. **Increased passive excretion**
     a. **Altering the urinary pH** increases the excretion of ionizable drugs by ion-trapping, preventing their reabsorption from tubular urine.
        (1) **Urinary alkalinizers** (e.g., sodium bicarbonate) increase the excretion of acidic drugs.
        (2) **Urinary acidifiers** (e.g., ammonium chloride) increase the excretion of basic drugs.
     b. **Increasing urine flow** (e.g., with diuretics) hastens the excretion of many drugs by decreasing their reabsorption from the nephron.

III. PHARMACODYNAMIC INTERACTIONS

A. Antagonistic effects

  1. Specific receptor antagonists are available for certain classes of drugs (e.g., α- and β-adrenergics, cholinergics, opiates, and H_1 and H_2 histaminergics). These antagonists are used therapeutically to block or reverse agonist activity; however, antagonism may result in reduced efficacy. For example:
     a. Antihistamine drugs have weak anticholinergic actions that reduce the effect of miotics in glaucoma.
     b. Phenothiazine tranquilizers have an α-adrenergic blocking action that nullifies the vasopressive action of epinephrine and may produce hypotension by unmasking the β-adrenergic action of epinephrine. This effect is known as **epinephrine reversal.**

  2. Bacteriostatic antibiotics (e.g., tetracycline) slow bacterial growth; therefore, these agents may antagonize the action of bactericidal cell wall inhibitors (e.g., penicillins, cephalosporins), which are most effective against rapidly growing organisms.

B. **Additive effects.** Drugs with similar mechanisms of action may exhibit additive effects when administered in combination.

  1. The end point of the pharmacologic effect is the algebraic sum of each drug's action.

  2. Additive interactions are observed with many classes of drugs, including hypnotics, sedatives, tranquilizers, and the individual sulfonamides in triple sulfonamide preparations.

C. **Synergistic effects.** Drug combinations that produce a therapeutic or toxic effect that is greater than the sum of each drug's action are termed synergistic.

  1. **Therapeutic synergism** is observed with sulfonamide–trimethoprim combinations.

  2. **Potentiation of toxicity** results from the combination of aminoglycosides and furosemide or tetracyclines and methoxyflurane.

IV. PHARMACEUTIC INTERACTIONS (DRUG INCOMPATIBILITIES). Physical or

chemical incompatibility, or both, between drugs is common and may result in inactivation or increased toxicity. Drugs should never be mixed in a syringe or added to parenteral solutions unless the components are known to be compatible. Visual indicators of incompatibilities (e.g., cloudiness) may not be evident.

A. **Physical incompatibilities** are usually manifested as insolubility. For example:

1. The addition of sodium bicarbonate to calcium gluconate solutions produces a precipitate of calcium carbonate.

2. Amphotericin B precipitates in electrolyte solutions; therefore, it must first be dissolved in 5% dextrose.

B. **Chemical incompatibilities**

1. **pH.** The stability of many drugs in solution is pH-dependent.
   a. Alkaline solutions such as those containing sulfonamides, aminophylline, or barbiturates inactivate penicillin G, cephalosporins, and alkaloid salts (e.g., atropine).
   b. Ampicillin and furosemide are inactivated in acidic media (e.g., Ringer's solution, solutions of B-complex vitamins).

2. **Oxidation–reduction.** Redox reactions may result in loss of drug potency. For example, tetracyclines are oxidized by riboflavin and phenothiazine tranquilizers are oxidized by ferric salts.

3. **Complex formation.** Multivalent cations may form insoluble complexes with anionic drugs or poorly soluble chelates with tetracyclines. For example, cisplatin should not be administered using aluminum needles because aluminum inactivates cisplatin.

■STUDY QUESTIONS

DIRECTIONS: Each of the numbered items or incomplete statements in this section is followed by answers or by completions of the statement. Select the **one** numbered answer or completion that is **best** in each case.

1. A dog that is maintained on phenobarbital for the control of epilepsy may not respond to antifungal therapy with griseofulvin because phenobarbital:

(1) forms an insoluble complex with griseofulvin.
(2) blocks uptake of griseofulvin by keratin precursor cells.
(3) increases renal blood flow, hastening the excretion of griseofulvin.
(4) induces hepatic microsomal enzymes, increasing griseofulvin metabolism.

2. The efficacy of pilocarpine, a miotic, may be reduced in the presence of:

(1) phenytoin.
(2) antihistamines.
(3) glucocorticoids.
(4) salicylates.

3. A pharmacodynamic interaction resulting in drug antagonism may be caused by the concurrent administration of penicillin G and:

(1) cephalexin.
(2) gentamicin.
(3) tetracycline.
(4) enrofloxacin.

DIRECTIONS: Each of the numbered items or incomplete statements in this section is negatively phrased, as indicated by an italicized word such as *not, least,* or *except*. Select the **one** numbered answer or completion that is **best** in each case.

4. Drugs that inhibit hepatic microsomal metabolism (type I metabolism) include all of the following *except:*

(1) phenylbutazone.
(2) cimetidine.
(3) chloramphenicol.
(4) organophosphate insecticides.

5. All of the following are examples of combinations that would result in pharmaceutic interactions *except:*

(1) amphotericin B—Ringer's solution.
(2) tetracyclines—riboflavin.
(3) ampicillin—Ringer's solution.
(4) penicillin G—sulfonamide solutions.
(5) cephalexin—Ringer's solution.

ANSWERS AND EXPLANATIONS

1. The answer is 4 [II C 2].
Phenobarbital is a potent inducer of hepatic microsomal enzymes involved in the oxidative metabolism of many drugs, including griseofulvin. The resulting rapid metabolism may reduce or eliminate drug effects on target tissues or organisms. Phenobarbital does not alter the uptake, excretion, or solubility of griseofulvin.

2. The answer is 2 [III A 1 a].
Antihistamines have weak anticholinergic actions that may antagonize the miotic action of the cholinomimetic drugs used in the treatment of glaucoma (e.g., pilocarpine). This is an example of a pharmacodynamic drug interaction.

3. The answer is 3 [III A 2].
Concurrent administration of a penicillin and a tetracycline can reduce the efficacy of the penicillin. The bactericidal action of penicillins is greatest in rapidly dividing organisms. Tetracyclines, which are bacteriostatic antibiotics, inhibit protein synthesis, slowing bacterial growth. Cephalexin, gentamicin, and enrofloxacin are bactericidal.

4. The answer is 1 [II C 1].
Phenylbutazone induces enzymes of the cytochrome P-450 system, thus increasing the rate of metabolism of drugs inactivated by this pathway. Cimetidine, chloramphenicol, and organophosphate insecticides inhibit hepatic microsomal enzymes and may prolong the action of drugs that are metabolized by microsomes (e.g., digoxin).

5. The answer is 5 [IV A, B 1–2].
Cephalexin is not incompatible with the acidic to neutral pH of Ringer's solution, but it is inactivated by alkaline solutions. Amphotericin B is precipitated by the electrolytes in Ringer's solution. Tetracyclines are oxidized by riboflavin. Ampicillin is unstable in acidic media, such as Ringer's solution, and penicillin G is inactivated by alkaline media, such as sulfonamide solutions.

Chapter 15

Treatment of Poisoning

Franklin A. Ahrens

I. GENERAL CONSIDERATIONS

A. **Sources of poisoning.** Accidental ingestion of poisons by animals is common.

1. Many insecticides and rodenticides contain sugars to enhance their effectiveness as baits and are readily eaten or licked by animals.

2. Other poisons (e.g., lead salts, ethylene glycol) are naturally sweet-tasting.

3. Poisonous plants are a major source of toxicoses in large animals. Improper use or disposal of agricultural chemicals such as pesticides, herbicides, or fertilizers may also result in accidental poisoning of livestock.

B. **Poisoning is a medical emergency** and rapid treatment is often the difference between life and death. Specific antidotes are available for only a few poisons and thus, nonspecific therapy is essential in poison management.

II. NONSPECIFIC THERAPY AND SUPPORTIVE TREATMENT

A. **Reducing absorption of poisons**

1. **Emetics.** Parenteral administration of **apomorphine in dogs** or **xylazine in cats** is effective if the drugs are given within 2 hours of poison ingestion. Emetics must not be given if the animal is unconscious or convulsing or if the poison is corrosive or is a petroleum hydrocarbon.

2. **Gastric lavage.** In unconscious or anesthetized dogs or cats, an endotracheal tube is placed prior to passage of the stomach tube. Water or saline (10 ml/kg) is gently infused and removed from the stomach. This process is repeated until the withdrawn fluid is clear.

3. **Gastrointestinal adsorbents**
   a. **Activated charcoal** adsorbs a wide range of organic compounds and toxins and prevents their absorption from the gastrointestinal tract.
      (1) Heavy metal salts, halides, nitrates, nitrites, and fertilizers are not effectively adsorbed by charcoal.
      (2) Other carbon compounds (e.g., burnt toast) are not effective adsorbents.
   b. **Administration**
      (1) Activated charcoal is administered orally as a slurry (1–3 g/kg).
      (2) A saline cathartic (see II A 4 a) should be administered following charcoal administration to hasten fecal excretion of adsorbed poisons and prevent the formation of charcoal concretions in the intestinal lumen.

4. **Laxatives and cathartics.** The absorption of ingested poisons may be decreased by the administration of laxatives or cathartics that act in the small intestine and thus have a rapid onset of action.
   a. **Saline laxatives** (e.g., **sodium sulfate, magnesium sulfate**) exert a cathartic effect by osmotically retaining water in the lumen. They are the **laxatives of choice for poison therapy.**

   b. Bulk laxatives (e.g., **methylcellulose**) **are not effective** for poison therapy because they act in the large intestine and have a slow onset of action.

B. **Increasing elimination of poisons**

   1. Forced diuresis. The elimination of poisons that are excreted by the kidneys can be
   hastened by the intravenous administration of osmotic diuretics such as **5% mannitol.** The hydration status and urinary output of the animal should be monitored.

   2. Alteration of urinary pH. The urinary excretion of ionizable poisons may be increased by acidifying or alkalinizing the urine.
      a. Acidic compounds (e.g., **acetylsalicylic acid, barbiturates, sulfonamides**) are ion-
      ized and trapped in alkaline urine. **Sodium bicarbonate** is an effective urinary al-
      kalizer.
      b. Basic compounds (e.g., **amphetamine**) are ionized in an acidic urine. **Ammo-
      nium chloride** administered orally acidifies the urine.

   3. Peritoneal dialysis. Diffusible poisons may be removed from the systemic circulation in small animals by peritoneal dialysis.
      a. Sterile physiologic solutions (e.g., **Ringer's solution**) are infused into the perito-
      neal cavity, removed after 30–60 minutes, and replaced with fresh solution. The
      process is repeated as required.
      b. If the poison is ionizable, dialysate **solutions may be buffered** to facilitate ion
      trapping.

C. **Supportive treatment**

   1. Maintenance of cardiovascular function
      a. Intravenous administration of **lactated Ringer's solution or plasma** is necessary
      when shock occurs as the result of poisoning.
      b. Glucocorticoids may improve tissue perfusion.

   2. Maintenance of respiratory function
      a. Endotracheal intubation and **mechanical ventilation** may be required in an un-
      conscious animal with severe respiratory depression.
      b. Small animals may benefit from being placed in a **chamber supplied with
      40%–50% oxygen.**

   3. Maintenance of body temperature. Prevention of hypothermia is essential in coma-
   tose animals or in animals that have been sedated to control seizures.
      a. Heating pads, lamps, or blankets may be used.
      b. The animal should be repositioned frequently.

III. **ANTIDOTAL THERAPY OF POISONING**

A. **General mechanisms of antidotal action**

   1. Complex formation (chelation). Some antidotes bind to the toxicant, rendering it unable to cross cell membranes or bind to receptors. The resultant compound is stable
   and inactive.

   2. Detoxification. Some antidotes metabolically convert the toxicant to a less toxic metabolite.

   3. Prevention of biotransformation. Antidotes that work in this manner prevent the formation of toxic metabolites.

   4. Facilitation of excretion. These antidotes promote more rapid or complete elimination of the toxicant by altering its structure.

5. **Competitive antagonism.** Some antidotes compete with the toxin for receptor sites.

6. **Restoration of normal function.** Some antidotes supply a missing component or enhance a function that corrects the effects of the toxicant.

B. Acetaminophen toxicosis

1. **Sources.** Acetaminophen is a common household analgesic. It is occasionally administered by owners to cats but is very toxic to this species (see Chapter 9 I C 5 b).

2. **Mechanism of toxicity**
   a. In humans and most animal species, acetaminophen is metabolized by hepatic conjugation to inactive glucuronides or sulfates. In cats, however, levels of glucuronyl transferase and sulfonyl transferase are low, and the drug is very slowly inactivated by glutathione conjugation.
   b. Depletion of hepatic glutathione results in the accumulation of reactive, oxidative metabolites that covalently bind to cell proteins, causing cell death.

3. **Clinical signs.** Salivation, vomiting, and depression progress to severe cyanosis, methemoglobinemia, and dyspnea. Death may occur.

4. **Therapy. N-Acetylcysteine** is used to treat acetaminophen poisoning.
   a. **Mechanism of antidotal action.** N-Acetylcysteine, a precursor of glutathione, replenishes hepatic levels of glutathione.
   b. **Administration.** N-Acetylcysteine is administered orally every 4–8 hours. Three to five treatments are usually necessary.

C. Cyanide toxicosis

1. **Sources**
   a. **Plants.** *Sorghum* species (Sudan grass, Johnson grass) and fruit seeds (e.g., cherry, apricot, peach) contain cyanogenic glycosides that may accumulate under stressed plant growing conditions (e.g., frost).
   b. **Rodenticides** may contain cyanide.

2. **Mechanism of toxicity**
   a. Normally, small amounts of cyanide are detoxified to thiocyanate ion by **sulfurtransferase,** an enzyme that is abundant in well-perfused tissue. However, sulfur donors (e.g., cysteine) are required to initially contribute sulfur to the enzyme and these are not abundant.
   b. Cyanide accumulates and binds to the ferric iron (Fe^{3+}) of ferricytochrome oxidase in mitochondria, inhibiting cellular respiration.

3. **Clinical signs.** Muscle tremors, dyspnea, and salivation are followed by collapse, convulsions, and death. Venous blood and mucous membranes are bright red because tissue oxygen use is reduced.

4. **Therapy.** Rapid administration of **sodium nitrite (4%)** and **sodium thiosulfate (6%)** is effective even for severely poisoned animals.
   a. **Mechanism of antidotal action**
      (1) **Sodium nitrite** converts a fraction of the circulating hemoglobin (Fe^{2+}) to methemoglobin (Fe^{3+}), which binds the cyanide ion and reduces its binding to ferricytochrome oxidase.
      (2) **Sodium thiosulfate** serves as a sulfur donor for sulfurtransferase.
   b. **Administration.** Sodium nitrite and sodium thiosulfate are administered intravenously.

D. Ethylene glycol toxicosis

1. **Sources.** Ethylene glycol is the major ingredient of automotive **antifreeze.** It has a sweet taste and is readily ingested by dogs and cats from spills or radiator leaks. The minimum lethal dose for cats is 1.5 ml/kg.

2. **Mechanism of toxicity.** Ethylene glycol is converted to a series of metabolites, including **glycolic acid** and **oxalic acid**. These metabolites produce severe acidosis and renal tubular damage.

3. **Clinical signs**

   a. In the **acute phase** (1–6 hours following ingestion), vomiting, polydipsia, polyuria, depression, and incoordination are observed.
   b. Subacute phase. The animal appears to recover until renal failure develops, in 1–3 days.
   (1) Clinical signs of this subacute phase include depression, anorexia, oliguria, and uremic coma.
   (2) Calcium oxalate crystals accumulate in the renal tubules but are not the primary cause of nephrosis.

4. **Therapy. Ethanol (20% in saline)** is used to treat ethylene glycol toxicosis. **4-Methylpyrazole (4-MP)** is an alternative antidote for use in dogs. (In cats, 4-MP is less effective than ethanol.)
   a. Mechanism of antidotal action. The first and rate-limiting step of ethylene glycol metabolism is the formation of glycolaldehyde; this reaction is catalyzed by alcohol dehydrogenase. Ethanol and 4-MP **competitively inhibit alcohol dehydrogenase,** preventing the formation of toxic metabolites.
   b. Administration
   (1) Ethanol is administered to dogs and cats intravenously every 4–6 hours for five treatments, and then every 6–8 hours for five treatments.
   (a) Ethanol may **also** be **administered intraperitoneally to dogs.**
   (b) Sodium bicarbonate (5%) is administered concurrently to reduce metabolic acidosis.
   (2) 4-MP is administered intravenously at 12-hour intervals for a total of four doses. The antidotal action is not accompanied by the central nervous system (CNS) depression observed with ethanol.

E. **Nitrate/nitrite toxicosis**

1. **Sources**
   a. Plants. Nitrates may accumulate in cereal grasses, corn, sorghums, or weeds (e.g., pigweed, Jimson weed), especially under cool, damp growing conditions.
   b. Contamination of livestock feeds or water with **nitrate fertilizer** may occur.

2. **Mechanism of toxicity**
   a. Nitrates are reduced to nitrites by ruminal microflora. Bacteria in the equine cecum and the intestine of young (but not adult) pigs may also convert nitrates to nitrites, but poisoning is less common in these species.
   b. Absorbed nitrite oxidizes hemoglobin to methemoglobin, which cannot carry oxygen.

3. **Clinical signs**
   a. Clinical **signs of anoxia** (i.e., dyspnea, cyanosis, muscle weakness, collapse, and coma) develop when 40% or more of the hemoglobin is converted to methemoglobin.
   b. The vasodilatory effects of nitrite ion may contribute to the clinical signs.
   c. The **blood is chocolate-brown in color.**

4. **Therapy. Methylene blue (1%)** is the antidote for nitrate/nitrite poisoning. It **should not be used in cats.**
   a. Mechanism of antidotal action
   (1) Methylene blue (oxidized) is rapidly converted to **leucomethylene blue** (reduced) by nicotinamide adenine dinucleotide phosphate (NADPH)-linked reductase in the blood. Leucomethylene blue **reduces methemoglobin (Fe^{3+}) to hemoglobin (Fe^{2+}).**
   (2) Because feline hemoglobin is more susceptible to oxidative denaturation than that of other species, methylene blue should not be used in cats. Denatured hemoglobin precipitates and coalesces to intracellular inclusions called Heinz bodies, which accumulate and cause fragmentation of erythrocyte membranes.
   b. Administration. Methylene blue is administered by slow intravenous infusion. If required, the dose may be repeated in 30 minutes.

F. **Lead toxicosis**

1. **Sources.** Lead is contained in old paints, batteries, solder, glazing compounds, greases, and other industrial products.
   a. Poisoning is most common in cattle because of their penchant for licking painted surfaces or lead-containing lubricants.
   b. Dogs and cats may ingest paint chips, putty, lead shot, or other lead compounds.
   c. Waterfowl may ingest spent lead shot from lakes and waterways.

2. **Mechanism of toxicity.** Lead, which binds to the sulfhydryl groups of cellular constituents and inhibits enzyme activity, biosynthesis, and membrane function, affects the hematopoietic, gastrointestinal, musculoskeletal, renal, and nervous systems. Lead encephalopathy is the most frequent consequence of lead ingestion in young animals.

3. **Clinical signs.** Neurologic signs predominate and may be accompanied by gastrointestinal signs. Cattle exhibit ataxia, blindness, bellowing, colic, grinding of teeth, muscle twitching, and convulsive seizures.

4. **Therapy. Calcium disodium ethylenediaminetetraacetic acid (EDTA)** is used to treat lead poisoning (Figure 15-1).
   a. **Mechanism of antidotal action.** Calcium disodium EDTA is a chelating agent that forms a stable, multiringed structured complex with divalent metals. The ligand affinity for lead is much greater than that for calcium; therefore, the chelate binds the lead, forming a complex that is excreted by the kidneys.
   b. **Administration.** Calcium disodium EDTA is administered subcutaneously or by slow intravenous infusion every 6 hours in dogs or every 12 hours in cattle, for 3–4 days.
      (1) Calcium disodium EDTA **should not be administered orally** because oral administration may increase intestinal lead absorption.
      (2) Repeated doses of calcium disodium EDTA are often necessary because tissue storage sites for lead are not readily accessible to chelators and a slow redistribution/equilibrium between these sites and the extracellular fluid is required between treatments.
      (3) D-**Penicillamine,** an orally effective chelator, may be used as an adjunct to calcium disodium EDTA therapy in dogs. It is administered once daily for 2 weeks.

G. **Arsenic toxicosis**

1. **Sources.** Inorganic arsenic salts may be used in orchard sprays, rodenticides, and wood preservatives.

2. **Mechanism of toxicity.** Arsenic combines with the sulfhydryl groups of enzymes and enzyme cofactors such as **thioctic acid,** an essential cofactor of the pyruvic oxidase system. As a result, **glycolysis, the tricarboxylic acid cycle, and oxidative phosphorylation are inhibited.** Tissues with a high rate of metabolism (e.g., the intestines, liver, and cardiovascular system) are affected most severely.

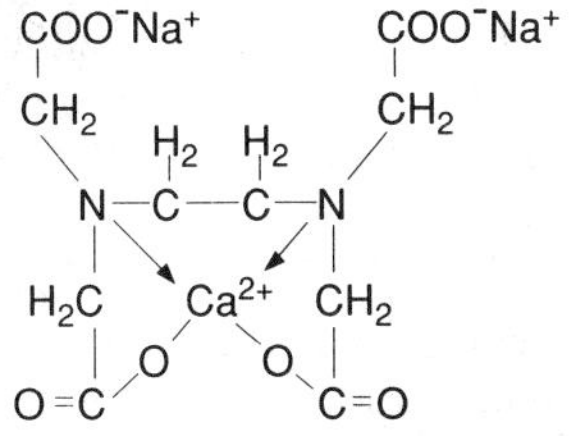

FIGURE 15-1. Calcium disodium ethylenediaminetetraacetic acid (EDTA). When EDTA and cations such as calcium (Ca^{2+}) form a complex, a very stable multiringed chelate is formed.

3. **Clinical signs.** Depression, gastrointestinal pain, hemorrhagic diarrhea, staggering, and collapse are characteristic signs of acute arsenic poisoning.

4. **Therapy. Dimercaprol [British antilewisite (BAL)]** is effective for treating arsenic poisoning.
   a. **Mechanism of antidotal action.** Dimercaprol is a dithiol chelating agent that forms a dimer complex with arsenic to remove it from essential enzymes and hasten its excretion. Because the complex tends to dissociate, an excess of dimercaprol must be maintained by frequent dosing.
   b. **Administration**
      (1) Dimercaprol is administered intramuscularly every 4 hours for 2 days, then every 6 hours for 1 day, and every 12 hours for the next 10 days.
      (2) The concurrent intramuscular administration of thioctic acid, which restores essential coenzyme function, greatly enhances the effectiveness of treatment.

H. Copper toxicosis

1. **Sources**
   a. **Chronic hepatic copper accumulation in dogs.** Some breeds, such as Bedlington terriers and West Highland white terriers, have an inherited defect that results in defective copper-binding proteins.
   b. **Chronic copper toxicosis in ruminants**
      (1) **Plants.** Copper poisoning occurs in sheep and, less commonly, cattle, from plants such as subterranean clover, *Heliotropium* species, or *Senecio* species.
      (2) Low dietary levels of molybdenum or sulfate predispose to copper toxicosis.

2. **Mechanism of toxicity.** Copper accumulates in the lysosomes of hepatocytes.
   a. The accumulated copper damages lysosomal membranes, causing hydrolytic enzymes to be released and leading to liver cell necrosis.
   b. In ruminants, the release of large amounts of copper and oxidative products from the liver precipitates a **hemolytic crisis** (i.e., the sudden and massive destruction of erythrocytes).

3. **Clinical signs**
   a. Copper accumulation in dogs produces clinical signs associated with hepatitis and liver necrosis (e.g., anorexia, vomiting, diarrhea, lethargy, and icterus).
   b. Clinical signs in sheep and calves are related to the hemolytic crisis and include weakness, exhaustion, hemoglobinemia, dyspnea, and shock.

4. **Therapy.** D-Penicillamine and **tetramine** are chelating agents used to treat copper toxicosis in dogs. **Ammonium molybdate** administered with **sodium sulfate** is the preferred treatment for affected lambs and calves. In ruminants, copper chelating drugs are effective only if administered during the early stages of the disease.
   a. **Mechanism of antidotal action**
      (1) D-Penicillamine and **tetramine** bind copper and hasten its urinary excretion.
      (2) **Ammonium molybdate** and **sodium sulfate** react with copper in the rumen to form a copper–thiomolybdate complex that is poorly absorbed. In addition, thiomolybdates interfere with the mobilization of copper from the liver.
   b. **Administration**
      (1) D-Penicillamine or **tetramine** is administered orally twice a day. Prolonged therapy is required for chronic hepatic toxicosis in dogs.
      (2) **Ammonium molybdate** and **sodium sulfate** are administered orally, once daily for 3 weeks. Alternatively, ammonium molybdate and sodium sulfate may be added to the feed for 3 weeks.

I. Organophosphates and carbamate toxicosis

1. **Sources.** Organophosphates and carbamates are widely used as topical and systemic insecticides and parasiticides in animals and plants. Accidental ingestion or excessive topical application are common causes of poisoning in animals.

2. **Mechanism of toxicity.** Organophosphates and carbamates inhibit acetylcholinester-

ase (AChE) by binding and phosphorylating or carbamylating the esteratic site of the enzyme. Phosphorylation is reversible, but carbamylation is not. The resultant accumulation of acetylcholine (ACh) neurotransmitter causes excessive stimulation of muscarinic and nicotinic cholinergic receptors and cholinergic synapses in the CNS.

3. **Clinical signs**
   a. The earliest signs of poisoning are related to muscarinic stimulation and include profuse salivation, lacrimation, bronchial secretions, diarrhea, urination, bradycardia, and pupillary constriction.
   b. These signs are followed by signs of nicotinic and CNS stimulation (e.g., muscle tremors, spasms, and hyperexcitability) that may progress to clonic or clonic–tonic convulsions.

4. **Therapy. Atropine sulfate** and **pyridine aldoxime methiodide (2-PAM)** are used to counteract organophosphate and carbamate poisoning.
   a. **Mechanism of antidotal action**
      (1) **Atropine sulfate** competitively blocks the binding of ACh to muscarinic receptors.
      (2) **2-PAM,** a nucleophilic oxime, reactivates AChE by forming an oxime–phosphonate complex at the phosphorylated site. The complex is split off, leaving the regenerated enzyme.
   b. **Administration**
      (1) **Atropine sulfate** is administered intravenously ($^1/_4$ of the dose) and intramuscularly or subcutaneously ($^3/_4$ of the dose). The dose is repeated at 3–6-hour intervals until the symptoms subside.
      (2) **2-PAM** should be administered intramuscularly or by slow intravenous infusion after the initial dose of atropine if nicotinic signs (e.g., muscle twitching, rigidity) are severe. The dose may be repeated if necessary.

J. **Thiaminase toxicosis**

1. **Sources.** Ferns (e.g., bracken fern) may contain thiaminase, which produces thiamine deficiency in nonruminants. Poisoning is most common in horses fed hay contaminated with young fronds.*

2. **Mechanism of toxicity.** Thiaminase destroys thiamine in the alimentary tract, resulting in a deficiency of this vitamin, which functions as a coenzyme in carbohydrate metabolism.

3. **Clinical signs.** Clinical signs in horses include abnormal gait, staggering, arching of the back, crouching, and blindness.

4. **Therapy. Thiamine** is administered intravenously or intramuscularly 2–4 times daily for 1 day, and then 1–2 times daily for 7 days.

K. **Warfarin toxicosis**

1. **Sources**
   a. Warfarin and other coumarin derivatives are common ingredients of **rodent poisons.** Ingestion of baits or poisoned rodents by dogs, cats, or pigs will produce toxicity.
   b. Coumarins also occur in **spoiled sweet clover forage** and may produce a hemorrhagic syndrome in ruminants.

2. **Mechanism of toxicity.** Warfarin and other anticoagulant rodenticides antagonize vitamin K, which is required for the hepatic synthesis of clotting factors I, II, VII, IX, and X. Capillary permeability is increased by unknown mechanisms.

---

* Bracken fern poisoning occurs in ruminants, but not as a result of thiamine deficiency, because thiamine is synthesized by rumen microflora. Poisoning in ruminants results from ptaquiloside, a glucoside that produces aplastic anemia and an acute hemorrhagic syndrome.

3. **Clinical signs** are related to internal hemorrhage and include anemia, hematomas, melena, hemothorax, and hematuria.

4. **Therapy**
   a. **Vitamin K_1** restores depleted endogenous levels of K_1, allowing resumption of clotting factor synthesis.
      (1) Vitamin K_1 is administered subcutaneously twice daily for 2 days and then orally, twice daily for 2–4 weeks.
      (2) Because vitamin K_1 is lipid-soluble, **oral absorption is increased by dietary fats.**
   b. **Blood transfusions** are necessary in severe cases.

STUDY QUESTIONS

DIRECTORS: Each of the numbered items or incomplete statements in this section is followed by answers or by completions of the statement. Select the **one** numbered answer or completion that is **best** in each case.

1. How does sodium nitrite counteract cyanide poisoning?

(1) It activates sulfurtransferase within cells.
(2) It forms methemoglobin to compete with cytochrome oxidase for the cyanide ion.
(3) It converts thiocyanate ion to a less toxic metabolite.
(4) It inhibits glycosidase, thus reducing cyanide release from plant glycosides.
(5) It reduces sodium thiosulfate to an inactive form in the blood.

2. Copper toxicity arising from a genetic abnormality of copper binding proteins in Bedlington terriers may be treated by chelation of copper with:

(1) tetramine.
(2) dimercaprol [British antilewisite (BAL)].
(3) calcium disodium ethylenediaminetetraacetic acid (EDTA).
(4) 4-methylpyrazole (4-MP).

3. Hay contaminated with bracken fern and fed to horses produces a deficiency of:

(1) vitamin K_1.
(2) thioctic acid.
(3) thiamine.
(4) ferric iron.

4. Which one of the following statements is true regarding calcium disodium ethylenediaminetetraacetic acid (EDTA) therapy of lead poisoning?

(1) Therapy is most effective when calcium disodium EDTA is administered orally.
(2) Therapy is usually restricted to single-dose administration because of calcium disodium EDTA toxicity.
(3) Calcium disodium EDTA forms a stable complex with lead that is excreted by the kidneys.
(4) Calcium disodium EDTA rapidly reduces the body burden of lead.

5. The specific antidote for organophosphate or carbamate poisoning is:

(1) 4-methylpyrazole (4-MP).
(2) dimercaprol.
(3) sodium thiosulfate.
(4) atropine sulfate.

6. Which toxicosis may be prevented by oral administration of ammonium molybdate and sodium sulfate?

(1) Copper
(2) Coumarin
(3) Thiaminase
(4) Arsenic

7. Which agent is administered intramuscularly to treat arsenic poisoning?

(1) D-Penicillamine
(2) Dimercaprol
(3) Calcium disodium ethylenediaminetetraacetic acid (EDTA)
(4) Acetylcysteine

8. Acetaminophen poisoning in cats may produce methemoglobinemia. However, methylene blue should not be administered to this species because:

(1) cats are unable to reduce methylene blue to its active form, leucomethylene blue.
(2) methylene blue inhibits hepatic metabolism of acetylcysteine in cats.
(3) methylene blue induces Heinz body formation and hemolysis in cats.
(4) methylene blue is nephrotoxic in cats.

9. Thioctic acid restores enzyme activity in the pyruvic oxidase system when this system has been inhibited by poisoning with:

(1) lead.
(2) arsenic.
(3) copper.
(4) molybdenum.

10. Decreased hepatic synthesis of clotting factors essential for the conversion of prothrombin to thrombin results from ingestion of warfarin rodenticides. The antidote is:

(1) thiamine.
(2) vitamin A.
(3) vitamin B_6.
(4) vitamin K_1.

11. Which one of the following is an orally effective chelating agent that may be used as an adjunct to calcium disodium ethylenediaminetetraacetic acid (EDTA) in the treatment of lead poisoning?

(1) D-Penicillamine
(2) Tetramine
(3) Dimercaprol
(4) Ptaquiloside

DIRECTIONS: Each of the numbered items or incomplete statements in this section is negatively phrased, as indicated by an italicized word such as *not, least,* or *except.* Select the **one** numbered answer or completion that is **best** in each case.

---

12. Which one of the following statements is *not* true concerning nitrate poisoning in ruminants?

(1) The venous blood of poisoned animals is bright red.
(2) Nitrates are reduced to nitrites by rumen microflora.
(3) Clinical signs include dyspnea, muscle weakness, and collapse.
(4) Methylene blue converts methemoglobin to hemoglobin.

13. Activated charcoal prevents absorption of many ingested poisons. Which of the following statements is *not* true?

(1) Its efficacy results from the adsorption of organic molecules to the large surface area of carbon particles.
(2) It is especially effective for ingested heavy metals or halides, because these bind covalently to carbon.
(3) Its use should be followed by administration of a saline cathartic (e.g., sodium sulfate) to hasten fecal excretion of adsorbed poisons.
(4) Carbon particles from burnt toast are not effective.

■ ANSWERS AND EXPLANATIONS

1. The answer is 2 [III C 4 a].
Sodium nitrite converts a fraction of the circulating hemoglobin to methemoglobin, which contains ferric iron (Fe^{3+}). The cyanide binds to the ferric iron of the methemoglobin, instead of binding to the ferric iron of cytochrome oxidase, an enzyme essential to cellular respiration. Sulfurtransferase is activated by sulfur donors such as sodium thiosulfate. Sulfurtransferase converts cyanide to nontoxic thiocyanate ion. Glycosidase activity is not affected by sodium nitrite.

2. The answer is 1 [III H 4].
Chelation of copper with tetramine or with D-penicillamine is effective in reducing hepatic stores of copper in Bedlington terriers afflicted with a genetic defect for copper metabolism. Dimercaprol and calcium disodium ethylenediaminetetraacetic acid (EDTA) are chelating agents for arsenic and lead, respectively. 4-Methylpyrazole (4-MP) inhibits alcohol dehydrogenase and slows the formation of the toxic metabolites of ethylene glycol.

3. The answer is 3 [III J 2].
Bracken fern contains a thiaminase that produces thiamine deficiency in horses. Vitamin K_1 deficiency is produced by coumarin derivatives, which may be present in spoiled sweet clover. Arsenic poisoning produces a deficiency of thioctic acid, an essential coenzyme for pyruvic oxidase. Nitrites oxidize ferrous iron to ferric iron to produce methemoglobinemia.

4. The answer is 3 [III F 4 a].
Lead has a much greater affinity than calcium for calcium disodium ethylenediaminetetraacetic acid (EDTA). Calcium disodium EDTA and lead form a multi-ring, stable complex that is excreted by the kidneys. Calcium disodium EDTA should not be administered orally because oral administration may increase lead absorption from the intestine. Removal of lead by chelation therapy is relatively slow and requires multiple doses of calcium disodium EDTA because tissue storage sites of lead are not readily accessible to the circulating drug.

5. The answer is 4 [III I 4].
Atropine sulfate is the specific antidote for organophosphate or carbamate poisoning. Atropine sulfate competitively blocks the binding of acetylcholine (ACh) to muscarinic receptors to prevent the excessive stimulation caused by acetylcholinesterase (AChE) inhibition. Dimercaprol, 4-methylpyrazole (4-MP), and sodium thiosulfate are antidotes for arsenic, ethylene glycol, and cyanide, respectively.

6. The answer is 1 [III H 4].
Lambs, and to a lesser extent, calves are susceptible to copper toxicosis. Ammonium molybdate and sodium sulfate react with copper in the rumen to form a thiomolybdate complex that is poorly absorbed. Thiomolybdates also block mobilization of copper from the liver, helping to prevent the hemolytic crisis that arises when large amounts of stored copper are suddenly released by the liver. Vitamin K_1, thiamine, and dimercaprol are antidotes for coumarin, thiaminase, and arsenic poisoning, respectively.

7. The answer is 2 [III G 4].
Dimercaprol chelates arsenic by forming a dimer in which two molecules of dimercaprol combine with one molecule of arsenic. D-Penicillamine and calcium disodium ethylenediaminetetraacetic acid (EDTA) are chelating agents for copper and lead, respectively. Acetylcysteine is the antidote for acetaminophen poisoning.

8. The answer is 3 [III E 4 a (2)].
Methylene blue should not be administered to cats because it causes oxidative denaturation of hemoglobin, Heinz body formation, and erythrocyte lysis.

9. The answer is 2 [III G 4 b (2)].
Arsenic combines with the sulfhydryl groups of thioctic acid and inhibits this essential coenzyme of the pyruvic oxidase system. Administration of thioctic acid restores enzyme function. The pyruvic oxidase system is not affected by lead, copper, or molybdenum.

10. The answer is 4 [III K 4].
Warfarin rodenticides antagonize vitamin K,

which is required for the hepatic synthesis of clotting factors. Administration of vitamin K_1 restores clotting factor synthesis and corrects the anticoagulant effects of warfarin.

11. The answer is 1 [III F 4 b (3)].
D-Penicillamine is not as effective as calcium disodium ethylenediaminetetraacetic acid (EDTA) in chelating lead from tissues. However, it is absorbed orally and will remove lead when used as an adjunct to parenteral calcium disodium EDTA therapy. It is especially useful when long-term removal of lead is required. Dimercaprol is used to treat arsenic poisoning. Tetramine is used as an alternative to D-penicillamine in the treatment of copper toxicosis. Ptaquiloside is a glycoside that causes bracken fern poisoning in ruminants; in nonruminants, bracken fern poisoning results from thiamine deficiency.

12. The answer is 1 [III E 3 c].
Absorbed nitrite oxidizes hemoglobin to methemoglobin, which cannot carry oxygen. The venous blood of nitrate poisoned ruminants is chocolate-brown because of methemoglobinemia, not bright red. Venous blood is bright red in cyanide poisoning because oxygen cannot be used by tissues. Nitrates are converted to nitrites by rumen microflora. Clinical signs of anoxia (i.e., dyspnea, muscle weakness, and collapse) are reversed by administration of methylene blue, which converts methemoglobin to hemoglobin.

13. The answer is 2 [II A 3 a–b].
Activated charcoal is less effective for adsorbing heavy metals or halides than for adsorbing organic compounds from the gastrointestinal tract. Organic compounds are effectively adsorbed on the large surface area of carbon particles of activated charcoal and are eliminated following saline catharsis with sodium sulfate. Commercial preparations of activated charcoal are prepared by heating selected vegetable carbons to high temperatures and then exposing them to oxidizing gases. This process vastly increases the adsorptive surface to $1000–3000$ m^2/g of powdered charcoal. Other carbon compounds, such as burnt toast, are not effective.

Comprehensive
Examination

DIRECTIONS: Each of the numbered items or incomplete statements in this section is followed by answers or by completions of the statement. Select the **one** numbered answer or completion that is **best** in each case.

1. Which one of the following statements regarding methotrexate is true?

(1) Methotrexate stops neoplastic cell division in metaphase.
(2) Methotrexate blocks purine synthesis by inhibiting dihydrofolate reductase.
(3) Methotrexate is used primarily for adrenal tumors.
(4) Methotrexate is not cell-cycle specific.

2. The drug of choice to treat status epilepticus in dogs is:

(1) diazepam.
(2) acepromazine.
(3) phenobarbital.
(4) primidone.
(5) potassium bromide.

3. A syndrome characterized by blindness, ataxia, colic, grinding of the teeth, and convulsions in calves is suggestive of poisoning with:

(1) nitrates.
(2) arsenic.
(3) copper.
(4) lead.

4. Which one of the following would be most likely to produce dilation of the bronchiolar smooth muscle following oral administration?

(1) Epinephrine
(2) Ephedrine
(3) Norepinephrine
(4) Isoproterenol

5. Which one of the following corticosteroids can be used in the alternate-day therapy for control of an allergic condition?

(1) Betamethasone
(2) Paramethasone
(3) Prednisolone
(4) Fludrocortisone
(5) Flumethasone

6. A 20-kg dog is dosed with 5 mg of drug X. If the half-life of drug X is 30 minutes, how long will it take for the animal to have less than 1 mg of the drug remaining in the body?

(1) 90 minutes
(2) 120 minutes
(3) 150 minutes
(4) 180 minutes
(5) 210 minutes

7. Poloxalene relieves ruminant bloat by:

(1) stimulating the eructation reflex.
(2) inhibiting growth of gas-forming bacteria.
(3) altering the surface tension of froth.
(4) stimulating rumen motility.

8. How does digoxin exert its positive inotropic effect?

(1) Direct stimulation of the Na^+-Ca^{2+} pump
(2) Competitive inhibition of Na^+-K^+-adenosine triphosphatase (ATPase)
(3) Activation of G_s regulatory protein
(4) Peripheral and central sympathetic stimulation
(5) Inhibition of phosphodiesterase activity

9. Considering efficacy, anthelmintic spectrum, and safety, which one of the following is the preferred anticestodal drug?

(1) Dichlorophen
(2) Fenbendazole
(3) Mebendazole
(4) Praziquantel

10. Which of the drugs listed below inhibits the release of histamine?

(1) Betazole
(2) Cimetidine
(3) Pyrilamine
(4) Cromolyn sodium

11. A dog is being given oral digoxin for heart failure. Which of the following approaches would yield the best absorption?

(1) Use of the tablet form
(2) Use of the elixir form
(3) Giving the drug with food
(4) Concurrent kaolin-pectin use
(5) Concurrent antacid use

12. What is the mechanism of action of tetracyclines?

(1) Binding to the 30S ribosome to inhibit the addition of amino acids to the growing peptide chain
(2) Binding to phospholipids in bacterial cell membranes to increase permeability
(3) Binding to the 50S ribosome to inhibit peptidyl transferase
(4) Inhibition of deoxyribonucleic acid (DNA) gyrase

13. The plasma concentration of drug X in a dairy cow is 5 μg/ml. Assume that drug X is a weak base with a pK_a of 8.4. The milk pH is 6.4 and the pH of the plasma is 7.4. What is the concentration of drug X in the milk?

(1) 5 μg/ml
(2) 30 μg/ml
(3) 45 μg/ml
(4) 55 μg/ml
(5) 500 μg/ml

14. Which one of the following combinations of drugs would be used to induce neuroleptanalgesia?

(1) Xylazine and zolazepam
(2) Acepromazine and diazepam
(3) Midazolam and azaperone
(4) Fentanyl and droperidol
(5) Detomidine and acepromazine

15. Which of the following anesthetics has the lowest blood:gas partition coefficient?

(1) Methoxyflurane
(2) Nitrous oxide
(3) Isoflurane
(4) Enflurane
(5) Halothane

16. By what primary mechanism is dopamine useful for treating certain types of shock?

(1) It increases blood flow to the skin.
(2) It causes vasodilation in skeletal muscle vascular beds.
(3) It increases blood flow to the kidneys.
(4) It increases systemic blood pressure.

17. The high concentration of tubulin protein in neural tissue may be the basis for neuromuscular weakness and constipation observed with which antineoplastic drug?

(1) Vincristine
(2) Doxorubicin
(3) Chlorambucil
(4) Methotrexate
(5) 5-Fluorouracil (5-FU)

18. Which one of the following statements is true regarding tylosin?

(1) It inhibits the first step of cell wall synthesis and thus is bactericidal in growing bacteria.
(2) It may produce anemia by blocking iron uptake in erythroblasts.
(3) It is effective against *Mycoplasma* species.
(4) It is usually effective against organisms resistant to erythromycin.

19. Aspirin may increase the toxicity of methotrexate in cancer chemotherapy patients by:

(1) inhibiting the hepatic metabolism of methotrexate.
(2) slowing active renal excretion of methotrexate.
(3) acting synergistically with methotrexate to inhibit dihydrofolate reductase.
(4) increasing intestinal absorption of methotrexate.

20. Stanozolol and boldenone are steroids closely related to:

(1) aldosterone.
(2) cortisol.
(3) estradiol.
(4) progesterone.
(5) testosterone.

21. Which of the following is the most common side effect of antihistaminics?

(1) Bronchoconstriction
(2) Sedation
(3) Excessive salivation
(4) Constipation

22. The most common complication of chronic treatment of dogs with anticonvulsants is:

(1) loss of appetite.
(2) renal failure.
(3) hepatotoxicity.
(4) vomiting.
(5) diarrhea.

23. A 9-year-old beagle has an irregular heartbeat and lethargy. Radiographs show moderate cardiomegaly, and an electrocardiogram (ECG) shows second-degree heart block. Based on the information given, appropriate therapy would include:

(1) digoxin.
(2) propranolol.
(3) procainamide.
(4) propantheline bromide.
(5) diltiazem.

24. Which one of the following statements is true regarding bile acids?

(1) Bile acids increase fat absorption and bile secretion.
(2) Bile acids are lipotropic agents useful for preventing fatty liver degeneration.
(3) Bile acids are used mainly as appetite stimulants in lactose-intolerant patients.
(4) Bile acids are usually combined with aluminum salts to prevent rebound hydrochloric acid secretion.

25. Which one of the following is a true statement about organophosphate antiparasitics?

(1) Pralidoxime is effective in reactivating cholinesterase 48 hours after onset of the poisoning.
(2) Trichlorfon must be biotransformed to dichlorvos in order to exert anticholinesterase activity.
(3) Trichlorfon must be encapsulated to slow down gastrointestinal absorption.
(4) Dichlorvos is used in ponds to control fish nematodes.

26. Which one of the following statements concerning the use of drugs in the nonspecific treatment of poisoning in dogs and cats is true?

(1) Methylcellulose laxatives are frequently used because they are inert and have a rapid onset of action.
(2) Apomorphine should be used to induce emesis in a dog that has ingested oven cleaner.
(3) Alkalinization of urine with sodium bicarbonate hastens the elimination of acidic compounds.
(4) Xylazine is a useful central-acting emetic in the unconscious cat.

27. Weekly monitoring of renal function [e.g., by evaluating blood urea nitrogen (BUN) levels] is necessary in antifungal therapy with:

(1) amphotericin B.
(2) ketoconazole.
(3) flucytosine.
(4) griseofulvin.

28. The function of sodium thiosulfate in the treatment of cyanide poisoning is:

(1) to reduce hemoglobin to the ferric state.
(2) to increase the breakdown of thiocyanate ion.
(3) to provide sulfur donors for sulfurtransferase.
(4) to bind to cytochrome and prevent attachment of cyanide.

29. The drug of choice for converting atrial fibrillation in horses without heart failure is:

(1) procainamide.
(2) quinidine.
(3) propranolol.
(4) diltiazem.
(5) phenytoin.

30. The renal clearance of a weak organic base is favored if the drug:

(1) has a high solubility in fat.
(2) reduces renal blood flow.
(3) has a high degree of binding to plasma protein.
(4) is put in the ionized form by acidifying the urine.
(5) is put in the nonionized form by alkalinizing the urine.

31. Which one of the following statements is true regarding the high-ceiling (loop) diuretics (e.g., furosemide, ethacrynic acid, bumetanide)?

(1) They have a slow onset of action because they are bound to plasma albumin.
(2) They are the diuretics of choice in acute pulmonary edema.
(3) They are useful in treating aminoglycoside toxicity because they increase renal excretion of these antibiotics.
(4) Their action is potentiated by carbonic anhydrase (CA) inhibitors such as acetazolamide or dichlorphenamide because they require an alkaline urine for their diuretic action.

32. Excessive sodium (Na^+) retention and potassium (K^+) excretion resulting from aldosterone-secreting adrenal gland tumors may be treated with:

(1) furosemide.
(2) chlorothiazide.
(3) triamterene.
(4) spironolactone.

33. Ivermectin is most effective against which one of the following larval stages of *Dirofilaria immitis*?

(1) L_1
(2) L_2
(3) L_3
(4) L_4
(5) L_5

34. A veterinarian sees a dog that is exhibiting signs of diabetes insipidus that do not respond to desmopressin [a synthetic analog of pituitary antidiuretic hormone (ADH)]. Which one of the following diuretics may paradoxically decrease urine output?

(1) Amiloride
(2) Aminophylline
(3) Chlorothiazide
(4) Acetaxolamide
(5) Ammonium chloride

35. How is pyridine aldoxime methiodide (2-PAM) useful in the treatment of organophosphate poisoning?

(1) It blocks cholinergic receptor sites.
(2) It reactivates acetylcholinesterase (AChE).
(3) It serves as a catalyst for acetylcholine (ACh) breakdown.
(4) It stimulates microsomal metabolism of the poison.

36. In the presence of renal disease, hyperkalemia might occur following administration of:

(1) mannitol.
(2) triamterene.
(3) furosemide.
(4) chlorothiazide.

37. Xylazine administration in the horse frequently results in which one of the following cardiac rhythms?

(1) Atrial fibrillation
(2) Sinus tachycardia
(3) Ventricular premature contractions
(4) Second-degree atrioventricular (A-V) block
(5) Premature atrial contractions

38. The primary reason for addition of glucose to oral rehydration solutions in treating diarrheal disease is:

(1) to correct severe hypoglycemia and weakness.
(2) to stimulate disaccharidase activity in the mucosal brush border.
(3) to stimulate sugar–sodium coupled uptake by enterocytes.
(4) to provide a hypertonic gradient for water absorption.

39. Which inhalant anesthetic would be contraindicated in a dog with severe pneumothorax?

(1) Nitrous oxide
(2) Methoxyflurane
(3) Enflurane
(4) Halothane
(5) Isoflurane

40. How do ethanol and 4-methylpyrazole (4-MP) counteract ethylene glycol (antifreeze) poisoning?

(1) They complex with ethylene glycol, rendering it inert.
(2) They accelerate the metabolic conversion of ethylene glycol to a nontoxic product.
(3) They inhibit the formation of toxic metabolites.
(4) They compete with ethylene glycol for essential cell membrane receptors.

41. Which inhalant anesthetic causes the greatest myocardial sensitization to epinephrine?

(1) Nitrous oxide
(2) Enflurane
(3) Methoxyflurane
(4) Halothane
(5) Isoflurane

42. Which one of the following analgesics has the strongest sedative effect?

(1) Acetaminophen
(2) Aspirin
(3) Phenylbutazone
(4) Flunixin meglumine
(5) Xylazine

43. Which one of the following drugs is considered the most potent analgesic among the inhibitors of prostaglandin (PG) synthesis?

(1) Aspirin
(2) Dipyrone
(3) Flunixin meglumine
(4) Naproxen
(5) Phenylbutazone

44. It is unwise to use acepromazine to sedate an acutely injured animal that has lost significant blood volume because severe hypotension may develop from:

(1) platelet function inhibition and further blood loss.
(2) myocardial depression as a result of β_1-adrenoreceptor blockade.
(3) reduced sympathetic nervous system tone secondary to α_2-adrenoreceptor blockade.
(4) α_1-adrenoreceptor blockade in peripheral arterioles and epinephrine reversal.
(5) enhanced γ-aminobutyric acid (GABA) activity in the brain leading to severe cardiovascular depression.

45. Which of the following laxatives exerts its action primarily in the large bowel and thus has a slow onset of action?

(1) Magnesium sulfate
(2) Cascara sagrada
(3) Castor oil
(4) Carbachol
(5) Sodium sulfate

46. Which anticonvulsant is excreted unchanged by the kidneys and acts by hyperpolarizing the cell membrane after entering the cell through the chloride channels?

(1) Valproic acid
(2) Phenobarbital
(3) Diazepam
(4) Phenytoin
(5) Potassium bromide

47. Which one of the following drugs renders amoxicillin effective against penicillinase-producing organisms?

(1) Phenethicillin
(2) Enrofloxacin
(3) Penicilloic acid
(4) Ampicillin
(5) Clavulanic acid

48. Which one of the following insecticides is an insect growth regulator?

(1) Carbaryl
(2) Diazinon
(3) Methoprene
(4) Pyrethrins
(5) Rotenone

49. Which one of the following statements concerning antineoplastic agents is true?

(1) They kill a constant number of undifferentiated cells with each dose.
(2) They are most effective against cells in the G_0 phase of the cell cycle.
(3) They kill malignant cells quickly; thus, resistance seldom develops.
(4) Their dosage calculations should be based on body surface area.

50. Which injectable anesthetic causes the least amount of direct myocardial depression?

(1) Pentobarbital
(2) Thiopental
(3) Ketamine
(4) Etomidate
(5) Propofol

51. Nematode species that are resistant to ivermectin are also likely to be resistant to:

(1) coumaphos.
(2) levamisole.
(3) milbemycin.
(4) phenothiazine.
(5) thiabendazole.

52. Which one of the following is used as the antidote for xylazine overdose?

(1) Atropine
(2) Naloxone
(3) Propranolol
(4) Yohimbine

53. Which of the following drugs is effective (at different doses) as both a heartworm preventative and a microfilaricide?

(1) Ivermectin
(2) Thiacetarsamide
(3) Diethylcarbamazine
(4) Melarsomine dihydrochloride
(5) Dithiazanine iodide

54. Which anesthetic is most commonly found in euthanasia products?

(1) Pentobarbital
(2) Phenobarbital
(3) Thiopental
(4) Ketamine
(5) Etomidate

55. Which of the following is a preferred drug for the treatment of equine colic?

(1) Aspirin
(2) Flunixin
(3) Acetaminophen
(4) Naproxen
(5) Meclofenamic acid

56. Which one of the following antineoplastic agents must be activated in the liver to cytotoxic metabolites?

(1) L-Asparaginase
(2) Chlorambucil
(3) Lomustine
(4) Cyclophosphamide

DIRECTIONS: Each of the numbered items or incomplete statements in this section is negatively phrased, as indicated by an italicized word such as *not, least,* or *except.* Select the **one** numbered answer or completion that is **best** in each case.

57. All of the following would be effective for producing closure of the esophageal groove in a calf *except*:

(1) water.
(2) milk.
(3) sodium bicarbonate, 10%.
(4) copper sulfate, 5%.

58. Plants are associated with specific toxic syndromes in ruminants and horses. Which of the following pairs is *not* correct?

(1) *Heliotropium* or *Senecio* species—copper poisoning
(2) Bracken fern—Vitamin K_1 deficiency
(3) Johnson grass or Sudan grass—cyanide poisoning
(4) Jimson weed or pigweed—nitrate poisoning

59. Which antineoplastic drugs should *not* be used in cats?

(1) Chlorambucil and methotrexate
(2) Cisplatin and 5-fluorouracil (5-FU)
(3) Vincristine and bleomycin
(4) Mitotane and 6-thioguanine (6-TG)

60. All of the following antinematodal drugs affect the nervous system of worms *except*:

(1) ivermectin.
(2) dichlorvos.
(3) piperazine.
(4) pyrantel.
(5) thiabendazole.

61. Trimethoprim or ormetoprim combined with a sulfonamide results in all of the following *except*:

(1) sequential blockade of folate synthesis in susceptible bacteria.
(2) decreased ability of sulfonamides to produce keratoconjunctivitis sicca.
(3) a decreased rate of development of resistant bacteria.
(4) an extended antibacterial spectrum.
(5) increased inhibition of purine and deoxyribonucleic acid (DNA) synthesis in susceptible bacteria.

62. The use of which one of the following anticoccidial drugs in chickens does *not* require preslaughter withdrawal?

(1) Sulfadimethoxine
(2) Nicarbazin
(3) Lasalocid
(4) Decoquinate
(5) Amprolium

63. All of the following statements concerning griseofulvin are true *except*:

(1) oral absorption is increased by dietary fats.
(2) distribution is to keratin precursor cells.
(3) its action is rapid and fungicidal.
(4) it inhibits mitosis in dermatophytes.

64. Which one of the following therapies is *not* correct?

(1) Metronidazole for anaerobic infection of the pelvis in cats
(2) Lincomycin for swine dysentery
(3) Apramycin for swine colibacillosis
(4) Tetracycline for psittacosis in birds
(5) Chloramphenicol for mycoplasmal pneumonia in swine

65. The antiemetic actions of metoclopramide include all of the following *except*:

(1) inhibition of H_1 receptors in the vomiting center.
(2) stimulation of gastric motility.
(3) inhibition of dopaminergic receptors in the chemoreceptor trigger zone.
(4) increased sensitivity of intestinal smooth muscle to acetylcholine (ACh).

66. Intravenous administration of xylazine produces all of the following pharmacologic effects *except*:

(1) bradycardia.
(2) increased gastrointestinal motility.
(3) transient hypertension.
(4) diuresis.

67. The pharmacologic effects of glucocorticoids include all of the following *except*:

(1) neutrophilia.
(2) increased vasomotor response.
(3) central nervous system (CNS) depression.
(4) wasting of skeletal muscle mass.

68. Progestins can be used for all of the following conditions *except*:

(1) follicular cysts.
(2) contraception.
(3) behavioral control.
(4) estrus synchronization.

69. Intravenous mannitol (5%) would be indicated in all of the following clinical situations *except*:

(1) oliguria arising from traumatic shock.
(2) ingestion of toxic amounts of cleaning solution containing potassium oxalate.
(3) generalized edema arising from congestive heart failure.
(4) cerebral edema resulting from trauma.
(5) increased intraocular pressure caused by narrow-angle glaucoma.

70. All of the following predispose to digoxin toxicity *except*:

(1) use of loading doses.
(2) hypokalemia.
(3) renal disease.
(4) quinidine.
(5) cholestyramine.

71. The α_2-agonist tranquilizer with the *most* selectivity for α_2 adrenoreceptors is:

(1) medetomidine.
(2) yohimbine.
(3) xylazine.
(4) acepromazine.
(5) tolazoline.

72. Which one of the following species is *least* likely to become hyperexcitable after administration of an opioid drug with mu-receptor agonist activity?

(1) Pig
(2) Horse
(3) Cat
(4) Cow
(5) Dog

DIRECTIONS: Each group of items in this section consists of numbered options followed by a set of numbered items. For each item, select the one numbered option that is most closely associated with it. Each numbered option may be selected once, more than once, or not at all.

Questions 73–77

For each of the following diuretic agents, choose the anatomic site in the renal nephron where the principal action of the agent occurs.
(1) Glomerulus
(2) Proximal tubule
(3) Ascending limb of the loop of Henle
(4) Distal tubule, early part
(5) Distal tubule, late part

73. Acetazolamide
74. Spironolactone
75. Furosemide
76. Chlorothiazide
77. Mannitol

Questions 78–81

Match each description with the appropriate drug.
(1) Tetracycline
(2) Probenecid
(3) Calcium gluconate
(4) Digoxin

78. Forms a precipitate with sodium bicarbonate

79. Concomitant administration of cimetidine prolongs this drug's action

80. Prolongs the plasma level of penicillins

81. Milk or antacids containing aluminum salts reduce absorption of this drug

ANSWERS AND EXPLANATIONS

1. The answer is 2 [*Chapter 12 III B 2, C 1*]. Methotrexate, an antimetabolite antineoplastic agent, inhibits the reductase required for conversion of dihydrofolic acid to tetrahydrofolic acid in purine biosynthesis. All antimetabolites are specific for the S phase of the cell cycle. Mitotane is specific for adrenal tumors.

2. The answer is 1 [*Chapter 4 II D 1 d (2)*]. Diazepam, administered intravenously, is the drug of choice to treat status epilepticus in dogs. Acepromazine is a phenothiazine tranquilizer, not an anticonvulsant, and may actually lower seizure threshold. Phenobarbital is too slow in its onset of action to be valuable in treating status epilepticus. Even with intravenous administration, it may take 20 minutes before phenobarbital exerts a significant anticonvulsant effect. Primidone and potassium bromide are oral anticonvulants with slow onset of action. Primidone needs to be metabolized by the liver ro produce phenylethylmalonamide (PEMA) and phenobarbital before it is effective.

3. The answer is 4 [*Chapter 15 III F 3*]. Lead poisoning in calves is characterized by neurologic damage, which produces clinical signs of blindness, ataxia, grinding of the teeth, and convulsions. Lead-induced colic is also observed. Clinical signs of nitrate poisoning result from methemoglobinemia and include dyspnea, cyanosis, muscle weakness, and collapse. Gastrointestinal hemorrhage is characteristic of arsenic poisoning, whereas hemolysis, hemoglobinura, and shock are observed in copper poisoning.

4. The answer is 2 [*Chapter 2 II B 3 b; Table 2-1*].
Ephedrine would be most likely to dilate the bronchiolar smooth muscle following oral administration. Bronchiolar smooth muscles are dilated by β_2-adrenoceptor agonists. Of the drugs listed, epinephrine, ephedrine, and isoproterenol have β_2-agonist activity. However, epinephrine and isoproterenol are inactivated following oral administration; therefore, they are ineffective by this route.

5. The answer is 3 [*Chapter 8 III E 3 e (1) (b)*].

Prednisolone is an intermediate-acting glucocorticoid that can be used in alternate-day therapy for allergy control. Betamethasone, flumethasone, and paramethasone are long-acting glucocorticoids. Fludrocortisone has potent glucocorticoid and mineralocorticoid activities; therefore, it is used in the treatment of hypoadrenocorticism.

6. The answer is 1 [*Chapter 1 II F 2*].
The dog will have less than 1 mg of the drug remaining in its body 90 minutes after administration. After 30 minutes (i.e., the half-life of the drug), 2.5 mg will remain in the body. After 60 minutes, 1.25 mg will remain in the body, and after 90 minutes, 0.62 mg will remain in the body.

7. The answer is 3 [*Chapter 10 X F*].
Poloxalene relieves bloat by altering the surface tension of rumen froth to break up and release entrapped gases. It does not alter rumen microflora or rumen motility. Breakup of froth permits normal functioning of the eructation reflex.

8. The answer is 2 [*Chapter 6 I D 1 a*].
Digoxin inhibits Na^+-K^+-ATPase at the myocardial cell membrane, allowing sodium to build up inside the cell, thereby enhancing its exchange with extracellular calcium. The resulting increase in intracellular calcium leads to a positive inotropic effect.

9. The answer is 4 [*Chapter 13 V D 5*].
Praziquantel and epsiprantel are the most effective and safest drugs against tapeworms. Dichlorophen's efficacy against *Echinococcus* and *Dypilidium* is variable. Febendazole and mebendazole are not effective against *Dypilidium*. The benzimidazoles may cause hepatotoxicity in dogs.

10. The answer is 4 [*Chapter 3 V A 1 b*].
Cromolyn sodium inhibits the release of histamine and other autacoids from mast cells. Betazole is an H_2-receptor agonist. Cimetidine is an H_2-receptor antagonist. Pyrilamine is an H_1-receptor antagonist.

11. The answer is 2 [*Chapter 6 I D 1 b (1) (a)*].
Absorption is better with the elixir than the tablet form. Administering digoxin with food, kaolin-pectin compounds, or antacids decreases absorption.

12. The answer is 1 [*Chapter 11 VII B*].
Tetracyclines inhibit bacterial protein synthesis by binding to the 30S ribosome of bacteria, preventing attachment of aminoacyl transfer ribonucleic acid (tRNA) to the ribosome and blocking the addition of amino acids to the peptide chain. Polymyxin B disrupts bacterial cell membranes. Chloramphenicol binds to the 50S ribosome and inhibits peptidyl transferase. Fluoroquinolones inhibit deoxyribonucleic acid (DNA) gyrase.

13. The answer is 3 [*Chapter 1 II A 1 b (2)*].
The concentration of the drug X in the milk is approximately 45 μg/ml. Knowledge of the Henderson-Hasselbalch equation is necessary to solve this problem. Because the drug is a weak base, the proper formula to use is:

$$pK_a = pH + \log \frac{\text{ionized drug (I)}}{\text{nonionized drug (U)}}$$

Only the nonionized form of the drug is lipid-soluble and able to cross the biologic membrane. At equilibrium, the concentration of nonionized drug will be the same on both sides of the biologic membrane. The drug will dissociate on both sides of the membrane based on the pH of the environment.

	Milk	Plasma
pH:	6.4	7.4
Substituting:	$8.4 = 6.4 + \log \frac{I}{U}$	$8.4 = 7.4 + \log \frac{I}{U}$
	$2 = \log \frac{I}{U}$	$1 = \log \frac{I}{U}$
Take the antilog of both sides:	$100 = \frac{I}{U}$	$10 = \frac{I}{U}$
If U = 1 drug unit, then:	I = 100	I = 10

Because the total amount of the drug equals the nonionized plus the ionized portion, the milk:plasma ratio equals 101:11, or 9.18. If the plasma concentration is 5 μg/ml, then the milk concentration can be determined as follows:

$$\frac{\text{milk } (\mu g/ml)}{\text{plasma } (\mu g/ml)} = \frac{101 \text{ drug units}}{11 \text{ drug units}}$$

$$\frac{X \, \mu g/ml}{5 \, \mu g/ml} = \frac{101}{11}; 11X = 505; X = 45.9 \, \mu g/ml$$

14. The answer is 4 [*Chapter 4 V B 3 c (2)*].
A neuroleptanalgesic combination is a neuroleptic (tranquilizer) plus an analgesic (opioid). Innovar-Vet is a commercial product consisting of 0.4 mg/ml fentanyl and 20 mg/ml droperidol. Fentanyl is an opioid agonist, and droperidol is a butyrophenone tranquilizer. The other four choices are tranquilizer–tranquilizer combinations.

15. The answer is 2 [*Chapter 5; Table 5-4*].
Nitrous oxide has a lower blood:gas partition coefficient than the other anesthetics listed (i.e., methoxyflurane, isoflurane, enflurane, halothane). The speed of induction and recovery is correlated with the blood:gas partition coefficient. The lower the blood:gas partition coefficient (i.e., the less soluble the agent), the faster the anesthetic agent acts.

16. The answer is 3 [*Chapter 2 II A 1 d (3)*].
Because dopamine dilates the renal vasculature via D_1 receptors, it is often used to treat cardiogenic and septic shock, which are characterized by a decrease in renal blood flow. Activation of α_1 adrenoceptors in the vasculature and β_1 receptors in the heart will increase systemic blood pressure. Other sympathomimetic amines will increase systemic blood pressure, but these also reduce renal blood flow.

17. The answer is 1 [*Chapter 12 IV F 1*].
Vincristine binds to tubulin in the mitotic spindle to inhibit mitosis. Neuronal tissue contains high concentrations of tubulin protein. This may explain the neuromuscular weakness and constipation observed as adverse effects of vincristine therapy. Doxorubicin is an antibiotic that inhibits deoxyribonecleic acid (DNA) replication. Chlorambucil is an alkylating agent that cross-links DNA. Methotrexate

and 5-fluorouracil (5-FU) are antimetabolites, which impair DNA synthesis.

18. The answer is 3 [*Chapter 11 IX D*].
Tylosin, a macrolide antibiotic, is effective against Gram-positive pathogens and infections caused by *Mycoplasma* species. It is also active against some Gram-negative bacteria, including *Pasteurella* and *Haemophilus* species. Like other macrolides (e.g., erythromycin) tylosin inhibits protein synthesis by binding to the 50S ribosome. Thus, cross-resistance would be expected.

19. The answer is 2 [*Chapter 14 II D 5*].
Salicylates slow the renal excretion of methotrexate by competing for the active tubular transport of organic acids into the urine. The resultant prolonged blood levels of methotrexate may hasten the development of bone marrow suppression.

20. The answer is 5 [*Chapter 8 III C 3 b*].
Boldenone and stanozolol are weak androgens and are called anabolic steroids. They are closely related to testosterone.

21. The answer is 2 [*Chapter 3 V A 1 a (1) (f)*].
Central nervous system (CNS) depression (e.g., sedation, lethargy, ataxia) is the most common side effect of antihistamine therapy. The newer H_1 blockers (e.g., terfenadine) tend to cause less sedation than their older counterparts. Antihistamines relieve the bronchoconstriction caused by histamine. Some antihistamines have antimuscarinic activity, causing side effects such as xerostomia. Anticholinergic actions may promote constipation, but this is not a common side effect of H_1 antagonists.

22. The answer is 3 [*Chapter 4 II A 5 d*].
In dogs, the chronic use of phenobarbital, phenytoin, and primidone either alone or in combination frequently elevates serum levels of the liver enzymes (e.g., alanine transaminase). In approximately 6%–15% of patients, hepatic pathology develops. The overall incidence of hepatic disease associated with long-term use of anticonvulsant drugs is relatively low.

23. The answer is 4 [*Chapter 6 II C 1 e (3)*].
Anticholinergic therapy (e.g., with propantheline bromide) is initially indicated for symptomatic second-degree heart block. Digoxin, propranolol, procainamide, and diltiazem are relatively or absolutely contraindicated with atrioventricular (A-V) nodal disease.

24. The answer is 1 [*Chapter 10 IV B*].
The bile acids (e.g., deoxycholic acid, chenodeoxycholic acid) emulsify lipids to enhance absorption and stimulate bile flow. Lipotropic agents (e.g., methionine) are methyl donors, which stimulate hepatic lipoprotein synthesis. Lactose intolerance is treated by eliminating dairy products from the diet. Bile acids may be administered as sodium salts, not aluminum salts.

25. The answer is 2 [*Chapter 13 III C 3 b*].
Trichlorfon is slowly converted to dichlorvos for action; thus, trichlorfon is one of the safest organophosphate agents that can be used in ponds to control fish nematodes. Pralidoxime is only effective in reactivating cholinesterase within 24 hours after organophosphate poisoning. Dichlorvos, not trichlorfon, is a lipophilic liquid that is incorporated into polyvinyl chloride resin pellets for slow release.

26. The answer is 3 [*Chapter 15 II B 2*].
Acidic compounds are ionized in alkaline urine; therefore, they are more rapidly excreted. Bulk laxatives such as methylcellulose are not effective in poisoning because they act in the large intestine and have a slow onset of action. Emetics such as apomorphine or xylazine should never be used in unconscious animals or if a corrosive poison (e.g., oven cleaner) has been ingested.

27. The answer is 1 [*Chapter 11 XII C 7*].
Amphotericin B is nephrotoxic, and renal function must be monitored weekly during long-term therapy for systemic mycoses.

28. The answer is 3 [*Chapter 15 III C 4 a (2)*].
Sodium thiosulfate serves as a sulfur donor for the endogenous enzyme, sulfurtransferase. This enzyme converts cyanide to the nontoxic thiocyanate ion. Sodium nitrite is administered concomitantly to reduce hemoglobin to the ferric state. Sodium thiosulfate does not bind to cytochrome to prevent attachment of cyanide.

29. The answer is 2 [*Chapter 6 II B 1 e (1)*].
Quinidine is often successful in converting atrial fibrillation in horses without heart failure or significant underlying cardiac disease. Procainamide is much less effective for supra-

ventricular arrhythmias. Propranolol along with digoxin is sometimes used if heart failure is present; these drugs would be expected to slow the ventricular response rate but not convert the rhythm to sinus rhythm. Likewise, diltiazem might slow the ventricular response rate, but it is usually not used clinically. Phenytoin is not used in horses.

30. The answer is 4 [*Chapter 1 II E 1*].
Acidification of the urine increases the percent of the weak base that exists in an ionized form. The ionized form of a drug crosses biologic membranes poorly and thus is not able to be passively reabsorbed from the tubule once filtration has taken place. In the nonionized form, the drug would be reabsorbed to its greatest extent, thus decreasing excretion. Drugs that are bound to plasma proteins are filtered poorly. A high lipid solubility enhances passive reabsorption in the renal tubule, reducing renal clearance. A reduction in renal blood flow reduces glomerular filtration volume, thereby reducing renal clearance.

31. The answer is 2 [*Chapter 7 II E 1*].
Loop (high-ceiling) diuretics are the diuretics of choice in life-threatening conditions such as pulmonary edema because they effect the rapid mobilization of accumulated fluid. They have a rapid onset of action and produce a peak diuresis that is greater than that produced by other classes of diuretics. They may potentiate the ototoxicity of the aminoglycoside antibiotics and should not be used with this class of antimicrobials. The action of loop diuretics is independent of urinary pH.

32. The answer is 4 [*Chapter 7 VI B 2, D 3*].
Spironolactone, a potassium (K^+)-sparing diuretic, is used to counter the aldosterone-induced sodium (Na^+) and K^+ changes produced by adrenal gland tumors. Mineralocorticoids such as aldosterone are secreted in large amounts by adrenal gland tumors and produce excessive Na^+ retention and K^+ excretion by the kidneys. Spironolactone, a competitive antagonist of aldosterone, blocks the effects of the hormone. Furosemide, chlorothiazide, and triamterene do not affect aldosterone actions.

33. The answer is 4 [*Chapter 13 IV D 2*].
Both ivermectin and milbemycin are effective against stage L_4 microfilariae. Because it takes 2.5 months for L_4 microfilariae to develop into L_5 microfilariae, the elimination of L_4 mi-

crofilariae once monthly using these drugs will prevent heartworm infection.

34. The answer is 3 [*Chapter 7 III C 2, E 2*].
The thiazide diuretics (e.g., chlorothiazide) decrease urine volume in nephrogenic diabetes insipidus. The mechanism is not completely understood, but sodium (Na^+) depletion, increased Na^+ and chloride (Cl^-) absorption in the proximal tubule, and reduced volume delivered to the distal nephron may enhance the action of antidiuretic hormone (ADH). This effect is not observed with other classes of diuretics.

35. The answer is 2 [*Chapter 15 III I 4 a (2)*].
The action of pyridine aldoxime methiodide (2-PAM) in organophosphate poisoning is to reactivate acetylcholinesterase (AChE) by forming an oxime–phosphonate complex at the phosphorylated site. The complex is then split off, leaving the regenerated enzyme. The drug has no direct action on muscarinic receptor sites or microsomes. 2-PAM does not serve as a catalyst for acetylcholine (ACh) breakdown.

36. The answer is 2 [*Chapter 7 VI F 1*].
Triamterene is a potassium (K^+)-sparing diuretic that inhibits active sodium (Na^+) reabsorption in the distal tubule and collecting duct. K^+ retention may produce hyperkalemia in the presence of renal disease. Mannitol, furosemide, and chlorothiazide are not K^+-sparing diuretics.

37. The answer is 4 [*Chapter 4 III D 1 c (1) (b)*].
Sinus bradycardia and second-degree atrioventricular (A-V) block frequently occur in horses following intravenous injection of xylazine. The other arrhythmias listed would not be associated with α_2-adrenoreceptor stimulation.

38. The answer is 3 [*Chapter 10 VIII A*].
Glucose stimulates sodium absorption by enterocytes via a coupled transport mechanism. Sodium uptake then secondarily provides the osmotic force for water absorption. Increased glucose absorption may be beneficial, but it is not essential for rehydration. Disaccharidase activity is not altered by monosaccharides.

39. The answer is 1 [*Chapter 5 III D 1 F (2)*].
Nitrous oxide is contraindicated in animals with trapped pockets of gas (e.g., pneumothorax, an accumulation of gas in the pleural

space). Because this gas is most likely to be room air, the primary component would be nitrogen. Nitrous oxide will diffuse into the trapped gas space faster than the nitrogen will diffuse out. Thus, the gas space will expand, causing the lungs to collapse further. The other inhalant anesthetics listed will also diffuse into the space, but because they are administered at a much lower concentration (1%–3%) than nitrous oxide (50%–67%), they will not result in significant expansion of the pneumothorax.

40. The answer is 3 [*Chapter 15 III D 4 a*]. Ethanol and 4-methylpyrazole (4-MP) competitively inhibit alcohol dehydrogenase, the first and rate-limiting step in the conversion of ethylene glycol to its toxic metabolites, glycolic acid and oxalic acid. The antidotes do not form a complex with the poison, or compete for membrane receptors. Ethanol and 4-MP do not accelerate the metabolic conversion of ethylene glycol to a nontoxic product.

41. The answer is 4 [*Chapter 5 III D 2 c (1) (c)*].
Very low doses of epinephrine administered to a halothane-anesthetized animal will result in serious ventricular arrhythmias (e.g., premature ventricular contractions, ventricular tachycardia, or ventricular fibrillation). Nitrous oxide, enflurane, methoxyflurane, and isoflurane also sensitize the myocardium to catecholamines, but to a much lower degree.

42. The answer is 5 [*Chapter 9 II A 1 b*].
Xylazine is an α_2-adrenergic agonist, which has a much stronger sedative effect than acetaminophen, aspirin, phenylbutazone, and flunixin meglumine, which are inhibitors of prostaglandin (PG) synthesis.

43. The answer is 3 [*Chapter 9 I E*].
Flunixin meglumine is considered to be a more potent analgesic than other inhibitors of prostaglandin synthesis. It is considered a more potent analgesic than even opioids, pentazocine, meperidine, or codeine.

44. The answer is 4 [*Chapter 4 IV A 3 a (1)*].
The phenothiazine tranquilizers cause a dose-related α_1-adrenoreceptor blockade, which leads to vasodilation. If the sympathetic tone of the animal is high secondary to blood loss, the hypotension caused by α_1 blockade may be profound. Likewise, if circulating levels of epinephrine are high (as would occur follow-ing blood loss) and the α receptors are partially blocked, then the β_2 effect of epinephrine would become physiologically apparent and its vasodilating effect would lower the arterial blood pressure even more. This effect is called epinephrine reversal.

45. The answer is 2 [*Chapter 10 VII C 2 b*]. Cascara sagrada contains glycosides, which are hydrolyzed in the large intestine to liberate irritant anthraquinones, which stimulate myenteric plexuses. Anthraquinones must traverse the intestinal tract for activation in the large intestine and, thus, they have a slower onset of action than osmotic cathartics, castor oil, or carbachol, which act on the small intestine.

46. The answer is 5 [*Chapter 4 II E 1*]. Potassium bromide is not bound to protein and not metabolized but is excreted unchanged by the kidneys. Bromide and chloride can both enter neurons through existing chloride channels such as those associated with γ-aminobutyric acid (GABA) receptors. When GABA stimulates the receptor, the ion channels open and bromide competes with chloride for passage into the cell. Because both ions have a negative charge, their movement into the cell makes the membrane potential more negative. Apparently, when bromide enters the cell, it affects membrane potential for a longer period of time than chloride. The hyperpolarized cell has a membrane potential more negative than normal and further from threshold; thus, the cell is less likely to fire on its own or when stimulated, thereby preventing seizures.

47. The answer is 5 [*Chapter 11 IV E 4 a*]. Clavulanic acid inhibits beta-lactamases and prevents inactivation of amoxicillin by otherwise resistant organisms. Phenethicillin, enrofloxacin, and ampicillin do not inhibit penicillinases. Penicilloic acid, which acts as an antigenic determinant in penicillin allergy, is a degradation product of penicillinase action.

48. The answer is 3 [*Chapter 13 II E 1*]. Methoprene affects the action of the juvenile hormone of insects. Carbaryl and diazinon are cholinesterase inhibitors. Pyrethrins and rotenone are "knockdown" insecticides.

49. The answer is 4 [*Chapter 12 I A 2, B 1, D*].
Antineoplastic drug dosage is based on body

surface area because antineoplastic agents have a narrow therapeutic index. Drug amounts based on body weight tend to produce overdosage in large or heavy individuals. A constant percentage, not a constant number, of malignant cells are killed by antineoplastic drugs. Cells in the G_0 (resting) phase are generally not susceptible to antineoplastic drugs. Resistance to antineoplastic drugs is common.

50. The answer is 4 [*Chapter 5 IV D 2 a*].
Etomidate causes minimal cardiovascular and respiratory depression. Pentobarbital, thiopental, propofol, and ketamine are all direct depressants of myocardial function. Ketamine is unique in that it increases sympathetic nervous system tone, which usually counteracts the direct effect of ketamine on the heart. Thus, the increased heart rate, blood pressure, and cardiac output associated with ketamine are secondary to increased sympathetic autonomic tone.

51. The answer is 3 [*Chapter 13 III D 1–2*].
Both ivermectin and milbemycin activate the GABA-receptor–chloride channel macromolecular complex, thus inhibiting neurotransmission of arthropods. Cross-resistance between these two drugs has been recently reported.

52. The answer is 4 [*Chapter 9 II A 3 b*].
Yohimbine is an α_2-adrenergic antagonist that blocks α_2 receptors activated by xylazine. Atropine should not be used to antagonize the bradycardia and heart block induced by α_2-adrenergic agonists because it may change the α_2-adrenergic agonist–induced bradycardia into a tachycardia while potentiating the α_2-adrenergic agonist–induced hypertension. Naloxone and propranolol block opioid and β-adrenergic receptors, respectively; therefore they are not useful in this situation.

53. The answer is 1 [*Chapter 6 IV A 1 b, C 1 b*].
Ivermectin is commonly used as both a preventative and, at single higher doses, as a microfilaricide after adulticide therapy, except in the collie breed. Thiacetarsamide is only effective as an adulticide. Diethylcarbamazine is contraindicated in dogs with circulating microfilariae because of potentially fatal adverse reactions. Melarsomine has only been evaluated as an adulticide. Dithiazanine is only useful as a microfilaricide.

54. The answer is 1 [*Chapter 5 IV A 2 b (1)*].

Pentobarbital is used to euthanize animals. Very concentrated solutions are rapidly injected intravenously, resulting in severe central nervous system (CNS) and cardiopulmonary depression.

55. The answer is 2 [*Chapter 9 I E 3*].
Flunixin is widely used to treat equine colic and gastrointestinal spasm or hypermotility; however, the latter use has been challenged.

56. The answer is 4 [*Chapter 12 II C 1 a (1) (b)*].
Cyclophosphamide is activated in the liver to phosphoramide mustard and acrolein; therefore, it is not effective if injected directly into tumors. Chlorambucil and lomustine are alkylating agents that are active as parent compounds. L-Asparaginase acts by depleting circulating levels of L-asparagine.

57. The answer is 1 [*Chapter 10 X B*].
Water is not an effective stimulus for esophageal groove closure. Milk, sodium bicarbonate, and copper sulfate are effective stimuli.

58. The answer is 2 [*Chapter 15 III K 2*].
Bracken fern contains a thiaminase and thus produces thiamine deficiency, not vitamin K_1 deficiency, in nonruminants ingesting contaminated forage. Vitamin K_1 deficiency may result from ingestion of spoiled sweet clover forage. *Heliotropium* and *Senecio* species are associated with copper poisoning. Johnson grass and Sudan grass, of the *Sorghum* species, are associated with cyanide poisoning. Jimson weed and pigweed are associated with nitrate poisoning.

59. The answer is 2 [*Chapter 12 III C 2 f; VII*].
In cats, cisplatin produces severe pulmonary lesions and 5-fluorouracil (5-FU) produces severe central nervous system (CNS) toxicity; therefore, these drugs cannot be used in cats. Chlorambucil, methotrexate, vincristine, bleomycin, mitotane, and 6-thioguanine (6-TG) may be used in feline chemotherapy.

60. The answer is 5 [*Chapter 13 III A 1 a, B 3 c, C 2, D 1 a, E 2 c*].
Thiabendazole inhibits fumarate reductase, thereby preventing adenosine triphosphate (ATP) formation. Piperazine and invermectin act on the γ-aminobutyric acid (GABA) system to inhibit neurotransmission. Dichlorvos

and pyrantel have a stimulatory effect on the cholinergic system.

61. The answer is 2 [*Chapter 11 II D; Figure 11-2*].
The ocular toxicity of sulfonamides, especially the sulfapyrimidines, is not reduced by combination with trimethoprim or ormetoprim. Potentiated sulfonamides, which sequentially block folate synthesis in susceptible bacteria, have an extended spectrum of activity and reduce the rate of bacterial resistance development.

62. The answer is 5 [*Chapter 13 VII A 2 c (3) (b)*].
Amprolium is a quaternary drug that is poorly absorbed through the gastrointestinal tract; thus, no preslaughter withdrawal period is necessary when amprolium is used in broilers. Decoquinate, lasalocid, nicarbazin, and sulfadimethoxine all have a preslaughter period of 4–5 days.

63. The answer is 3 [*Chapter 11 XII A*].
Griseofulvin is fungistatic, and its action is slow. Griseofulvin inhibits mitosis in dermatophytes (ringworm) by binding to microtubules to prevent spindle formation. It is widely distributed to keratin precursor cells. Infected cells are slowly shed and replaced with uninfected cells. Oral absorption is increased by dietary fats.

64. The answer is 5 [*Chapter 11 VIII E, H 1 b*].
Chloramphenicol use in food-producing animals is illegal because of the potential danger of residue-induced aplastic anemia in humans.

65. The answer is 1 [*Chapter 10 VI B 2 a*].
The central antidopaminergic actions of metoclopramide do not include blockade of H_1 receptors. Metoclopramide inhibits dopaminergic receptors in the chemoreceptor trigger zone and stimulates gastric and intestinal motility and gastric emptying by increasing the sensitivity of intestinal smooth muscle to acetylcholine (ACh).

66. The answer is 2 [*Chapter 9 II A*].
The intravenous administration of xylazine induces bradycardia, transient hypertension followed by hypotension, diuresis, and decreased (not increased) gastrointestinal motility.

67. The answer is 3 [*Chapter 8 III E 3 d (1) (b)*].
Glucocorticoids cause central nervous system (CNS) stimulation, not depression. Neutrophilia, increased vasomotor response, and wasting of muscle mass can occur with pharmacologic doses of glucocorticoids.

68. The answer is 1 [*Chapter 8 III C 2 b (2)*].
Luteinizing hormone (LH) and human chorionic gonadotropin (HCG), not progestins, are used for treatment of follicular cysts because they induce ovulation. Progestins are used as contraceptive agents, for behavioral control, and estrus synchronization.

69. The answer is 3 [*Chapter 7 IV E*].
Osmotic diuretics produce an initial increase in blood volume, which can cause decompensation in animals with congestive heart failure. In addition, they are not effective in reducing generalized edema because their saluretic action is weak. They are effective in treating oliguria, forcing diuresis in cases of poisoning, and treating cerebral edema and glaucoma.

70. The answer is 5 [*Chapter 6 I D 1 f (1) (b)–(c)*].
Cholestyramine will bind digoxin in the gut and may be helpful immediately after oral overdose. Loading doses, hypokalermia, renal disease, and quinidine predispose to toxicity.

71. The answer is 1 [*Chapter 4 IV D 1 a (1)*].
Detomidine has the least selectivity for α_1 adrenoreceptors. The ratios of α_2 to α_1 activity are: xylazine, 160:1; detomidine, 260:1; and medetomidine, 1620:1. Yohimbine and tolazoline are α_2 antagonists used to reverse the effects of the α_2 agonists. Acepromazine is a phenothiazine derivative tranquilizer that has α_1-antagonist activity but no α_2-agonist activity.

72. The answer is 5 [*Chapter 4 V B 1 e (1)*].
Dogs are least likely to experience hyperexcitability following the administration of mu-receptor agonist drugs (e.g., morphine). Horses, cows, cats, and pigs are all very susceptible to developing hyperexcitability following the administration of a mu-receptor agonist, unless it is administered after or with adequate doses of a tranquilizer (e.g., acepromazine, diazepam, xylazine).

73–77. The answers are: 73–2 [*Chapter 7 V C; Table 7-1*], **74–5** [*Chapter 7 VI B 2; Table 7-1*], **75–3** [*Chapter 7 II C 1; Table 7-1*], **76–4** [*Chapter 7 III C 1; Table 7-1*], **77–2** [*Chapter 7 IV C 1; Table 7-1*].

Although acetazolamide acts on both the proximal and distal convoluted tubules, its diuretic effects are strongest in the proximal tubules because carbonic anhydrase (CA) concentrations are highest in this segment.

Spironolactone, a potassium (K^+)-sparing diuretic, acts as a competitive antagonist of aldosterone. The receptor for aldosterone is located in the distal convoluted tubule; and thus, this is the site of action for spironolactone.

Furosemide is a loop (high-ceiling) diuretic. Like ethacrynic acid, it inhibits reabsorption in the ascending limb of the loop of Henle.

Chlorothiazide is one of several thiazide diuretics. The thiazides act primarily on the early part of the distal convoluted tubule to block sodium (Na^+) and chloride (Cl^-) resorption.

Osmotic diuretics (e.g., mannitol) act at the proximal convoluted tubule, where 65% of the filtered water normally is reabsorbed isosmotically.

78–81. The answers are: 78-3 [*Chapter 14 IV A 1*], **79-4** [*Chapter 14 II C 1*], **80-2** [*Chapter 14 II D 1*], **81-1** [*Chapter 14 II A 3*].

The addition of sodium bicarbonate to calcium gluconate results in the precipitation of calcium carbonate. This is an example of physical incompatibility.

Cimetidine inhibits the microsomal enzymes that metabolize digoxin and thus prolongs the cardiac effects of digoxin.

Probenecid competes with penicillin for active renal tubular secretion and thus slows the rate of urinary elimination of penicillin.

Tetracyclines form insoluble chelates with calcium, magnesium, and aluminum ions. These complexes are poorly absorbed from the gastrointestinal tract.

Index

Note: Page numbers in italics denote illustrations, those followed by (*t*) denote tables, those followed by Q denote questions, and those followed by E denote explanations

A

Abdominal distention, treatment of, 34
Abnormal heart rhythms, 122
Abortifacients, 157
Abortion, early, 159
Absolute refractory period, 85
Absorption, drug interactions affecting, 265
Acepromazine, 66, 194–195, 289Q, 297E
Acetaminophen, 174–175, 184Q, 186E
  adverse effects, 175
  intoxication from, 185Q, 186E
  mechanism of action, 174–175
  pharmacokinetics, 174–175
  pharmacologic effects, 175
  therapeutic uses, 175
  toxicosis, 273, 279Q, 281E
Acetazolamide, 147Q, 149E, 291Q, 300E
Acetylcholine (ACh), 33, 42Q, 44E
  antagonists, 34
  chemistry and biosynthesis, 33, *33*
  mechanism of action, 34
  pharmacologic effects, 34
  therapeutic uses, 34
Acetylcholinesterase (AChE), 288Q, 296E
Acetylsalicylic acid, 272
Acid-base disturbances, 174
α_1-acid glycoprotein, 4
Acidifying salts, 146
Acids, weak, 1, 16Q, 18E
Acquired growth hormone deficiency, 153
Acromegaly, 153
ACTH (corticotropin), 151, 159
  adverse effects, 159
  mechanism of action, 159
  preparations, 159
  therapeutic uses, 159
Actinomycin D, 234–235, 239Q, 241E
Activated charcoal, 271, 280Q, 282E
Active transport, 3
  and drug excretion, 8
  mechanisms for, 5
Active tubular secretion, 7, 8(t)
Acute glaucoma, 143
Acute lymphocytic leukemia, 232
Acute renal failure, 141
Acute thromboembolism, 135Q, 137E
Administration, 211, 232
  adverse effects, 211
  bacterial resistance, 211
  routes of, 16Q, 18E
Administrator, 144
Adrenal dysfunction, 153
Adrenal gland, tumors of, 145
Adrenal steroid inhibitors, 162–163
Adrenergic agonists, 23, 24(t)
  adverse effects, 28

catecholamines, 23–24, 24(t), 25
  pharmacokinetics, 25–26
  pharmacologic effects, 26–27
  therapeutic uses, 27
α_2-adrenergic agonists, 69, 178–180, 185Q, 187E
  administration, 71
  detomidine (Dormosedan), 180
  mechanism of action, 70, *70*
  pharmacologic effects, 70–71, 173(t), 178–179
  preparations, 69
  reversal, 71
  therapeutic uses, 71
  xylazine, 179–180
α-adrenergic antagonists, 31
  phenoxybenzamine, 31
    adverse effects, 31
    mechanism of action, 31
    pharmacologic effects, 31
    therapeutic uses, 31
  phentolamine, 31
    adverse effects, 32
    mechanism of action, 31
    pharmacologic effects, 31
    therapeutic uses, 32
  prazosin, 31
    adverse effects, 31
    mechanism of action, 31
    pharmacologic effects, 31
    therapeutic uses, 31
  yohimbine, 32
    adverse effects, 32
    mechanism of action, 32
    pharmacologic effects, 32
    therapeutic uses, 32
β-adrenergic antagonists, 32
  atenolol, 32
    adverse effects, 32–33
    mechanism of action, 32
    pharmacologic effects, 32
    therapeutic uses, 32
  propranolol, 32
    adverse effects, 32
    contraindications, 32
    mechanism of action, 32
    pharmacokinetics, 32
    pharmacologic effects, 32
    therapeutic uses, 32
α-adrenergic antagonists (α_2-receptor blockers), 179
β-adrenergic receptors, 134Q, 136E
Adrenergic receptors (adrenoceptors), 21
β_1-adrenoceptor antagonists, 57
Adulticides, 132, 253–255
Adverse effects, 29
  and contraindications, 144
Agar, 197
Age, and drug metabolism, 7
Agonist-antagonist opioid, 81Q, 83E
Agonists, 11

Air
  and drug excretion, 8
  expired, 8
Albendazole, 248, 257
Albumin, 4
Alcohol dehydrogenase, 6
Alcuronium, 39, 41
Aldehyde dehydrogenase, 6
Aldosterone, 159, 162
Aldosterone-secreting adrenal gland tumors, 288Q, 296E
Alkylating agent, 230, 238Q, 240E
  chemistry, 230, *230*
  mechanism of actions, 230
  preparations, *230*, 230–231
Alkylsulfonate, 231
Allergic reactions to penicillin, 213, 214
Allethrin, 246
All-or-none response, 14, 85
Aloe, 197
α-blockers, 132
Aluminum hydroxide, 201
Amebiasis, 260
Amikacin, 215
Amiloride, 144
Aminocyclitols, 220
Aminoglycosides, 214
  administration, 215
  adverse effects, 215–216
  as antibiotics, 225–226Q, 227E, 228E
  bacterial resistance, 215
  chemistry, 214
  mechanism of action, 214
  pharmacokinetics, 215
  preparations and therapeutic uses, 215
  spectrum of activity, 215
Aminopentamide, 196, 198
Aminophylline, 145
Amiodarone, 128
  adverse effects, 129
  pharmacologic effects, 129
  therapeutic uses, 129
Amitraz, 32, 247, 261Q, 263E
Amlodipine besylate, 132
Ammonium carbonate, 201
Ammonium chloride, 146, 272
Ammonium molybdate, 276, 279Q, 281E
Amoxicillin, 212, 289Q, 297E
Amphotericin B, 223–224, 287Q, 295E
  administration, 224
  adverse effects, 224
  chemistry, 223
  mechanism of action, 224
  pharmacokinetics, 224
  spectrum of activity, 224
  therapeutic uses, 224
Ampicillin, 212